Clinical Work with Traumatized Young Children

Clinical Work with Traumatized Young Children

■ ■ ■ ■

Edited by
Joy D. Osofsky

Foreword by
Alicia F. Lieberman

THE GUILFORD PRESS
New York   London

© 2011 The Guilford Press
A Division of Guilford Publications, Inc.
72 Spring Street, New York, NY 10012
www.guilford.com

Paperback edition 2012

Printed in the United States of America

This book is printed on acid-free paper.

Last digit is print number: 9 8 7 6 5 4 3 2

Library of Congress Cataloging-in-Publication Data

Clinical work with traumatized young children / edited by Joy D. Osofsky.
    p. ; cm.
  Includes bibliographical references and index.
  ISBN 978-1-60918-206-9 (hardback : alk. paper)
  ISBN 978-1-4625-0964-5 (paperback: alk. paper)
  1. Post-traumatic stress disorder in children.   2. Stress (Psychology)   I. Osofsky,
Joy D.
  [DNLM: 1. Stress Disorders, Traumatic—therapy.   2. Stress, Psychological—
psychology.   3. Child.   4. Parent–Child Relations.   5. Psychotherapy—
methods.   WM 172]
  RJ506.P55C55 2011
  618.92'8521—dc22
                                                            2010051671

About the Editor

Joy D. Osofsky, PhD, a clinical and developmental psychologist and psychoanalyst, is Barbara Lemann Professor of Pediatrics and Psychiatry at Louisiana State University Health Sciences Center, where she is also Head of the Division of Pediatric Mental Health. Dr. Osofsky is Codirector of the Louisiana Rural Trauma Services Center, part of the National Child Traumatic Stress Network, and Director of the Harris Program for Infant Mental Health. Her research, consulting, and clinical work focus on infants, children, and families exposed to trauma as a result of disasters, community and domestic violence, maltreatment, and military deployment. Dr. Osofsky is past president of Zero to Three and of the World Association for Infant Mental Health. She is a recipient of, among other honors, the Sarah Haley Award for Clinical Excellence from the International Society for Traumatic Stress Studies and of the Presidential Commendation from the American Psychiatric Association, for her work in the aftermath of Hurricane Katrina.

Contributors

Marilyn Augustyn, MD, Department of Pediatrics, Boston University School of Medicine, Boston, Massachusetts

Kristin Bernard, MA, Department of Psychology, University of Delaware, Newark, Delaware

Johanna Bick, MA, Department of Psychology, University of Delaware, Newark, Delaware

Stacey R. Bromberg, PhD, Department of Psychiatry, University of Colorado Denver School of Medicine, Aurora, Colorado

Jeri B. Cohen, JD, 11th Judicial Circuit, Juvenile Division, Miami, Florida

Stephen J. Cozza, MD, Col, U.S. Army (Ret.), Center for the Study of Traumatic Stress, Department of Psychiatry, Uniformed Services University of the Health Sciences, Bethesda, Maryland

Gayle A. Dakof, PhD, 11th Judicial Circuit, Juvenile Division, Miami, Florida

Amy Dickson, PsyD, Department of Psychiatry, Louisiana State University Health Sciences Center, New Orleans, Louisiana

Mary Dozier, PhD, Department of Psychology, University of Delaware, Newark, Delaware

Eliette Duarte, LMHC, 11th Judicial Circuit, Juvenile Division, Miami, Florida

Natalia Estassi, PsyD, Safe Start Program, San Carlos, California

Margaret M. Feerick, PhD, Center for the Study of Traumatic Stress, Department of Psychiatry, Uniformed Services University of the Health Sciences, Bethesda, Maryland

Lynette Fraga, PhD, Zero to Three: National Center for Infants, Toddlers, and Families, Washington, DC

Karen A. Frankel, PhD, Department of Psychiatry, University of Colorado Denver School of Medicine, Aurora, Colorado

Chandra Ghosh Ippen, PhD, Child Trauma Research Program, University of California, San Francisco, San Francisco, California

Lili Gray, LCSW, Adult Child and Family Counseling Center, Jewish Child and Family Services, Arlington Heights, Illinois

Betsy McAlister Groves, LCSW, Department of Pediatrics, Boston Medical Center, Boston, Massachusetts

Alisa Hathaway, LCSW, Mt. Hope Family Center, Rochester, New York

Donna J. Hitchens, JD, San Francisco Superior Court, San Francisco, California

Douglas F. Johnson, JD, Douglas County Juvenile Court, Omaha, Nebraska

Sandra J. Kaplan, MD (deceased), The Florence and Robert A. Rosen Family Wellness Center for Law Enforcement and Military Personnel and Their Families, Division of Trauma Psychiatry, Department of Psychiatry, North Shore–Long Island Jewish Health System, Manhasset, New York

Mindy Kronenberg, PhD, Department of Psychiatry, Louisiana State University Health Sciences Center, New Orleans, Louisiana

Marva L. Lewis, PhD, School of Social Work, Tulane University, New Orleans, Louisiana

Alicia F. Lieberman, PhD, Child Trauma Research Project, Department of Psychiatry, University of California, San Francisco, and San Francisco General Hospital, San Francisco, California

Jody Todd Manly, PhD, Mt. Hope Family Center, Rochester, New York

Jennifer M. Newman, PhD, The Florence and Robert A. Rosen Family Wellness Center for Law Enforcement and Military Personnel and Their Families, Division of Trauma Psychiatry, Department of Psychiatry, North Shore–Long Island Jewish Health System, Manhasset, New York

Mary O'Grady, MSW, Zero to Three: National Center for Infants, Toddlers, and Families, Washington, DC

Joy D. Osofsky, PhD, Departments of Pediatrics and Psychiatry, Louisiana
State University Health Sciences Center, New Orleans, Louisiana

Beth Pettinelli, LCSW, Jewish Child and Family Services, Northbrook,
Illinois

Gwynneth Smith, JD, PhD, Child Trauma Research Project, University of
California, San Francisco, and San Francisco General Hospital,
San Francisco, California

Sheree L. Toth, PhD, Mt. Hope Family Center, Rochester, New York

Patricia Van Horn, PhD, Child Trauma Research Program, San Francisco
General Hospital, San Francisco, California

Juliet M. Vogel, PhD, The Florence and Robert A. Rosen Family Wellness
Center for Law Enforcement and Military Personnel and Their
Families, Division of Trauma Psychiatry, Department of Psychiatry,
North Shore Hospital, Zucker Hillside Hospital, North Shore–Long
Island Jewish Health System, Manhasset, New York

Dorinda Silver Williams, MSW, LCSW-C, Zero to Three: National Center
for Infants, Toddlers, and Families, Washington, DC

Foreword

The innocence of young children is a recurrent theme in the public imagination that has also found a favored place in myth and in the arts. Yet the tenderness at the heart of this perception has a dark side as well, because it can render adults oblivious to the violations that routinely befall the very young and rob them of the essence of their innocence—their trust in the benevolence of the parents and caregivers who are expected to protect them.

Every year our national statistics show alarmingly high rates of traumatization in young children, primarily through physical and sexual abuse, and through the violence they witness in their homes and communities. Epidemiological studies consistently demonstrate that although victimization is not distributed evenly, the rate is high not only among social groups traditionally considered "at risk" but also in the general population, and the United States is routinely ranked among the industrialized countries with the highest rates of violence overall. There is a steady accumulation of research studies documenting the adverse sequelae of exposure to violence on children's physical health and biological, emotional, social, and cognitive functioning. The urgent public health implications of this situation are underscored by repeated statements from leaders in academia and public policy comparing the effects of violence on children's mental health to the effects of tobacco on physical health, and warning that violence has reached the proportions of a public health epidemic.

Violence and trauma are not isolated phenomena. They create and reinforce each other, they have consequences that generate new stresses and compound existing adversities, and they are jointly engendered by circumstances that make the individual feel embattled, exploited, oppressed, and embittered. Extreme poverty, social marginalization, cultural dislocation, political instability, severe economic disparities, and the traumas inflicted by war have been consistently identified as environmental factors that spawn and exacerbate the conditions for family and community violence and trauma across societies. These conditions are also conducive to a pervasive absence of well-functioning institutional supports and protective resources such as safe streets and communities, adequate housing, access to education, reliable jobs, and living wages. In this context, stressful and traumatic events are not discrete and isolated phenomena in an otherwise predictable interpersonal and social environment but become chronic and cumulative, affecting the capacity to respond adaptively to environmental challenges ranging from everyday frustrations to natural disasters. Healthy development and functioning of individuals across the age range are derailed when the social contract between the state and its citizens is perceived as faltering or failed. Traumatized adults become parents who are more likely to traumatize their children, creating an intergenerational cycle of psychopathology. This understanding is at the root of the ecological–transactional model of development that represents one of the major advances in psychology in the past 25 years (Bronfenbrenner, 1977; Cicchetti & Lynch, 1993; Rutter, 2003; Sameroff & Fiese, 2000).

In spite of the voluminous evidence documenting the mental health sequelae, and the social and financial costs of childhood trauma, the public health and public policy responses fall far short of the need in mobilizing trauma resources for children and their families. Changes that are pivotal in creating momentum toward substantial and lasting change include moving beyond the confines of the mental health system to offer trauma-focused, integrated interventions to children and families in the environments where they spend their time and receive services, including military family institutions, pediatric care clinics, child care settings, residential and domestic violence shelters, substance abuse programs, the welfare system, and the courts (Harris, Putnam, & Fairbank, 2006).

We are fortunate that Joy Osofsky has pioneered groundbreaking initiatives that implement this vision, creating new models of collaboration with the law enforcement, child welfare, and judicial systems; bringing trauma-informed infant mental health interventions to systems of care, as well as natural disaster zones; and creating partnerships with agencies and institutions already involved with the family in order to expand the reach of mental health interventions to include the children as well. In this timely and invaluable book, she also deploys her academic gifts as scholar, educator, and editor in bringing together a collection of chapters that, when read as a whole, redefine the landscape of what is needed to intervene effectively in transforming the impact of trauma and, when read individually, convey extraordinary devotion, insight, and know-how in creating the conditions to alleviate suffering and instill hope. This book will become a "must-read" resource for all who are committed to the well-being of children, and will be an indispensable companion and guide in pursuing this most important of endeavors.

ALICIA F. LIEBERMAN, PHD

REFERENCES

Bronfenbrenner, U. (1977). Toward an experimental ecology of human development. *American Psychologist, 32,* 513–531.

Cicchetti, D., & Lynch, M. (1993). Toward an ecological/transactional model of community violence and child maltreatment: Consequences for children's development. *Psychiatry, 53,* 96–118.

Harris, W. W., Putnam, F. W., & Fairbank, J. A. (2006). Mobilizing trauma resources for children. In A. F. Lieberman & R. DeMartino (Eds.), *Interventions for children exposed to violence* (pp. 311–340). New York: Johnson & Johnson Pediatric Institute.

Rutter, M. (2003). Poverty and child mental health: Natural experiments and social causation. *Journal of the American Medical Association, 290*(15), 2063–2064.

Sameroff, A. J., & Fiese, B. H. (2000). Transactional regulation: The developmental ecology of early intervention. In J. P. Shonkoff, S. J. Meisels, & E. F. Zigler (Eds.), *Handbook of early childhood intervention* (pp. 135–159). Cambridge, UK: Cambridge University Press.

Preface

The effects of trauma on young children are profound and often unrecognized. High rates of traumatization have become commonplace in our country, recurring year after year, with the greatest impact on the youngest, most vulnerable children. Adults, including professionals working with young children, need to learn much more about the significant effects of different types of trauma exposure on young children, and about interventions and treatments that work. Education should include increasing awareness and training in different settings such as classrooms, communities, hospitals, schools, and courts. This book is designed to expand understanding and knowledge in this important area for prevention, intervention, and treatment services. In raising awareness about the impact of trauma on children, it is crucial to recognize and acknowledge that infants, toddlers, and young children are more vulnerable than older children, because they are dependent on care, support, and nurturance from adults to protect them and, if they are exposed, to help them recover. At the same time, it is important to understand that if stability can be created in their environment, including safety, support, and routines, they often have the flexibility to recover quickly. We have observed and experienced the amazing capacity of young children, when they are supported by caregivers, to resume play in the midst of adversity that weighs heavily on older children and adults.

This volume is designed to provide "state-of-the-art" new knowledge on young children and trauma, with an emphasis on intervention, best practice, and treatment approaches and services. Given the fact that information on interventions, evaluation, and treatment in work with young traumatized children and their families is not included in educational training for most disciplines, this book, from a variety of different perspectives, will inform the reader about the impact of trauma at many different levels in the lives of young children. Even more important, the book provides strategies to mitigate the effects of trauma exposure.

The book is divided into five topically focused sections: Part I describes perspectives related to trauma and the impact of trauma on young children; Part II presents evaluation and treatment models for young children exposed to trauma; Part III introduces an important area in which little has been written—the impact of the stress of deployment on young children from military families; Part IV focuses on different perspectives related to working with abused and neglected young children, including children of substance-abusing parents in juvenile court; and Part V identifies special issues for those who work with high-risk infants, young children, and families, including the effects of disasters, work in pediatric settings, and vicarious traumatization that can be experienced by both professional and nonprofessional helpers, using examples from the different perspectives presented in the book.

The book covers a broad array of relevant topics, with examples from those who work in juvenile court in different capacities, interveners for children in military families during deployments and with combat-injured parents, therapists who work with abused and neglected children and substance-abusing parents in the child welfare system, pediatric health practitioners, and those who respond to children traumatized by disasters. All of this work can be not only very satisfying but also frustrating and potentially traumatizing. Therefore, it is important to conclude a book focusing on young children and trauma with an emphasis on self-care and the need for helpers to take care of themselves in order to help our most vulnerable young children and their families.

As the reader approaches this volume to learn more about and to gain skill in helping young children exposed to trauma, I want to share a question posed to us several years ago by our close friend Dr. William (Bill) Harris: "Do we really have free will in all of our choices, particularly in the work that we do and how we spend our lives?" His question is very profound and I have thought about it a great deal over the years. Many of us who work with traumatized young children and families in an effort to help make a difference in their lives recognize that we do not have a choice. We are passionately committed to helping these young children. Through our work, we find ourselves serving as their "voice" to help them get "back on track," regain their developmental trajectory, and achieve their long-term potential.

Acknowledgments

In this book, my colleagues and I have written about experiences of young children in different, and often difficult, settings—military families, the judicial system, the child welfare system, pediatric settings, those exposed to substance abuse, those impacted by disasters—and elaborated on ways to provide support, intervention, evaluation, and treatment services. I have also emphasized the need to recognize the risk of vicarious traumatization and the need for self-care for all individuals who work with young children exposed to trauma.

An extremely important component of working effectively with traumatized young children and their families and caregivers relates to being in a supportive environment. I am very appreciative of the Department of Psychiatry Trauma Team and the Harris Program for Infant Mental Health at the Louisiana State University Health Sciences Center (LSUHSC), which has provided a "holding environment" for all of our work with traumatized young children, including maltreated infants and toddlers, those exposed to domestic and community violence, those impacted by disasters, and the many young children we see who grow up in poverty and in families suffering with mental illness and substance abuse. I am fortunate to work with programs and individuals who are committed to prevention, early intervention, and providing services for young children who very often "fall between the cracks" of both the heath care and mental health systems. The important infant mental health training, consultation, and supervision provided at LSUHSC in New Orleans not only helps support young children and families locally but also—through collaboration with the National Child Traumatic Stress Network; Zero to Three/National Center for Infants, Toddlers, and Families; and the Irving Harris Foundation Professional Development Network—we have been able to provide such support for individuals and programs both nationally and internationally. I am grateful for these relationships and the opportunity to work with individuals who believe that we can make a difference in the lives of traumatized young children and their families.

I want to thank my supportive and loving husband, Howard, who has always provided a very important "secure base" for me and my three wonderful children. As I have undertaken this very difficult work with young children exposed to trauma, I have been so fortunate to always have someone to listen and also believe in what I am doing, and to see my children—Hari, Justin, and Michael—grow up to be sensitive, responsible young adults with a commitment to helping others.

Finally, I thank Kathryn Moore, Senior Editor at The Guilford Press, who has been so supportive and extremely helpful as this book evolved. She has worked with me in conceptualizing the most effective ways to communicate this material so that it will be most helpful to the readers. I appreciate her openness, sensitivity, and creativity. Guilford Press has been a pleasure to work with on this book, showing much careful preparation and efficiency at each stage in the production of the final product.

Contents

CHAPTER 1

■ ■ ■ ■

Introduction

Trauma through the Eyes
of a Young Child

Joy D. Osofsky

Despite much evidence to the contrary, many continue to believe that very young children are not significantly impacted by exposure to trauma. Although people believe that early adversity has a deleterious effect on children, a common misunderstanding continues that if they are affected, they will "grow out of" the behavioral and emotional problems that may result from traumatic exposure (Osofsky, 2004; Shonkoff & Phillips, 2000). In the field of mental health, infancy is often not included as part of the regular curriculum, and the result is a lack of understanding about infant development—and how it can be derailed. For those who want to help young children impacted by trauma, relatively few are familiar with ways to evaluate, intervene, and treat these young children. We try to redress that imbalance by offering a comprehensive picture of how to understand the effect of exposure to trauma on infants and toddlers, and exploring the many exciting new interventions that have been researched and developed to help these vulnerable children get back on track.

A critical first step in supporting children exposed to trauma is understanding developmental issues. Emotional and behavioral reactions to trauma vary tremendously, of course, depending on the child's capacity to comprehend and internalize his or her experiences, both of which depend on cognitive and emotional development. Given their innate and adaptive desire to maintain control over their world, young children often feel responsible for the traumatic event, as if they caused the "badness" to occur, believing that they did something, either through their actual behavior or even simply through their thoughts. It is important to recognize that young children are exquisitely sensitive to the adults in their environment, and that their reactions and behaviors resonate with those of their caregivers. Therefore, to help support young children exposed to trauma, it is imperative also to attend to adults in their caregiving environment, which is one of the major reasons all treatments need to address the relationship between the parent or caregiver and child.

WHAT ARE THE EFFECTS
OF TRAUMA ON YOUNG CHILDREN?

Young children suffer trauma from many different sources, and in different ways. The statistics related to abuse and neglect speak for themselves: approximately one million cases of child abuse and neglect substantiated in the United States each year (U.S. Department of Health and Human Services, Administration of Children, Youth, and Families, 2005, *www.acf.hhs.gov*). The Centers for Disease Control and Prevention (CDC; 2008) estimates that 1 of 7 children between 2 and 17 years is a victim of maltreatment. However, it is likely that the actual rate of abuse and neglect is considerably higher (Theodore et al., 2005). In 2006, more than 100,000 children under the age of 3 entered the child welfare system in the United States (State of Child Welfare in America: 2010, 2009), and infants under the age of 1 were the largest cohort. In the United States in 2006, 1 of 43 infants less than 1 year of age suffered abuse and neglect. Furthermore, young children are more likely to be abused or neglected and to remain in care longer (Wulczyn, Hislop, & Harden, 2002). Children under the age of 4 are more vulnerable; 79% of child fatalities occur in this age range, with children under age 1 accounting for 44% (U.S. Department of Health and Human Services, Administration on Children, Youth, and Families, 2005, *www.acf.hhs.gov*). Solid evidence points to the negative effect of abuse and neglect on children's physical, intellectual and cognitive, and social and emotional development, as well as their brain development (Center for the Developing Child at Harvard, 2007, *developingchild.harvard.edu*). Developmental delays are four to five times greater for abused than for nonabused children, and abused children have a much higher incidence of behavioral problems and risk for mental health problems (Dore, 2005; Leslie et al., 2005). There is strong evidence that the social and educational consequences of maltreatment start early in childhood and continue into later development (Anda et al., 2006; Edwards, Dube, Felitti, & Anda, 2007). Substance abuse and mental illness among parents contributes substantially to abuse and neglect (Boris, 2009). Multiple traumatization related to concurrent exposure to domestic and/or community violence substantially increases the risk and vulnerability for young children (Osofsky, 2004; Putnam, 2006).

Different life events can also result in traumatization of young children. For example, deployment of parents in the military, while not typically thought of as a traumatic event, has been shown to have a significant effect on development because of the suddenness of the event, uncertainty created for often newly married or young parents not knowing how long their loved one will be away and whether he or she will be safe, and often limited support for the home-front parents. For military families, it is important to recognize that over half (52.3%) of Active Duty enlisted personnel are 25 years old or younger and married (Department of Defense, 2008). Furthermore, the age of the largest group of children in the military is between birth and 5 years. Therefore, young children are frequently exposed to and impacted by deployment, and sometimes multiple deployments. They are also exposed to resultant combat-related injuries of a parent, as well as the impact of such injuries and the effects of the recovery process on family function. Relatively little attention has been paid to the potentially traumatizing effects of such experiences on the young child and the family. Only recently have interventions and treatments been developed for young children in military families, and several new and innovative models are included in this book.

Disasters of all types also profoundly affect young children. These events—including hurricanes, earthquakes, floods, terrorist attacks, and other major disruptions—are characterized by the fact that they seemingly come out of the blue. Since disasters by their very nature are often unpredictable, families and communities are rarely well enough prepared, which can leave children exposed to situations in which the parents may be unable to protect them. In some cases, during or following disasters, if parents are able to protect their children from direct traumatic exposure, keep some type of routines, and avoid separations, the children are frequently less effected. Again, young children who are particularly vulnerable will be more significantly impacted if they are separated from parents, or if their parents or caregivers are themselves traumatized during and in the aftermath of disasters.

THE IMPORTANCE OF CREATING TRAUMA-INFORMED SYSTEMS

Many agencies and service systems in a range of areas—such as health, mental health, education, child welfare, law enforcement, and juvenile justice—are responsible for providing a safe and secure environment for everyone;

however, children are especially vulnerable if they have been traumatized. Each one of these systems has different levels of training and awareness, knowledge, and skills in dealing with trauma. The challenge is in creating a system of care both to maintain children's safety and to be able to provide the nurture and support that are so important for children exposed to trauma. The National Child Traumatic Stress Network (NCTSN, 2007) emphasizes the need to create trauma-informed systems, acknowledging the critical importance of the role of trauma in the development of emotional, behavioral, educational, and physical difficulties in the lives of children and adults. A trauma-informed system recognizes and avoids inflicting secondary trauma or retraumatizing young children through uniformed policies and procedures. Within all of the different systems of care, it is important that professionals learn more about policies and procedures in systems that serve children but continue to retraumatize them—and also be shown new ways to intervene to decrease this risk. Developing trauma-informed systems begins with educating professionals in the system about the impact of trauma on infants and toddlers, and showing them how to recognize the signs and symptoms in children of different ages. In addition, critically important is showing how long- and short-term decisions can have the unintended effect of retraumatizing children. An example of a potentially retraumatizing situation for young children is separation from primary caregivers, and its potentially damaging effects. Even in cases in which a caregiver has been abusive or neglectful, separation can nonetheless still be traumatic and stressful because this may be the only primary caregiver an infant or toddler has known, with the child attached to and seeking love from that individual. Another common decision made daily in the child welfare and judicial systems that is often retraumatizing to children relates to foster care or other placements, or changing placements. Even if these placements are made for good reason, the net effect can traumatize the child even further. Visitations can also retraumatize, depending on the consistency of the meetings, as well as the level and type of support given to the child when visitations occur.

THE IMPORTANCE OF SENSITIVITY TO CULTURE

All systems personnel who interact with young children need to recognize the importance of culture. Interventions and services for young children and families are most effective if they take into account cultural competence, within both individuals and systems. Cultural competence relates both to individual recognition and sensitivity to cultural differences among racial and ethnic groups, and to understanding the need for cultural sensitivity about systems that impact vulnerable young children. Thus, there needs to be cultural competence within the judicial, legal, and child welfare systems that impact abused and neglected children, the military system that impacts on families when service members are deployed or injured, the health care system that may be the first to identify trauma in a young child, the mental health system that provides evaluations and services for young children, and the substance abuse system that recognizes vulnerabilities for young children and their caregivers.

PREVENTION, INTERVENTIONS, AND TREATMENT FOR YOUNG CHILDREN EXPOSED TO TRAUMA

Work with young children exposed to trauma is crucial for many reasons. The Adverse Childhood Experiences Study (Dube et al., 2003) has shown clearly that childhood adversity is cumulative, with increases in mental health symptoms as a child develops related to the amount of exposure to childhood adversities. Adversities may begin with family dysfunction, such as abuse and neglect, mental health problems, substance abuse, and domestic violence. These problems can lead to neurobiological effects in the infant and young child (brain abnormalities, stress hormone dysregulation), psychosocial effects (poor attachment, socialization, and self-esteem), and health risk behaviors (smoking, substance abuse, risky sexual behaviors) (*www.acestudy.org*). Evidence is compelling that the effects of such adversities on the brain, without early intervention, can result in serious cognitive and learning problems, as well as social and emotional difficulties (Center for the Developing Child at Harvard, 2007). The problems have been referred to as a developmental cascade of transgenerational child maltreatment risk (Trickett, Noll, & Putnam, in press).

A very important area for prevention and intervention is within the family system, where support is crucial for parents and caregivers who may also be traumatized by events similar to those impacting on the child, for example, domestic violence, separation from a military spouse, or exposure to disasters. When a young child is traumatized, it is likely the parent or caregiver is also traumatized, and less able to be sensitive and emotionally available to the child. Even under typical circumstances, parenting is a complex and challenging process. The added stress related to supporting a child who is traumatized, while coping with issues such as domestic violence, separation from and worry about a spouse who has been deployed, or coping with loss of property and family–community support following a disaster, can affect the parent's relationship with the child and the child's capacity to form a healthy attachment relationship. Such stresses can lead to additional problems such as depression, substance use, or other behaviors that can result in the parent being less physically and emotionally available to the child. Exposure to trauma of any of these types can also interfere with normal developmental transitions for both the child and parent. With exposure to trauma, a young child may lose trust in the safety of the environment (Erikson, 1950). Therefore, supports outside the family may be very important. Furthermore, it is necessary for parents to cope with their own traumatization before they can effectively support their children.

In young children, reactions to a traumatic event or experience may be difficult to predict. Changes in behaviors and emotions may occur right after the event, days, or even weeks later. Young children are much more vulnerable and dependent on the reactions, responses, and availability of consistent, nurturant caregivers. As discussed earlier, one level of intervention for young children is through parents, extended family, and other caregivers. When the traumatization goes beyond the support, care, and nurturance that a parent or caregiver can provide, professional intervention and treatment are important to help the child before the unaddressed traumatization leads to more serious and difficult problems. Because, in general, young children communicate through play rather than language, behavioral observations and interventions during play and parent–child interactions provide an important way to understand the young child's conflicts and what he or she may be experiencing internally. The work of relationship-based psychotherapy is to uncover, discover, and support strengths in the relationship; recognize and work with weaknesses; and build a stronger, more positive relationship. An important part of the work involves learning more about the child's internal world through observation, and helping the caregiver and child understand that behaviors have meaning. A number of different approaches to intervention and treatment are presented in this book.

In summary, recognizing the needs of young traumatized children and understanding that interventions and treatment can make a difference lead to more effective programs and practice. This book presents "state-of-the-art" information on ways to understand and help young children exposed to trauma and their families across systems and disciplines. The hope is that researchers, clinicians, educators, and policymakers will become better informed, in order to influence and implement the important changes needed to help the most vulnerable young children.

REFERENCES

Anda, R. F., Felitti, V. J., Walker, J., Whitfield, C. L., Bremner, J. D., Perry, B. D., et al. (2006). The enduring effects of abuse and related adverse experiences in childhood: A convergence of evidence from neurobiology and epidemiology. *European Archives of Psychiatry and Clinical Neurosciences, 56*(3), 174–186.

Boris, N. W. (2009). Parental substance abuse. In C. H. Zeanah, Jr. (Ed.), *Handbook of infant mental health* (3rd ed., pp. 171–179). New York: Guilford Press.

Center for the Developing Child at Harvard. (2007). The foundations of lifelong health. Cambridge, MA: Harvard University. Available at *www.developing child.harvard.edu.*

Dore, M. (2005). Child and adolescent mental health. In G. Malon & P. Hess (Eds.), *Child welfare for the twenty-first century: A handbook of practices, policies, and programs* (pp. 148–172). New York: Columbia University Press.

Dube, S. R., Felitti, V. J., Dong, M., Chapman, D. P., Giles, W. H., & Anda, R. F. (2003). Childhood abuse, neglect, and household dysfunction and the risk of illicit drug use: The Adverse Childhood Experiences Study. *Pediatrics, 111,* 564–572.

Edwards, V. J., Dube, S. R., Felitti, V. J., & Anda, R. F. (2007). It's OK to ask about past abuse. *American Psychologist, 62*(4), 327–328.

Erikson, E. (1950). *Childhood and society.* New York: Norton.

Leslie, L. K., Gordon, J. N., Lambros, K., Premji, K., Peoples, J., & Gist, K. (2005). Addressing the developmental and mental health needs of young children in foster care. *Journal of Developmental and Behavioral Pediatrics, 26,* 140–151.

National Child Traumatic Stress Network (NCTSN). (2007). Creating trauma-informed child-serving systems. *NCTSN Service System Briefs, 1*(1). Available at *www.NCTSN.org.*

Osofsky, J. D. (Ed.). (2004). *Young children and trauma: Intervention and treatment.* New York: Guilford Press.

Putnam, F. W. (2006, Winter). The impact of trauma on child development. *Juvenile and Family Court Journal, 57*(1), 1–11.

Shonkoff, J., & Philips, D. (2000). *From neurons to neighborhoods: The science of early childhood development.* Washington, DC: National Academies Press.

State of Child Welfare in America: 2010. (2009). Columbia: Center for Family Policy and Research, University of Missouri. Retrieved March 15, 2010, from *cfpr. missouri.edu/statechildwelfare10.pdf.*

Theodore, A., Chang, J., Runyan, D., Hunter, W., Shrikant, I., & Agans, R. (2005). Epidemiological features of physical and sexual maltreatment of children in the Carolinas. *Pediatrics, 115,* 331–337.

Trickett, P. K., Noll, J. G., & Putnam, F. W. (in press). The impact of sexual abuse on female development: Lessons from a multigenerational longitudinal research study. *Development and Psychopathology.*

U.S. Department of Defense. (2008). 2008 Demographic Report. Washington, DC: Author. Retrieved December 15, 2010, from *prhome.defense.gov/mcfp/reports. aspx.*

Wulczyn, F., Hislop, K., & Harden, B. (2002). The placement of children in foster care. *Infant Mental Health Journal, 23,* 454–475.

PART I

■ ■ ■ ■

PERSPECTIVES RELATED TO TRAUMA AND ITS IMPACT ON YOUNG CHILDREN

INTRODUCTION TO PART I

Children ages 0–5 experience disproportionately high rates of abuse and neglect, and these result in both short-term developmental problems and longer-term effects on their physical well-being and mental health. All domains of development are negatively affected with exposure to trauma, and often a child is derailed from a normal developmental trajectory. The role of interventions and clinical treatment is to help the young child get back on track. To understand and help young traumatized children, it is important to focus on clinical practice that includes the three components of prevention, intervention, and treatment. This volume, with authors discussing different systems that impact on young children, provides important information on the effects of trauma on infants, toddlers, young children, and their parents or caregivers, as well as how providers and other professionals can take the lead in creating trauma-informed, child-serving systems.

An area that has received increased attention in the past decade is the impact of trauma on brain development and physiological responses to stress. The brain incorporates experiences into its developing architecture, including those that are positive and negative, such as chronic, overwhelming stress (Shonkoff & Phillips, 2000; Thompson, 2008). With excess stress, the young child's physiological responses remain activated at high levels over long periods of time, with adverse effects on brain architecture that forms the basis for learning, behavior, and health (Carrión, Weems, Ray, & Reiss, 2002; De Bellis et al., 1999; Gunnar, 2003). On the positive side, evidence also shows that while flexibility in the developing brain declines over time, some plasticity remains, particularly in young children, such that the potential for recovery and change from both prevention and early intervention approaches is remarkable. Patricia Van Horn introduces the reader to groundbreaking research in the past decade on the impact of trauma and stress on the brain, with significant implications for early development, intervention, and clinical treatment services. She discusses and analyzes new research on the development of the social brain and the ways that stress and trauma may disproportionately impact on young children's social, emotional, and physiological development. Recognizing the importance for early development, she emphasizes the need to understand relationship security as a moderator of the impact of stress and trauma.

This book emphasizes that within systems impacting on young children, sensitivity to individual differences and culture is crucial. Chandra Ghosh Ippen and Marva L. Lewis develop a sensitive approach to this very important issue by discussing factors that may interfere with engagement and retention in clinical services for young children at risk and their caregivers. Ethnicity, socioeconomic status, and environmental context can play a role in lack of engagement. In a creative way, these authors elaborate on the importance of developing a diversity-informed approach to engagement. Sensitivity to culture is crucial for building relationships and delivering clinical services to young children and families from all racial, ethnic, and cultural backgrounds.

REFERENCES

Carrión, V. G., Weems, C. F., Ray, R., & Reiss, A. L. (2002). Toward an empirical definition of pediatric PTSD: The phenomenology of PTSD symptoms in youth. *Journal of American Academy of Child and Adolescent Psychiatry, 41,* 166–173.

De Bellis, M. D., Baum, A. S., Birmaher, B., Keshavan, M. S., Eccard, C. H., Boring, A. M., et al. (1999). Developmental traumatology: Part I. Biological stress systems. *Biological Psychiatry, 45*(10), 1259–1270.

Gunnar, M. R. (2003). Integrating neuroscience and psychological approaches in the study of early experiences. *Annals of the New York Academy of Sciences, 1008,* 238–247.

Shonkoff, J., & Philips, D. (2000). *From neurons to neighborhoods: The science of early childhood development.* Washington, DC: National Academies Press.

Thompson, R. A. (2008, December). Connecting neurons, concepts, and people: Brain development and its implications (National Institute for Early Education Research Policy Brief). Retrieved September 10, 2010, from *www.nieer.org.*

CHAPTER 2

■ ■ ■ ■

The Impact of Trauma on the Developing Social Brain

Development and Regulation in Relationship

Patricia Van Horn

It is by now accepted wisdom that a baby's brain development begins before birth; continues to unfold rapidly during the first years of life; is dependent, both before and after birth, on the environment in which the baby and young child is developing; and that the environment of development includes the child's significant relationships (Cozolino, 2006; Schore, 1994). Primary caregiving relationships have special significance in shaping the child's environment, sense of self, and physiology. Researchers have long been interested in pathways of intersubjective exchange between infant and mother and their contribution to development (Trevarthan, 1989). When development takes place in an optimal relational environment, there is a synchronistic interplay between mother and baby in which each matches the other's affective patterns, allowing re-creation in the other of their own inner psychobiological states (Reynolds, 2003; Schore, 2002). Tronick and his colleagues (1998, p. 292) make a similar point in stating his "dyadic expansion of consciousness hypothesis": "Each individual, in this case the infant and mother, ... is a self-organizing system that creates his or her own states of consciousness (states of brain organization), which can be expanded into more coherent and complex states in collaboration with another self-organizing system."

Optimal development depends on a "good-enough" fit between the organizing and regulating systems of the mother and baby. It also depends on myriad other variables, including the quality of care the child receives, the quality and quantity of stimulation that is present in the environment, and the quality of social supports that hold the baby and his caregivers. These variables interact with the baby's developing brain, which in turn interacts with the caregiver's brain to shape the baby's and growing child's capacity to regulate, translate the sensory world into integrated experience, make meaning of that experience, and engage in flexible action (Lillas & Turnbull, 2009).

It is also widely accepted that traumatic experiences, and the secondary stresses that follow them, interrupt these developmental trajectories, resulting in challenges to the capacity to trust relationships and regulate affect, distortions in sensory perception and meaning, and constrictions in action (Pynoos, Steinberg, & Piacentini, 1999). As with all else in development, relationships with caregivers are of central importance in an infant's or young child's experience of a traumatic event. Frightening, overwhelming caregiver behavior is the most potent source of stress a young child can experience; a secure relationship with a caregiver provides the most potent defense against overwhelming stress (Gunnar & Quevedo, 2007), and caregivers and family systems that function well are the best predictors of good adjustment over time for children traumatized in their early years (Laor, Wolmer, & Cohen, 2001).

This chapter examines the stresses that, often disproportionately, affect young children and the social, emotional, and physiological consequences of stress and trauma. It focuses on the impact of extreme stress and trauma on the developing brain and central nervous system, and on understanding relationship security as a moderator of that impact.

TRAUMATIC EVENTS THAT AFFECT YOUNG CHILDREN

Perhaps because, as a culture, we tend to idealize infancy and early childhood as a safe and carefree time of life, there has been little systematic study of the incidence of stress and trauma exposure among infants, toddlers, and preschoolers. Thus, none of the 12 studies included in one review of the literature on children's exposure to community violence had data about children under age 6 (Jenkins & Bell, 1997).

The available empirical evidence, however, shows that the youngest children are routinely exposed to a range of stressors. In one study, a pediatric sample of 305 children between ages 2 and 5 showed that 52.5% of the children had experienced a severe traumatic stressor in their lifetimes, including the loss of a loved adult, extended hospitalization, severe motor vehicle accidents, serious falls, and severe burns. Over 17% of these young children met criteria for a DSM-IV emotional or behavioral disorder, with a strong association between the number of stressors experienced and the likelihood of disorder (Egger & Angold, 2004). A study with a different pediatric sample found that children under age 6 are also commonly exposed to intentional violence: 47% of the mothers surveyed in the waiting room of the Boston Medical Center pediatric clinic reported that their children had heard gunshots, and 94% of this subset of mothers reported more than one such episode. In addition, 10% of the children had witnessed a knifing or a shooting, and nearly 20% had witnessed an episode of hitting, kicking, or shoving between adults (Taylor, Zuckerman, Harik, & Groves, 1994). Indeed, some traumatic stressors disproportionately affect children under age 5, including hospitalization or death from drowning and submersion, burning, falls, suffocation, choking, and poisoning (Grossman, 2000), and exposure to domestic violence (Fantuzzo, Brouch, Beriama, & Atkins, 1997).

Young children disproportionately are also the direct victims of violence, with children from birth to age 3 having the highest rates of morbidity and mortality due to physical abuse (U.S. Department of Health and Human Services, 2007). Poor children, ethnic minorities, and children living in single-parent and stepfamily households experience greater lifetime exposure to most forms of intentional victimization, including physical abuse, sexual abuse, and witnessing family violence (Turner, Finkelhor, & Ormrod, 2006), and this risk begins in early childhood. All of these events have profound and lasting effects on children and their relationships, as does neglect, the most prevalent of all forms of child maltreatment and one that, like trauma, can have a distinct impact on brain development (De Bellis, 2005).

THE CONTINUA OF STRESSES AND STRESS RESPONSES

Efficient, effective response to stress is essential to survival. Disparate theorists (Freud, 1920/1959a, 1926/1959b; Lazarus, 1991; Lazarus & Folkman, 1984) have formulated strikingly similar cognitive–affective processing models to explain human reactions to stresses ranging from normative to extreme. These models involve a three-step process: (1) recognition of potential danger; (2) appraisal of the threatening event to determine level of risk and identify coping strategies; and (3) deployment of coping resources and strategies. It is in cases of trauma and complex trauma that the individual's capacity to identify and deploy coping strategies is overwhelmed.

Although this basic model of stress appraisal and response is universal, it does not unfold identically across individuals or at every age. New stresses that arise and new skills acquired in the course of development impact an individual's ability to cope. Appraisal of external danger intersects with children's perception of dangers emerging from within themselves. These perceived dangers reflect conflicts that also shift with development: basic anxieties about annihilation, losing the parent, not being loved, body damage, and failing to meet the moral standards and expectations of the culture. Parents are intimately bound up with young children's sense of what is dangerous and what is safe, and parents' own stresses and traumas can have a major role in derailing their ability to protect their children (Osofsky, 1995).

The Stress Continuum

Stresses range from mild demands that may enhance performance, daily hassles that may dampen performance, and hardships that may challenge development, to the overwhelming stress of trauma that derails coping responses. Traumatic stress responses themselves lie along a continuum and are associated with a range of changes in functioning that depend on whether the trauma was an isolated incident or a pattern of chronic maltreatment or violence exposure. Isolated traumatic events are more likely to produce discrete, conditioned biological and behavioral responses to trauma reminders. These reminders both reinforce avoidance strategies and render the individual fearful and helpless when he or she is confronted with traumatic reminders that cannot be avoided (Bremner, 2005; Foa, Steketee, & Olasov-Rothbaum, 1989). In contrast, chronic or complex trauma interferes more profoundly with development, especially when the child is very young at the onset of traumatic experience, when the experiences are chronic, and when they occur in the context of the child's primary caregiving environment (Bremner, 2005; Herman, 1992a, 1992b; van der Kolk, 2005).

The Stress–Response Continuum

The effectiveness of response to real and perceived danger also exists along a continuum that ranges from healthy adaptation to pathological dysregulation, including severe constriction or derailment of the ability to relate to others and to explore the environment and learn. Responses to particular stressors are determined by a variety of factors, including environmental, experiential, and genetic characteristics that shape the individual's developmental pathways (National Research Council and Institute of Medicine, 2000; Pynoos et al., 1999).

For infants and very young children, effective coping with danger involves maintaining proximity to caregivers who can appraise danger on the infant's behalf and mount an appropriate protective response. Adaptive responses to stress depend on the adult's or child's ability to read cues accurately and choose effective self-protective strategies that match the level of objective danger. Maladaptive responses involve inaccurate appraisal and/ or response to danger cues either by underestimating danger and engaging in risky behaviors or overreacting to neutral stimuli as if they involve danger. In early childhood, these maladaptive responses—recklessness versus constriction of exploration—are often associated with distortions in secure base behavior and may be indices of disorders of attachment (Lieberman & Zeanah, 1995; Zeanah & Smyke, 2009).

The effects of parental maltreatment are more global. When parents are the source of danger, young children are unable to turn to them for help and become compromised in their ability to process and integrate the traumatic event. As a result, subsequent traumatic reminders evoke globally helpless and fearful states rather than discrete conditioned responses. This failure of emotional and cognitive integration is associated with dysfunction in multiple domains of functioning, including attachment security, affective and behavioral regulation, self-concept, and cognition (Cook, Blaustein, Spinazzola, & van der Kolk, 2003). Maltreated children have higher rates of insecure and disorganized attachment, and are less able to rely on their caregivers for emotional and behavioral regulation (Cicchetti & Lynch, 1995; Lyons-Ruth & Jacobovitz, 1999; Schore, 1994, 2002). These relationship problems are in turn associated with dysregulation in children's stress hormone systems (Kaufman et al., 1997).

In addition to problems in emotional, behavior, and relationship functioning, there is increasing evidence favoring the hypothesis that repeated extreme stress, particularly at developmentally vulnerable times, changes a developing child's physiology in ways that are long-lasting and affect future appraisal of and response to threat and stress. Evidence that supports this hypothesis is reviewed in the sections that follow.

PHYSIOLOGICAL RESPONSES TO STRESS AND TRAUMA

The body responds to highly stressful stimuli with a dynamic process that involves multiple systems. These include the catecholamine, serotonin, and dopamine neurotransmitter systems, and multiple neuroendocrine axes. The hypothalamic–pituitary–adrenal (HPA) axis produces cortisol (Lipschitz, Rasmusson, & Southwick, 1998; McEwen, 1999). The sympathetic–adrenomedullary (SAM) axis of the sympathetic nervous system releases epinephrine from the medulla of the adrenal gland, facilitating rapid mobilization of the fight-or-flight response (Frankenhaeuser, 1986). Trauma-associated dysregulations have been described in all of these systems, including catecholamines (responsible for regulation of the sympathetic nervous system); serotonin (involved in the regulation and modulation of mood); and the HPA axis, which is central both to fear conditioning and to the production of stress hormones in response to fear (Southwick, Yehuda, & Morgan, 1995; Yehuda, Giller, Levengood, Southwick, & Siever, 1995).

The body responds to the visual, auditory, tactile, and kinesthetic information that make up a traumatic experience using the related SAM and HPA systems. The SAM response results in immediate mobilization of the sympathetic nervous system's fight-or-flight response via production of epinephrine; the HPA response, which takes longer to develop but is more long-lasting, sends the sensory input via the thalamus to the amygdala, a bilateral structure located in the limbic brain, whose function is to assess the aversive emotional significance of the sensory input, and set in motion the fear response and the release of stress hormones, including cortisol. The level of cortisol is controlled by a system of negative feedback loops, with high cortisol levels triggering a shutdown in production (Jacobson & Sopolsky, 1991). Simultaneously, the sensory information is transmitted along a slower path to the sensory prefrontal cortex, the seat of analysis, planning, and executive function (LeDoux, 1996, 1998). Survival is dependent upon the rapid physiological response to danger that is made possible by sympathetic nervous system arousal and by the shorter pathway to the amygdala.

Stimulus evaluation is critical even after the initiation of the stress response in order to determine whether the situation continues to present an overwhelming danger, or whether effective coping is possible. Continued interpretation of the event as dangerous results in the prolonged activation of the SAM and HPA systems (LeDoux, 1995), interfering with the negative feedback loop that, under conditions of mild or moderate stress, halts the production of cortisol. Cortisol and other stress hormones then continue to be secreted for extended periods of time, leading to the potential for chronic activation of the HPA axis. Preclinical animal models have established that long-term secretion of cortisol result in cell death and atrophy of specific parts of the brain. A recent study with 7- to 13-year-old children that confirmed this research found that baseline cortisol levels and posttraumatic stress disorder (PTSD) symptoms predicted decreased hippocampal volume, with higher levels of cortisol associated with greater decreases in volume (Carrión, Weems, & Reiss, 2007).

Although the nervous system may habituate even to high levels of predictable stress over time, such habituation does not occur if stresses are severe, unpredictable, uncontrollable, or novel. In these conditions, high levels of stress hormones continue to be secreted even in response to stimuli that are not inherently traumatic (Cullinan, Herman, Helmreich, & Watson, 1995; Yehuda, Giller, Southwick, Lowy, & Mason, 1991). This may be one mechanism explaining the discomfort that many traumatized people feel when they experience reminders of the trauma. Their physiological response to reminders may also serve to perpetuate the dysregulation of the HPA system.

The core neuroendrocrine response just described is experienced by both males and females (Allen, Stoney, Owens, & Matthews, 1993), and has been labeled the "fight-or-flight" response, reflecting two alternative ways of coping with threat, either fending it off (fight) or escaping it (flight) (Cannon, 1932). Some researchers are now proposing, however, that there are sex differences in the ways humans respond to danger based on oxytocin release during the stress response (Taylor et al., 2000, 2006). "Oxytocin," believed to enhance relaxation, decrease fearfulness, and lower sympathetic activity, is a pituitary hormone released by both men and women in response to stress (Uvnas-Moberg, 1997), but which may have more pronounced effects in women for several reasons: (1) Females may release more oxytocin under stress than males (Jezova, Jurankova, Mosnarova, Kriska, & Skultetyova, 1996); (2) male sex hormones appear to inhibit oxytocin release (Jezova et al., 1996); and (3) oxytocin effects are modulated by estrogen (McCarthy, 1995).

In animal models, oxytocin is implicated in maternal caregiving behaviors immediately following the birth of young, with high levels of licking and grooming behavior during lactation associated with higher oxytocin receptor levels in the brain (Francis, Champagne, & Meaney, 2000). The enduring effects of early caregiving behavior in the anxiety regulation and stress responsiveness are demonstrated by the finding that higher levels of maternal care after birth are associated with lower levels of stress reactivity in adult offspring (Leckman, Feldman, Swain, & Mayes, 2007; Weaver et al., 2004).

Taylor and her colleagues (2000, 2006) note that females are more involved than males in the immediate protection of offspring, and suggest that the gender differences observed in oxytocin production are explained by the demands of pregnancy, nursing, and care of young, all of which render females particularly vulnerable to attack. Neither a fight response that could end in her incapacitation or death nor a flight response that could entail the abandonment of vulnerable offspring would be adaptive for these females, who may adopt alternative behavioral patterns for coping with stress that involve protecting offspring and affiliation, particularly with other females. These behaviors are labeled "tend or befriend" by Taylor and colleagues (2000) as a counterbalance to the fight-or-flight alternatives. Some emerging evidence, however, indicates that early stress and trauma may have lasting effects on levels of oxytocin. One researcher studied adult women who were victims of child abuse and found their cerebral spinal fluid concentrations of oxytocin to be markedly reduced compared to those of nonabused women (Neigh, Gillespie, & Nemeroff, 2009). If the hypothesis of Taylor and her colleagues is correct, this hormonal difference may signal differences in coping strategies among women depending on whether they were maltreated as children, with maltreated women more vulnerable to coping with stress in a way that is less protective of self and of their children.

DEVELOPMENT AND THE NORMATIVE STRESS RESPONSE

Prenatal Development of the Stress Response

There are connections between child outcomes and levels of the mother's stress during pregnancy. Wadhwa (2005) found that mothers who reported high stress and anxiety during their pregnancies had lower birthweight infants. The low birthweight was also associated with mothers' increased HPA activity and upregulation in production of placental corticotropin-releasing hormone, a precursor of cortisol, and with shorter gestation. Another study revealed a direct association between maternal and fetal concentrations of cortisol, with maternal concentrations explaining 40% of the variance in fetal cortisol levels (Gitau, Cameron, Fisk, & Glover, 1998). This association between maternal and fetal cortisol levels continues into the neonatal period, indicating a lasting impact of stress during pregnancy (Lundy et al., 1999). Field and her colleagues (2003) found associations between the norepinephrine levels of mothers who experienced higher levels of anxiety, anger, and depression during pregnancy, and lower levels dopamine and serotonin, neuotransmitters that are decreased in patients with mood disorders, in their babies. The babies of these mothers were more active and grew more slowly before birth, had lower vagal tone, spent more time in deep sleep and less time in quiet and active alert states, and had less optimal performance in areas of motor maturity, autonomic stability, and withdrawal than did the babies of low-anxiety mothers. These studies, taken together, establish a link between maternal stress and fetal and neonatal outcomes. This link has been studied much more extensively in animal models, but bears further investigation in humans to understand more fully the factors responsible for the associations (Gunnar, Fisher, & the Early Experience, Stress, and Prevention Network, 2006).

The Stress Response in Infants, Toddlers, and Preschoolers

Newborns secrete high levels of cortisol in response to novel stimuli, whether those stimuli are invasive or noninvasive, and their cortisol elevations are positively associated with crying. There are, however, individual differences that are apparent within hours after birth. Healthy newborns also have the capacity to self-regulate by withdrawing into quiescent states that are associated with lower levels of stress hormone secretion. While healthy babies quickly habituate to stress, so that over time they cry less and secrete less cortisol in response to the same levels of stimulation, less healthy babies habituate less readily to stress. In these infants, crying is not an accurate index of their stress levels because they continue to have high cortisol levels even after they have been soothed (Gunnar, 1992).

By the time most infants are 3 months old, their diurnal pattern of cortisol production is related to the sleep–wake cycle, with the highest cortisol level occurring in the morning and declining throughout the day (White, Gunnar, Larson, Donzella, & Barr, 2000). Older infants secrete stress hormones on separation from their caregivers or in novel situations, but even temperamentally wary babies are able to habituate quickly to novel situations when they are between 2 and 6 months of age.

Later in the first year of life, and continuing at least through the preschool years, the HPA system becomes less responsive to stress; on average, cortisol levels in toddlers and preschoolers do not elevate in response to mildly threatening situations that nevertheless bring about behavioral wariness and distress. This diminished HPA response is thought to be protective of development and has been compared to the period of relative stress hyporesponsivity observed in rats and other mammalian species (Tarullo & Gunnar, 2006). Among these young children with no reported history of trauma, HPA hyporesponsiveness may be moderated by sensitive caregiving because when children in moderately stressful situations can turn to caregivers who respond to them with sensitivity, they exhibit behavioral distress but not a rise in cortisol production (Feldman, Singer, & Zagoory, 2010; Gunnar, Larson, Hertsgaard, Harris, & Brodersen, 1992; Nachmias, Gunnar, Mangelsdorf, Parritz, & Buss, 1996). Similarly, toddlers with disorganized attachments, often associated with frightening caregiver behavior (Main & Hesse, 1990), have stronger cortisol concentrations than do children whose attachment patterns are more organized (Hertsgaard, Gunnar, Erickson, & Nachmias, 1995).

Even stronger evidence of the power of relationships in regulating HPA arousal early in development is the finding that children who have been traumatized or who live in severely depriving environments, such as Russian or Romanian orphanages, have lasting dysregulations in diurnal cortisol rhythms (Carlson & Earls, 1997; Kroupina, Gunnar, & Johnson, 1997).

The Stress Response in School-Age Children

As the developmental trajectory moves into the school years, there is evidence that children continue to be somewhat HPA-hyporesponsive, at least in regard to laboratory stress challenges (Gunnar, Frenn, Wewerka, & Van Ryzin, 2009). Among nontraumatized populations, children who deploy moderate cortisol levels in response to stress tend to be more competent with peers, more involved in schoolwork, more cooperative, and more realistic in their appraisals of a stressful situation. Elevations in cortisol do not automatically signal stress or anxiety, but they may index children's active attempts to cope with both the stressor and their emotional responses to it (Gunnar, 1992; McEwen, 1999). Similar to infants, toddlers, and preschoolers, however, traumatized school-age children show dysregulations in the HPA axis, with higher levels of cortisol than matched, nontraumatized controls (Carrión, 2006; De Bellis, 2001; De Bellis, Baum, et al., 1999). As with younger children, there is some evidence that the HPA reactivity of school-age children is under social control; in one study, children's stress hormone levels were correlated with their mothers' depressive state and even socioeconomic level (Lupien, King, Meaney, & McEwen, 2000).

Adult Dysregulation

The empirical evidence is somewhat mixed, but most studies of adult trauma survivors (including one study of Holocaust survivors with PTSD, but without the substance abuse history that is so frequently comorbid with PTSD) point to hyporesponsiveness in the HPA axis, with low levels of cortisol (van der Vegt, van der Ende, Kirschbaum, Verhulst, & Tiemeier, 2009; Yehuda et al., 1995). This difference in the child and adult literature has led to the hypothesis that the low cortisol levels in adults, as opposed to the higher levels reported earlier for children, reflect a long-term adaptation to trauma because the body cannot sustain the hypersecretion of cortisol triggered in childhood by extreme stress and trauma (De Bellis, Baum, 1999; Gunnar & Vazquez, 2001). As in the child trauma literature, there is evidence that quality of relationship continues to moderate HPA dysregulation in adulthood, with disorganized states of mind regarding attachment predicting more marked dysregulation (Pierrehumbert et al., 2009).

STRUCTURAL BRAIN CHANGES
AND COGNITIVE IMPAIRMENT AFTER TRAUMA

There is also empirical evidence of changes in brain structure following trauma, although the findings are inconsistent. Some studies show that maltreated children have smaller frontal lobe volumes (De Bellis, Keshavan, 1999), while others show larger frontal cortex volume associated with increased grey matter in the left frontal lobe attenuating normal frontal cortex asymmetry (Carrión, 2006; Carrión et al., 2001). All of these changes are associated with earlier age of maltreatment, longer duration of mal-treatment, and greater severity of PTSD symptoms. Maltreated children also show pronounced asymmetry in left–right volumes of the superior tempo-ral virus, a brain center implicated in the cognitive processes of language production (De Bellis, 2001; De Bellis et al., 2002). Most studies have not found hippocampal atrophy among maltreated children (Carrión et al., 2001; De Bellis, Hall, Boring, Frustaci, & Moritz, 2001), although this atro-phy has been observed in several adult samples, including combat veterans with PTSD (Bremmer et al., 1997; Gurvits et al., 1996), PTSD sufferers who experienced childhood physical maltreatment (Bremmer et al., 1997), and women with a history of sexual abuse as children (Stein, Koverola, Hanna, Torchia, & McClarty, 1997). Hippocampal atrophy has also been observed in a single longitudinal sample of children ages 7–13 years (Carrión et al., 2007).

The area of structural brain differences associated with trauma requires further study, with larger samples and longitudinal designs to help explain whether developmental processes or other factors explain the discrepancies between child and adult findings, and whether accompanying functional changes appear with maturation (De Bellis, Hooper, & Sapia, 2005). Cur-rent literature makes clear that the changes in brain structure observed among maltreated children with PTSD are associated with limitations in cognitive functioning potentially affecting children's readiness to learn (Green, Voeller, Gaines, & Kubie, 1991). Maltreated children with PTSD showed greater deficits in attention, abstract reasoning, and executive func-tion than did a group of matched, nonmaltreated controls; among the mal-treated children, IQ was positively correlated with total brain volume and negatively correlated with duration of maltreatment (Beers & De Bellis, 2002; De Bellis, Keshavan, et al., 1999). Childhood exposure to domestic violence was associated with an 8-point IQ loss among monozygotic and dizygotic twins in a large study that controlled for genetic factors and direct maltreatment but did not measure brain volume (Koenen, Moffit, Caspi, Taylor, & Purcell, 2003). In a sample of 7- to 14-year-olds, verbal IQ was negatively correlated with the number of traumas experienced, the number of reexperiencing symptoms reported, and the level of functional impair-ment from symptoms (Saltzman, Weems, & Carrión, 2005). Among trau-matized adults, stress hormone dysregulation is also associated with deficits in verbal memory and intelligence (Bremner et al., 1993, 1997).

One reason for the frequently observed decrements in intelligence may be that individuals who have suffered traumatic life experiences tend to attend to cues that, in their minds, may be tied to risk and danger. Find-ings that lower IQ is linked to higher numbers of reexperiencing symptoms support that hypothesis. In laboratory conditions, traumatized adults and children attended selectively to negative emotions and negative situations

(Armony, Corbo, Clément, & Brunet, 2005; McPherson, Newton, Ackerman, Oglesby, & Dykman, 1997; Pollak, Cicchetti, Klorman, & Brumaghim, 1997). Although preferential attention to negative stimuli is protective in chronically dangerous environments because it promotes an early response to threat, selective attention to danger cues is likely to interfere with the traumatized person's ability to process emotionally neutral information in both learning situations and nonthreatening social situations.

A recent study underlines the importance of understanding the links between altered brain volume, HPA axis dysregulation, decrements in verbal intelligence, and preferential attention to danger cues. Lieberman and his colleagues (2007) found that linguistic processing of emotional stimuli was associated with diminished responsiveness in the amygdala and other limbic structures. Although the question was not addressed in the study, it is logical to assume that diminished amygdala responsiveness would also be associated with diminished activity in the HPA axis. Still, Lieberman's work reminds us of the importance of language as a moderator of emotional arousal, and brings us full circle because the prelinguistic verbal interplay between a mother and baby is one of the earliest ways in which infants and caregivers synchronize their affective states (Trevarthen, 1989). It is may be that in dyads disrupted by trauma, this synchronicity is not firmly established, with the result that the baby's brain, dependent on experience for its development, does not wire as richly as it might in the orbitoprefrontal cortex, an area of the brain implicated in empathy, concern for others, and the use of language to solve relationship problems (Schore, 1994, 2002). This failure may be one of the links responsible for the frequently observed decrements in Verbal IQ among trauma populations. Verbally impoverished individuals may, in turn, be less adept at the type of linguistic processing of emotional cues that Lieberman found to be associated with less activity in the amygdala, and children traumatized in their attachment relationships may grow into adults whose brain structure is ill-equipped to support regulation of their own emotional or empathic responses to their children. Thus, the intergenerational transmission of interpersonal trauma may be mediated by changes at the neural level.

CONCLUSION: THE PROMISE OF INTERVENTION

Even in cases of trauma, however, detrimental effects are not necessarily irreversible. The presence in the child's life of protective factors, particularly in the form of a close emotional relationship with a supportive adult, can ameliorate the impact of adversity and promote a positive developmental outcome (Lynch & Cicchetti, 1998). There is also emerging evidence that interventions that strengthen children's primary caregiving relationships also improve their physiological reactivity. The abnormally high cortisol level of infants and toddlers in foster care declined to the normal range after their foster parents took part in Attachment and Biobehavioral Catchup, a brief intervention designed to help foster parents provide more individually tailored, nurturing care (see Dozier, Bick, & Bernard, Chapter 5, this volume; Dozier et al., 2006). Child–parent psychotherapy (Lieberman & Van Horn, 2005, 2008), another relationship-based intervention used with traumatized children and their caregivers, also shows promise in helping with emotional regulation, in that it demonstrated diminished PTSD and other symptoms in both children and parents, though cortisol reactivity was not directly measured (see Van Horn, Gray, Pettinelli, & Estassi, Chapter 4, and Toth, Manly, & Hathaway, Chapter 6, this volume; Lieberman, Ghosh Ippen, & Van Horn, 2006; Lieberman, Van Horn, & Ghosh Ippen, 2005). This intervention has proven to be efficacious with parent–child dyads that have experienced multiple traumas (Ghosh Ippen, Harris, Van Horn, & Lieberman, 2010). The promise that relationship-based interventions may succeed in restoring greater physiological balance has important clinical implications because of the dramatic and enduring impact of traumatic stress on brain development.

REFERENCES

Allen, M. T., Stoney, C. M., Owens, J. F., & Matthews, K. A. (1993). Hemodynamic adjustments to laboratory stress: The influence of gender and personality. *Psychosomatic Medicine, 55,* 505–517.

Armony, J. L., Corbo, V., Clément, M. H., & Brunet, A. (2005). Amygdala response in patients with acute PTSD to masked and unmasked emotional facial expressions. *American Journal of Psychiatry, 162,* 1961–1963.

Bremner, J. D. (2005). *Does stress damage the brain?: Understanding trauma-related disorders from a mind–body perspective.* New York: Norton.

Bremner, J. D., Randall, P., Vermetten, E., Staib, L., Bronen, R. A., Mazure, C., et al. (1997). Magnetic resonance imaging-based measurement of hippocampal volume in posttraumatic stress disorder related to childhood physical and sexual abuse—a preliminary report. *Biological Psychiatry, 41,* 23–32.

Bremner, J. D., Scott, T. M., Delaney, R. C., Southwick, S. M., Mason, J. W., Johnson, D. R., et al. (1993). Deficits in short-term memory in posttraumatic stress disorder. *American Journal of Psychiatry, 150,* 1015–1019.

Cannon, W. B. (1932). *The wisdom of the body.* New York: Norton.

Carrión, V. G. (2006). Understanding the effects of early life stress on brain development. In A. F. Lieberman & R. DeMartino (Eds.), *Interventions for children exposed to violence* (pp. 45–64). New York: Johnson & Johnson Pediatric Institute.

Carrión, V. G., Weems, C. F., Eliez, S., Patwardhan, A., Brown, W., Ray, R. D., et al. (2001). Attenuation of frontal asymmetry in pediatric posttraumatic stress disorder. *Biological Psychiatry, 50,* 943–951.

Carrión, V. G., Weems, C. F., & Reiss, A. L. (2007). Stress predicts brain changes in children: A pilot longitudinal study on youth stress, PTSD and the hippocampus. *Pediatrics, 119,* 509–516.

Cicchetti, D., & Lynch, M. (1995). Failures in the expectable environment and their impact on individual development: The case of child maltreatment. In D. Cicchetti & D. J. Cohen (Eds.), *Developmental psychopathology: Vol. 2. Risk, disorder, and adaptation* (pp. 32–71). New York: Wiley.

Cook, A., Blaustein, M., Spinazzola, J., & van der Kolk, B. (2003). *Complex trauma in children and adolescents* [White paper]. Washington, DC: Complex Trauma Task Force, National Child Traumatic Stress Network.

Cozolino, L. (2006). *The neuroscience of human relationships: Attachment and the developing social brain.* New York: Norton.

Cullinan, W. E., Herman, J. P., Helmreich, D. L., & Watson, S. J. (1995). A neuroanatomy of stress. In M. J. Friedman, D. S. Charney, & A. Y. Deutch (Eds.), *Neurobiological and clinical consequences of stress: From normal adaptation to PTSD* (pp. 3–26). Philadelphia: Lippincott-Raven.

De Bellis, M. D. (2001). Developmental traumatology: The psychobiological development of maltreated children and its implications for research, treatment, and policy. *Development and Psychopathology, 13*(3), 539–564.

De Bellis, M. D. (2005). The psychobiology of neglect. *Child Maltreatment, 10,* 150–172.

De Bellis, M. D., Baum, A. S., Birmaher, B., Keshavan, M. S., Ecard, C. H., Boring, A. M., et al. (1999). Developmental traumatology, Part 1: Biological stress systems. *Biological Psychiatry, 9,* 1259–1270.

De Bellis, M. D., Hall, J., Boring, A. M., Frustaci, K., & Moritz, G. (2001). A pilot longitudinal study of hippocamal volumes in pediatric maltreatment-related posttraumatic stress disorder. *Biological Psychiatry, 50,* 305–309.

De Bellis, M. D., Hooper, S. R., & Sapia, J. L. (2005). Early trauma exposure and the brain. In J. J. Vasterling & C. R. Brewin (Eds.), *Neuropsychology of PTSD: Biological, cognitive, and clinical perspectives* (pp. 153–177). New York: Guilford Press.

De Bellis, M. D., Keshavan, M. S., Clark, D. B., Casey, B. J., Giedd, J. B., Boring, A. M., et al. (1999). Developmental traumatology, Part 2: Brain development. *Biological Psychiatry, 45,* 1271–1284.

De Bellis, M. D., Keshavan, M. S., Frustaci, K., Shifflett, H., Iyengar, S., Beers, S. R., et al. (2002). Superior temporal gyrus volumes in maltreated children and adolescents with PTSD. *Biological Psychiatry, 51,* 544–552.

Dozier, M., Peloso, E., Lindhiem, O., Gordon, M. K., Manni, M., Sepulveda, S., et al. (2006). Developing evidence-based interventions for foster children: An example of a randomized clinical trial with infants and toddlers. *Journal of Social Issues, 62,* 767–785.

Egger, H., & Angold, A. (2004). *Stressful life events and PTSD in preschool children.* Paper presented at the annual meeting of the American Academy of Child and Adolescent Psychiatry, Washington, DC.

Fantuzzo, J. W., Brouch, R., Beriama, A., & Atkins, M. (1997). Domestic violence and children: Prevalence and risk in five major U.S. cities. *Journal of the American Academy of Child and Adolescent Psychiatry, 36,* 116–122.

Feldman, R., Singer, M., & Zagoory, O. (2010). Touch attenuates infants' physiological reactivity to stress. *Developmental Science, 13,* 271–278.

Field, T., Diego, M., Hernandez-Reif, M., Schanberg, S., Kuhn, C., Yando, R., et al. (2003). Pregnancy anxiety and comorbid depression and anger: Effects on the fetus and neonate. *Depression and Anxiety, 17,* 140–151.

Foa, E. B., Steketee, G., & Olasov-Rothbaum, B. (1989). Behavioral/cognitive conceptualizations of post-traumatic stress disorder: An animal model. *Psychological Bulletin, 112,* 218–238.

Francis, D. D., Champagne, F. C., & Meaney, M. J. (2000). Variations in maternal behavior are associated with differences in oxytocin receptor levels in the rat. *Journal of Neuroendocrinology, 12,* 1145–1148.

Frankenhaeuser, M. (1986). A psychobiological framework for research on human stress and coping. In M. H. Appley & R. Trumbull (Eds.), *Dynamics of stress: Physiological, psychological, and social perspectives* (pp. 101–116). New York: Plenum.

Freud, S. (1959a). Beyond the pleasure principle. In J. Stachey (Ed. & Trans.), *The standard edition of the complete psychological works of Sigmund Freud* (Vol. 18, pp. 1–30). London: Hogarth Press (Original work published 1920).

Freud, S. (1959b). Inhibitions, symptoms and anxiety. In J. Strachey (Ed. & Trans.), *The standard edition of the complete psychological works of Sigmund Freud* (Vol. 20, pp. 87–156). London: Hogarth Press. (Original work published 1926).

Ghosh Ippen, C., Harris, W. W., Van Horn, P., & Lieberman, A. F. (2010). *Intervention with young children with multiple early childhood adversities.* Manuscript under review.

Gitau, R., Cameron, A., Fisk, N., & Glover, V. (1998). Fetal exposure to maternal cortisol. *Lancet 352,* 707–708.

Green, A. H., Voeller, K, Gaines, R., & Kubie, J. (1991). Neurological impairment in maltreated children. *Child Abuse and Neglect, 5,* 129–134.

Grossman, D. C. (2000). The history of injury control and the epidemiology of child and adolescent injuries. *The Future of Children, 10*(1), 4–22.

Gunnar, M. R. (1992). Reactivity of the hypothalamic–pituitary–adrenocortical system to stressors in normal infants and children. *Pediatrics, 90,* 491–497.

Gunnar, M. R., Fisher, P. A., & the Early Experience, Stress, and Prevention Network. (2006). Bringing basic research on early experience and stress neurobiology to bear on preventive interventions for neglected and maltreated children. *Development and Psychopathology, 18,* 651–677.

Gunnar, M. R., Frenn, K., Wewerka, S. S., & Van Ryzin, M. J. (2009). Moderate versus severe early life stress: Associations with stress reactivity and regulation in 10–12 year old children. *Psychoneuroendocrinology, 34,* 62–75.

Gunnar, M. R., Larson, M., Hertsgaard, L., Harris, M., & Brodersen, L. (1992). The stressfulness of separation among 9-month old infants: Effects of social context variables and infant temperament. *Child Development, 63,* 290–303.

Gunnar, M. R., & Quevedo, K. (2007). The neurobiology of stress and development. *Annual Review of Psychology, 58,* 145–173.

Gunnar, M. R., & Vazquez, D. M. (2001). Low cortisol and a flattening of expected daytime rhythm: Potential indices of risk in human development. *Development and Psychopathology, 13,* 515–538.

Gurvits, T. V., Shenton, M. E., Hokoma, H., Ohta, H., Lasko, N. B., Gilbertson, M. W., et al. (1996). Magnetic resonance imaging study of hippocampal volume in chronic, combat-related posttraumatic stress disorder. *Biological Psychiatry, 40,* 1091–1099.

Herman, J. (1992a). Complex PTSD: A syndrome in survivors of prolonged and repeated trauma. *Journal of Traumatic Stress, 5,* 377–391.

Herman, J. (1992b). *Trauma and recovery: The aftermath of violence—from domestic violence to political terror.* New York: Basic Books.

Hertsgaard, L., Gunnar, M., Erickson, M. F., & Nachmias, M. (1995). Adrenocortical response to the Strange Situation in infants with disorganized/disoriented attachment relationships. *Child Development, 66,* 1100–1106.

Jacobson, L., & Sopolsky, R. M. (1991). The role of the hippocampus in feedback regulation of the hypothalamic–pituitary–adrenocortical axis. *Endocrine Research, 12,* 118–134.

Jenkins, E. J., & Bell, C. C. (1997). Exposure and response to community violence among children and adolescents. In J. Osofsky (Ed.), *Children in a violent society* (pp. 9–31). New York: Guilford Press.

Jezova, D., Jurankova, E., Mosnarova, A., Kriska, M., & Skulteyova, I. (1996). Neuroendocrine response during stress with relation to gender differences. *Acta Neurobiologiae Experimentalis, 56,* 779–785.

Kaufman, J., Birmaher, B., Perel, J., Dahl, R. E., Moreci, P., Nelson, B., et al. (1997). The corticotropin-releasing hormone challenge in depressed abused, depressed nonabused, and normal control children. *Biological Psychiatry, 42,* 669–679.

Koenen, K. C., Moffitt, T. E., Caspi, A., Taylor, A., & Purcell, S. (2003). Domestic violence is associated with environmental suppression of IQ in young children. *Development and Psychopathology, 15,* 297–311.

Kroupina, M., Gunnar, M. R., & Johnson, D. E. (1997). *Report on salivary coritsol levels in a Russian baby home.* Minneapolis, MN: Institute of Child Development, University of Minnesota.

Laor, N., Wolmer, L., & Cohen, D. (2001). Mothers' functioning and children's symptoms 5 years after a SCUD missile attack. *American Journal of Psychiatry, 158,* 1020–1026.

Lazarus, R. S. (1991). *Emotion and adaptation.* New York: Oxford University Press.

Lazarus, R. S., & Folkman, S. (1984). *Stress, appraisal, and coping.* New York: Springer.

LeDoux, J. (1995). Setting "stress" into motion: Brain mechanisms of stimulus evaluation. In M. J. Friedman, D. S. Charney, & A. Y. Deutch (Eds.), *Neurobiological and clinical consequences of stress: From normal adaptation to posttraumatic stress disorder* (pp. 125–134). New York: Lippincott-Raven.

Leckman, J. F., Feldman, R., Swain, J. E., & Mayes, L. C. (2007). Primary parental preoccupation: Revisited. In L. Mayes, P. Fonagy, & M. Target (Eds.), *Developmental science and psychoanalysis: Integration and innovation* (pp. 89–108). London: Karnac.

LeDoux, J. (1996). *The emotional brain: The mysterious underpinnings of emotional life.* New York: Simon & Schuster.

LeDoux, J. (1998). Fear and the brain: Where have we been, and where are we going? *Biological Psychiatry, 44,* 1229–1238.

Lieberman, A. F., Ghosh Ippen, C., & Van Horn, P. (2006). Child–parent psychotherapy: Six month follow-up of a randomized control trial. *Journal of the American Academy of Child and Adolescent Psychiatry, 45,* 913–918.

Lieberman, A. F., & Van Horn, P. (2005). *Don't hit my mommy!: A manual of child–parent psychotherapy with young witnesses of family violence.* Washington, DC: Zero to Three Press.

Lieberman, A. F., & Van Horn, P. (2008). *Psychotherapy with infants and young children: Repairing the effects of stress and trauma on early attachment.* New York: Guilford Press.

Lieberman, A. F., Van Horn, P., & Ghosh Ippen, C. (2005). Towards evidence-based treatment: Child–parent psychotherapy with preschoolers exposed to marital violence. *Journal of the American Academy of Child and Adolescent Psychiatry, 44,* 1241–1248.

Lieberman, A. F., & Zeanah, C. H. (1995). Disorders of attachment in infancy. *Child and Adolescent Psychiatric Clinics of North America, 3,* 571–587.

Lieberman, M. D., Eisenberger, N. J., Crockett, M. J., Tom, S. M., Pfeifer, J. H., & Way, B. M. (2007). Putting feelings into words: Affect labeling disrupts amygdala activity in response to affective stimuli. *Psychological Science, 18,* 421–428.

Lillas, C., & Turnbull, J. (2009). *Infant/child mental health, early intervention, and relationship-based therapies: A neurorelational framework for interdisciplinary practice.* New York: Norton.

Lipschitz, D. S., Rasmusson, A. M., & Southwick, S. M. (1998). Childhood posttraumatic stress disorder: A review of neurobiologic sequelae. *Psychiatric Annals, 28,* 452–457.

Lundy, B., Jones, N. A., Field, T., Nearing, G., Davalos, M., Pietro, P., et al. (1999). Prenatal depression effects on neonates. *Infant Behavioral Development, 22,* 119–129.

Lupien, S. J., King, S., Meaney, M. J., & McEwen, B. S. (2000). Children's stress hormone levels correlate with mother's socioeconomic status and depressive state. *Biological Psychiatry, 48,* 976–980.

Lynch, M., & Cicchetti, D. (1998). Trauma, mental representation, and the organization of memory for mother-referent material. *Development and Psychopathology, 10,* 739–759.

Lyons-Ruth, K., & Jacobovitz, D. (1999). Attachment organization: Unresolved loss, relational violence, and lapses in behavioral and attentional strategies. In J. Cassidy & P. R. Shaver (Eds.), *Handbook of attachment: Theory, research and clinical application* (pp. 520–554). New York: Guilford Press.

Main, M., & Hesse, E. (1990). Parents' unresolved traumatic experiences are related to infant disorganized attachment status: Is frightened and/or frightening parental behavior the linking mechanism? In M. T. Greenberg, D. Cicchetti, & M. Cummings (Eds.), *Attachment in the preschool years: Theory, research and intervention* (pp. 161–182). Chicago: University of Chicago Press.

McCarthy, M. M. (1995). Estrogen modulation of oxytocin and its relation to behavior. In R. Ivell & J. Russell (Eds.), *Oxytocin: Cellular and molecular approaches in medicine and research* (pp. 235–242). New York: Plenum Press.

McEwen, B. (1999). Development of the cerebral cortex: XIII. Stress and brain development–II. *Journal of the American Academy of Child and Adolescent Psychiatry, 38,* 101–103.

McPherson, W. B., Newton, J. E. O., Ackerman, P., Oglesby, D. M., & Dykman, R. A. (1997). An event-related brain potential investigation of PTSD and PTSD symptoms in abused children. *Integrative Physiological and Behavioral Science, 32,* 31–42.

Nachmias, M., Gunnar, M. R., Mangelsdorf, S., Parritz, R., & Buss, K. (1996). Behavioral inhibition and stress reactivity: Moderating role of attachment security. *Child Development, 67,* 508–522.

National Research Council and Institute of Medicine. (2000). *From neurons to neighborhoods: The science of early childhood development.* (Committee on Integrating the Science of Early Childhood Development [J. P. Shonkoff & D. A. Phillips, Eds.], Board on Children, Youth, and Families, Commission on Behavioral and Social Sciences and Education). Washington, DC: National Academy Press.

Neigh, G. N., Gillespie, C. F., & Nemeroff, C. B. (2009). The neurobiological toll of child abuse and neglect. *Trauma, Violence and Abuse, 10,* 389–410.

Osofsky, J. D. (1995). The effects of exposure to violence on young children. *American Psychologist, 50,* 782–788.

Pierrehumbert, B., Torrisi, R., Glatz, N., Dimitrova, N., Heinrichs, M., & Halfon, O. (2009). The influence of attachment on perceived stress and cortisol response to acute stress in women sexually abused in childhood or adolescence. *Psychoneuroendocrinology, 34,* 924–938.

Pollak, S. D., Cicchetti, D., Klorman, R., & Brumaghim, J. T. (1997). Cognitive brain event-related potentials and emotion processing in maltreated children. *Child Development, 68,* 773–787.

Pynoos, R. S., Steinberg, A. M., & Piacentini, J. C. (1999). A developmental psychopathology model of childhood traumatic stress and intersections with anxiety disorders. *Biological Psychiatry, 46,* 1542–1554.

Reynolds, D. (2003). Mindful parenting: A group approach to enhancing reflective capacity in parents and infants. *Journal of Child Psychotherapy, 29,* 357–374.

Saltzman, K. M., Weems, C. F., & Carrión, V. G. (2005). IQ and posttraumatic stress symptoms in children exposed to interpersonal violence. *Child Psychiatry and Human Development, 36,* 261–272.

Schore, A. N. (1994). *Affect regulation and the origin of the self: The neurobiology of emotional development.* Hillsdale, NJ: Erlbaum.

Schore, A. N. (2002). Advances in neuropsychoanalysis, attachment theory, and trauma research: Implications for self-psychology. *Psychoanalytic Inquiry, 22,* 433–484.

Southwick, S. M., Yehuda, R., & Morgan, C. A. (1995). Clinical studies of neurotransmitter alterations in post-traumatic stress disorder. In M. J. Friedman, D. S. Charney, & A. Y. Deutch (Eds.), *Neurobiological and clinical conse-*

quences of stress: From normal adaptation to post-traumatic stress disorder (pp. 335–350). New York: Lippincott-Raven.

Stein, M. B., Koverola, C., Hanna, C., Torchia, M. G., & McClarty, B. (1997). Hippocampal volume in women victimized by childhood sexual abuse. *Psychological Medicine, 27,* 951–959.

Tarullo, A. R., & Gunnar, M. R. (2006). Child maltreatment and the developing HPA axis. *Hormones and Behavior, 50,* 632–639.

Taylor, S. E., Gonzaga, G. C., Klein, L. C., Hu, P., Greendale, G. A., & Seeman, T. E. (2006). Relation of oxytocin to psychological stress responses and hypothalamic–pituitary–adrenocortical axis activity in older women. *Psychosomatic Medicine, 68,* 238–245.

Taylor, S. E., Klein, L. C., Lewis, B. P., Gruenwald, T. L., Gurung, R. A. R., & Updegraff, J. (2000). Biobehavioral responses to stress in females: Tend and befriend, not fight-or-flight. *Psychological Review, 107,*411–429.

Taylor, L., Zuckerman, B., Harik, V., & Groves, B. (1994). Witnessing violence by young children and their mothers. *Journal of Developmental and Behavioral Pediatrics, 15,* 120–123.

Trevarthen, C. (1989). Development of early social interactions and the affective regulation of brain growth. In C. von Euler, H. Forssberg, & H. Lagercrantz (Eds.), *Neurobiology of early Infant behaviour.* (Wenner-Gren Center International Symposium Series, Vol. 55, pp. 191–216). New York: Stockton Press.

Tronic, E. Z., Bruschweiler-Stern, N., Harrison, A. M., Lyons-Ruth, K., Morgan, A.C., Nahum, J. P., et al. (1998). Dyadically expanded states of consciousness and the process of therapeutic change. *Infant Mental Health Journal, 19,* 290–299.

Turner, H. A., Finkelhor, D., & Ormrod, R. (2006). The effect of lifetime victimization on the mental health of children and adolescents. *Social Science and Medicine, 62,* 13–27.

U.S. Department of Health and Human Services. (2007). America's children: Key national indicators of well-being, 2007. Retrieved July 14, 2007, from *www.childstats.gov/americaschildren/famsoc7.asp.*

Uvnas-Moberg, K. (1997). Oxytocin linked antistress effects—the relaxation and growth response. *Acta Psychologica Scandinavica, 640*(Suppl.), 38–42.

van der Kolk, B. (2003). The neurobiology of childhood trauma and abuse. *Child and Adolescent Psychiatric Clinics of North America, 12,* 293–317.

van der Kolk, B. A. (2005). Developmental trauma disorder: Towards a rational diagnosis for children with complex trauma histories. *Psychiatric Annals, 35,* 401–408.

van der Vegt, E. J. M., van der Ende, J., Kirschbaum, C., Verhulst, F. C., & Tiemeier, H. (2009). Early neglect and abuse predict diurnal cortisol patterns in adults: A study of international adoptees. *Psychoneuroendocrinology, 34,* 660–669.

Yehuda, R., Giller, E. L., Levengood, R. A., Southwick, S. M., & Siever, L. J. (1995). Hypothalamic–pituitary–adrenal functioning in post-traumatic stress disorder: Expanding the concept of the stress response spectrum. In M. J. Friedman, D. S. Charney, & A. Y. Deutch (Eds.), *Neurobiological and clinical consequences of stress: From normal adaptation to post-traumatic stress disorder* (pp. 351–366). New York: Lippincott-Raven.

Yehuda, R., Giller, E. L., Southwick, S. M., Lowy, M. T., & Mason, J. W. (1991). Hypothalamic–pituitary–adrenal dysfunction in posttraumatic stress disorder. *Biological Psychiatry, 30,* 1031–1047.

Wadhwa, P. D. (2005). Psychoneuroendocrine processes in human pregnancy influence fetal development and health. *Psychoneuoendocrinology, 30,* 724–743.

Weaver, I. C., Cervoni, N., Champagne, F. A., D'Alessio, A. C., Sharma, S., Seckl, J. R., et al. (2004). Epigenetic programming by maternal behavior. *Nature Neuroscience, 7,* 847–854.

White, B. P., Gunnar, M. R., Larson, M. C., Donzella, B., & Barr, R. G. (2000). Behavioral and physiological responsivity, and patterns of sleep and daily salivary cortisol in infants with and without colic. *Child Development, 71,* 862–877.

Zeanah, C. H., Jr., & Smyke, A. T. (2009). Attachment disorders. In C. H. Zeanah, Jr. (Ed.), *Handbook of infant mental health* (3rd ed., pp. 421–434). New York: Guilford Press.

CHAPTER 3

■ ■ ■ ■

"They Just Don't Get It"

A Diversity-Informed Approach to Understanding Engagement

Chandra Ghosh Ippen
Marva L. Lewis

Rena walked slowly into the office of her supervisor Lorraine. It had been 3 weeks since she had seen Jesse and his mother Crystal. Things weren't going well. They'd missed several appointments. Rena was worried about Jesse. He was only 32 months old and might soon be expelled from his day care. He kicked other kids, hit a teacher, and his speech was very delayed. The day care staff thought he needed a different placement. Jesse was in need of serious intervention, but his mother just didn't seem to get it. Rena didn't understand Crystal. Why didn't she see Jesse's problems and recognize that he needed help? Why didn't she appreciate the fact that the services Rena was offering were free? Didn't she understand that without help Jesse's problems might get worse? Rena had been trying her hardest to see Crystal and Jesse. She didn't know what else she could do. She wondered what Lorraine would say.

This chapter begins with a vignette that is common in the field of infant mental health. A young child is in need of intervention. The family is referred to services, but somehow the family fails to engage. Research shows that 10–30% of families invited to participate in home visiting programs either fail to enroll or drop out early, in the first month of services (Ammerman et al., 2006; Duggan et al., 2000; Gomby, Culross, & Berhman, 1999). Similarly high attrition rates are seen for parenting programs and mental health interventions (Fernandez & Eyberg, 2009; Gross, Julion, & Fogg, 2001; Kazdin, Stolar, & Marciano, 1995; Miller, Southam-Gerow, & Allin, 2008; Staudt, 2007). Given that services are limited, that significant resources are expended to recruit and retain families, and that engagement failures have emotional costs for families and practitioners, it is critical that as a field and as individuals we understand the factors and processes that contribute to engagement and disengagement.

Emergent research in this area suggests that many factors associated with poor uptake and low retention are related to aspects of diversity, including ethnicity, socioeconomic status, and environmental context (Kazdin et al., 1995; Kummerer & Lopez-Reyna, 2006; McCurdy, Gannon, & Daro, 2003; McGuigan, Katev, & Pratt, 2003a; Snowden & Yamada, 2005). For example, community violence and poor community health, including higher infant mortality and accidental death rates, have been linked to lower participation in home visiting programs (McGuigan et al., 2003a, 2003b). African Americans are more likely than whites or Latinas to have zero home visits (Wagner, Spiker, Linn, Gerlach-Downie, & Hernandez, 2003), but research suggests that the context of service delivery may influence engagement; African Americans report greater comfort seeking help in disasters compared to nonemergency contexts (Kaniasty & Norris, 2000). Together, these findings suggest that a diversity-informed approach to understanding engagement may be useful.

This chapter examines how differences in experience, connected to differences in ethnicity and socioeconomic status, among other variables, influence interactions among individuals, perceptions of intervention, and engagement with services. We first briefly present a diversity awareness model (Ghosh Ippen, 2009) to provide a framework for examining this perspective. Then, because learning about and working with diversity involves dialogue and exploration of processes, not just assimilation of facts, the chapter is organized around interactions among Rena, Crystal, Lorraine, and Jesse. Vignettes involving these characters are presented, details regarding their lives are discussed, and questions are posed to stimulate discussion. We encourage the reader to pause and think about your response to these questions before reading further. An analysis of the interaction is presented, with current work in this area linked to to research on diversity and engagement, and to four selected core concepts related to diversity (see Ghosh Ippen, 2011). The core concepts highlight the following themes: (1) History and experience shape assumptions and interactions; (2) mismatches and conflict between practitioner and family perspectives affect engagement; (3) our emotional state influences our ability to hold in mind another person's perspective; and (4) reflective practice is critical to integrating a diversity-informed approach. We connect these concepts and reflect on how they apply to our understanding of diversity and engagement. The way this chapter is written is also a product of culture. We honor the tradition of holistic cultures, in which learning occurs through experience and example, at the same time that we offer core concepts and analysis, consistent with Western tradition (Nisbett, Peng, Choi, & Norenzayan, 2001).

DIVERSITY AWARENESS MODEL

Figure 3.1a depicts a diversity awareness model that can be used to enhance awareness of differences in perception and diversity-related conflicts (Ghosh Ippen, 2009). Each circle represents the experience and perspective of a person involved in the interaction. The intersections represents the overlap in perspectives. When the overlap is large (Figure 3.1b), the triad is more likely to agree on the goals of intervention. When there is less overlap (see Figure 3.1c and 3.1d), the potential for conflict and misunderstanding increases. As we explore interactions among Rena, Crystal, and Lorraine, this visual model may help the reader hold multiple perspectives in mind and reflect on their intersections and conflicts.

In returning to the original vignette, it is clear that it is incomplete in many ways. First, it focuses only on Rena's perspective (Figure 3.1a, area A). At this point, we do not know how Crystal, Jesse, and Lorraine feel about the situation. This is because, at this moment, Rena is absorbed in her own view. She is not aware of Crystal's perspective (Figure 3.1a, area B). The vignette also does not provide information about Rena's role (e.g., home visitor, therapist, speech–language pathologist, day care consultant). The chapter starts this way so that infant mental health interventionists from diverse disciplines can read the vignette, think about how it applies to them and the families they serve, and answer the following questions:

- How do you understand Rena's perspective? How do you think she feels?
- How does the vignette make you feel?
- How do you think Rena's emotions and perceptions affect her interactions with Crystal, the way Crystal perceives her, and the intervention Rena is offering?
- Have you worked with people like Crystal and Jesse?
- If you were Lorraine, and Rena shared this information with you, how might you react?
- What types of policies does your system have in place regarding families' engagement or lack of engagement with services?

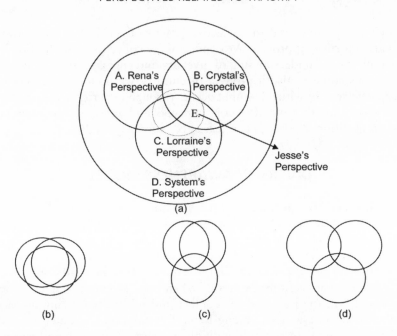

FIGURE 3.1. Diversity awareness model.

The vignette also provides no details, other than gender, about the individuals involved. We do not know their ethnicity, cultural or socioeconomic background (education and income, as well as professional status), religion, immigration status, age, or sexual orientation. These and other aspects of diversity contribute to each person's social identity (Lewis & Ghosh Ippen, 2004; Sue, Bingham, Porché-Burke, & Vasquez, 1999). Examples are presented below to illustrate a core diversity-related concept by experimenting and changing Rena's and Crystal's ethnicity and age.

Core Concept 1: Our assumptions influence our interactions with each other. Our assumptions are shaped by our personal and family history, and by the history of our cultural group.

This concept suggests that when Crystal first meets Rena, her perceptions of Rena and the services she is offering are shaped by her assumptions about people "like Rena." Even before Rena has said a word, Crystal is likely to have an opinion about "who she is." What Rena says and the ways she interacts with Crystal will either reinforce Crystal's assumptions or lead Crystal to form a new opinion. The same can be said of Rena's view of Crystal. Read through the following examples and reflect on how Rena and Crystal may view each other. While we do not want to make assumptions about them, how might their personal experience (including ethnicity, age, cultural values, immigration history, and treatment in the United States), the history of their cultural group, and interactions between their cultural groups influence their assumptions about the "other" and their interactions?

Example 1

Imagine for a moment that Rena is a 28-year-old African American woman and Crystal is a 39-year-old Vietnamese immigrant who speaks fluent English.

- How might Crystal's cultural background affect whether she engages in the type of services Rena can provide? Leong and Lau (2001), describe barriers to providing effective mental health services to Asian Americans, including cognitive barriers (e.g., different conceptualizations of illness and treatment) and affective barriers (e.g., feelings of shame and fear of stigma).
- How might Crystal's and Rena's beliefs about each other's ethnic group influence their interactions?
- If you were Lorraine, Rena's supervisor, how would you open a door to talking with Rena about how ethnicity culture, age, and other factors may affect her interactions with Crystal?
- Crystal is 39 years old. She was born in 1971. Is this an important fact? Wikipedia on the Internet provides an overview of the Vietnam War. How might awareness of this history affect your assessment of this mother? What questions might you have?

Example 2

Now imagine that Rena is a 28-year-old Vietnamese American and Crystal is a 19-year-old Chinese Vietnamese American; she is of Chinese ancestry, but her parents are from Vietnam. She has gang tattoos, and her son Jesse is half-Vietnamese and half-Latino. Rena and Crystal speak English, but both speak Vietnamese in the home. Ethnically they seem similar; they share the same country of origin and the same language; both are the children of immigrants, and both grew up in Orange County, California, which has one of the largest Vietnamese communities in the United States. The questions described following Example 1 can be applied to these individuals, along with additional questions that may be especially relevant to this dyad.

- In their community, each would be seen differently. Rena has her master's degree; she might be considered a success. Crystal has dropped out of high school. How might the way each is viewed in the community affect their interactions with one another?

- Is it possible that the history of their people in Vietnam and Orange County, California, might affect their current interactions? Trieu (2008) provides an excellent description of the dynamics among Vietnamese and Chinese Vietnamese youth from these ethnic subgroups.

Many of us are unaware of the history of the Chinese in Vietnam. Here are some facts that might inform our thinking (Trieu, 2008): (1) In the 1970s, anti-Chinese sentiments grew in Vietnam due to economic tension and clashes between the Vietnamese and Chinese governments; (2) many ethnic Chinese were forced to resettle into "new economic zones" and lose their land and means of subsistence; (3) there was a mass exodus of Chinese from Vietnam from 1978 to 1982, with many families leaving the country in small fishing boats. These people were called "boat people." Their journey away from Vietnam was often treacherous, with pirates attacking their boats, people dying along the way, and poor conditions in refugee camps once they were rescued from their boats. Children often immigrated without their parents. Imagine that Crystal's parents immigrated this way.

- How might Crystal's family history influence her desire to receive help from Rena?
- How might the history of Crystal's parents have affected the way they parented her and the way that Crystal in turn parents Jesse?
- What do we think about the role of historical trauma in terms of how it affects current relations between Crystal and Jesse, and between Rena and Crystal? Is this an important topic for supervision?

The answer to many of these questions is that we do not know. However, we do not want to ignore the history of the groups from which they came given that present-day and historical conflicts between groups can affect interactions among individuals. History should inform our hypotheses and lead us to open doors to dialogue about the possible role of culture, intercultural conflicts, and historical trauma. Although to Western eyes Rena and Crystal may seem "matched," they are part of subgroups that may be at odds with each other. Crystal's family was persecuted by the Vietnamese. Crystal and Rena were in two very different groups at school. Rena was in the group that excelled at school. Crystal was in the group that "ditched" school to hang out with their boyfriends. Crystal's parents wished she could be "like Rena." Rena knew people like Crystal at school. She felt that they were throwing away their chance to succeed.

- If this is their experience, how might it affect their interactions?
- If Rena is more "traditional," how might she view the fact that Crys-

tal has gang tattoos and a mixed-race child? Is it possible that Crystal may worry about how Rena perceives her?

- This seems like personal information. However, in supervision, is it important and safe for Rena to talk about how her upbringing and cultural values affect the way she perceives Crystal and the choices Crystal has made? Under what conditions might Rena discuss how their cultural groups have typically perceived each other, and how this may affect engagement?

These examples demonstrate that both the client's and the intervenor's ethnicity, culture, and history matter, in that they can shape assumptions and interactions. While much has been written about cultural conflicts between white–ethnic-minority dyads (Duan & Roehlke, 2001), these examples illustrate that cultural conflicts can also occur within ethnic-minority dyads, including those who share the same race and ethnic identity. A report from the American Psychological Association Office of Ethnic Minority Affairs (2008) suggests that more ethnic minorities are entering the mental health field. In 2004, 30% of associate's degrees, 29% of bachelor's degrees, 27% of master's degrees, and 20% of EdD and PhD degrees in psychology were awarded to members of ethnic minorities. As the field become more diverse, it will be increasingly important to understand and learn to address not only white–ethnic-minority practitioner–client cultural conflicts but also tensions that can occur between ethnic-minority dyads.

These examples, while focused on particular ethnic groups, are meant to illustrate core concepts that are applicable to practitioners of all ethnic groups. They illustrate a process for understanding how differences, whether they arise from culture or other factors (e.g., age, educational background, socioeconomic status), may shape our interactions. They also demonstrate how, as supervisors, we need to be aware of the way these processes may shape interactions, so we can facilitate dialogue in this area when it is clinically relevant.

Before we move on to explore other core concepts, let us return to Rena and Crystal. We have chosen another example for the remainder of the chapter in which both Rena, the therapist, and Crystal and Jesse, the clients, are African American, and the supervisor Lorraine is white. While we feel strongly that diversity conflicts are not limited to black–white interactions, we also feel there is much we can learn from interactions between these groups. Moreover, the research suggests that disparities within numerous service systems, child welfare, mental health, and education are greatest for African Americans (Farkas, 2003; Kazdin et al., 1995; Miller et al., 2008; van Ryn & Fu, 2003). Furthermore, African Americans have high dropout rates from services and are significantly less likely to engage in early intervention (Ammerman et al., 2006; Wagner et al., 2003). While some researchers have shown that poverty may contribute to lower engage-ment, others (e.g., Kazdin et al., 1995) have found reduced participation for African Americans even after accounting for socioeconomic differences. For the example, we chose to make Rena an African American because in the mental health field we often attempt to match ethnic-minority clients with practitioners of similar ethnic backgrounds. However, it is important to note that ethnic matching does not eliminate the need to integrate a focus on diversity-related issues.

Example 3

Introduction

Rena, a 26-year-old African American woman, grew up in a middle-class black neighborhood in Chicago that borders on a high crime public hous-ing area. When Rena was 8, her father died of a heart attack. Rena helped her mom raise her 3-year-old brother. In seventh grade, her mother became concerned about gangs in the public schools. They moved to a suburban neighborhood outside the city, and Rena and her brother attended an afflu-ent private school where there were few other black students. Rena excelled at school and ultimately decided to attend a historically black university in Washington, D.C. She obtained her master's degree in psychology and decided to return to Chicago for her psychology internship because she wanted to help her community, which she saw as riddled with racial dis-parities.

Crystal, age 19, was raised in the infamous public housing develop-ments of Chicago's South Side. The reality of her history fit the worse ste-reotypes about black people. She was removed from her mother's care at age 3 because her mother had significant substance abuse problems. Her father was in and out of her life and often violent to her mother. When Crystal was placed in foster care, her father visited her initially but soon stopped. Crystal lived in three different foster homes. There were allegations that she was abused in one of them. Crystal now lives with Jesse's father Marcus. Her mother is sober and helps care for Jesse, but Crystal and her mother often have serious arguments. Crystal and Jesse were referred for therapeu-tic services by their day care provider due to Jesse's aggressive behavior. The day care provider felt that if Jesse does not get help, they may not be able to keep him at their center. Jesse is very active and big for his age. The day care center personnel also note that Crystal has at times come in with bruises on her face.

Lorraine, Rena's 51-year-old supervisor, is of Irish and German ances-try. She grew up in a suburb outside of Boston. She earned a master's degree in social work and later a certificate in Infant Mental Health from the University of Michigan. She lives in Chicago's historic "rainbow" district, now gentrified, with her partner Gloria.

- In thinking again about the opening vignette and the questions raised in earlier sections, how do we begin to understand each person's perspective given the limited information provided about them?

"She Just Doesn't Get It"

Rena sat down in a chair opposite her supervisor Lorraine. She had all her case folders, with her notes neatly typed and well organized.

"Where would you like to start?" asked Lorraine.

"Well," said Rena, "we could start with Crystal and Jesse. That should go pretty fast. They didn't show again."

"No?" said Lorraine. "It seems like it's been a while since they've come in."

"Yes," said Rena, "I would just close their case, but his day care really wants me to see him. I was there consulting on another kid, and they told me that Jesse had just thrown a pencil, and it nearly hit a little girl in the eye. I called Jesse's mom and tried to explain the school's position; they just can't keep him, if she doesn't get help for him. But I don't think she gets it. She said she'd meet me, but she showed up half an hour late and said she only had 10 minutes because she had to go see her mom."

Lorraine listened to Rena and wondered if she should let her close the case. It was evident that Crystal and Jesse did not seem to be using the services Rena was offering. She thought further that Rena could just see Jesse at the day care center; however, it seemed that there might be problems at home linked to his behavior. She reminded herself that Crystal represented a hard client population to reach. Lorraine wondered how Rena felt about this. She was having a hard time engaging several other families in services and seemed to be getting frustrated. A week earlier during a case conference, Rena had remarked, "I don't think we can help people who don't want help." Lorraine reflected that she had often made this statement herself, but the way that Rena said it made Lorraine wonder. She could sense Rena's frustration. Instead of focusing on the facts of the case, Lorraine felt it would be important to process Rena's feelings about it.

Core Concept 2: The success of our interventions and our systems depends on whether those we serve share our assumptions and our perspective.

In beginning to process this interaction, it is important to return to the diversity awareness model (Figure 3.1) and think about how to visually depict interactions among Rena, Crystal, and Lorraine. As noted before, Rena appears to be focused on her own (circle A) and the day care provider's perspectives. All her efforts are geared toward changing rather than understanding Crystal. She does not appear to be holding Crystal's view (circle B). The intersection between Rena and Crystal seems small: "She just doesn't get it." This sentence applies as much to Rena as it may to Crystal. García Coll and Meyer (1993) offer questions that may help us reflect on the perspective of each person in the interaction: "Is there a problem? Why is there a problem? What can be done? And, who should intervene to address the problem?" (p. 61).

- How might Rena, Lorraine, and Crystal answer these questions?
- If they do not share the same answer, how might this influence their interactions?
- How might they begin to talk about this?

While Lorraine might help Rena explore the answers to these questions, any efforts to get Rena to reflect on Crystal's perspective may be less successful if Rena is in a charged emotional state. Right now, Rena is worried about Jesse. She is angry that Jesse's mom is not doing what she "should" to help Jesse. She feels helpless because she cannot change things for him, and she worries that Lorraine and the day care provider may view her as incompetent. Lorraine needs to be able to understand Rena's perspective in order to help her reach out more sensitively to this mother and child. In attempting to change Rena's perspective without understanding it, Lorraine would do exactly what Rena has done to Crystal. For Rena to "get it," Lorraine, as the supervisor, needs to "get it." To help and understand Rena, Lorraine will need to consider the role that emotion plays in influencing Rena's ability to see Crystal's perspective.

Core Concept 3: Our emotions influence our ability to see another person's perspective.

Visual diagrams (Figure 3.2), influenced by Fadiman (2008), illustrate this concept. To simplify, the graphic focuses only on Rena and Crystal. Figure 3.2a shows two overlapping circles representing Rena and Crystal's perspectives. When Rena is calm, she is able to travel, metaphorically, to the edges of her belief system and reflect on Crystal's perspective (see the calm position). When she is affectively aroused, however, her cognitive flexibility becomes more limited. She tends to return to her core beliefs, depicted in the center (see the aroused position), because it is here that she feels safest. The same process happens for Crystal. In Figure 3.2b, we see a dyad that has a

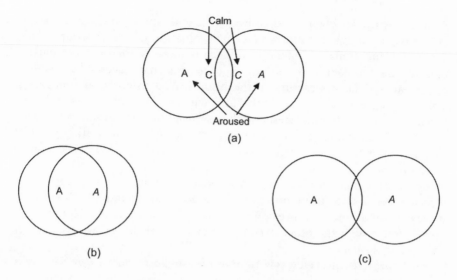

FIGURE 3.2. Affect and perception.

sizable overlap in terms of perspective and experience. When members of this dyad are aroused, and each goes to his or her "center," they still share perspective. In Figure 3.2c, the dyad members share little in common. When members of this dyad are aroused, they are more likely to be blind to each other's perspective.

The connection between affect and relationships is well documented. As Pawl (1995) noted, "It is not possible to work on behalf of human beings to try to help them without having powerful feelings aroused in yourself.... In working with families who are in great difficulty, rage can become the most familiar affect—at the system, at a world with too much violence that creates too much helplessness and also at a family who will not be better or even seem to try" (p. 24). The research shows that our emotions affect the way we process information and relationships. When we are angry, we are more likely to perceive people rather than situations as responsible for a problem (Keltner, Ellsworth, & Edwards, 1993). With anger, we are less likely to trust others (Dunn & Schweitzer, 2005) and more likely to make judgments based on stereotypes (Bodenhausen, Sheppard, & Kramer, 1994; DeSteno, Dasgupta, Bartlett, & Cajdrie, 2004; Tiedens & Linton, 2001). This happens even when the anger originates from an unrelated event or situation.

Ethnicity and race are linked to deep, unconscious feelings (Comaz-Díaz & Jacobsen, 1991). Strong emotions are linked to stereotypes (Lewis,

2000). A study by Phelps and colleagues (2000) shows an interesting link between physiology, emotions, and our evaluation of social groups. They conducted functional magnetic resonance imaging scans of white participants as they looked at black and white neutral male faces. They focused on the amygdala, a structure in the brain linked to emotion processing. They found greater activation of this area when white participants looked at black compared to white faces, and they showed that activation in this area was correlated with measures of unconscious racism. Interestingly, when they repeated the study but used famous and well-regarded black figures, the patterns did not hold. This study suggests that at a physiological level, emotions and judgments of others are connected. Our brains process social information. If one's brain notes that someone is different and less familiar, it may signal a potential threat. The resulting emotions may affect the way one interacts with the other person; the greater the difference, the greater the potential divides.

Qualitative interviews with parents suggest that anger and fear related to being judged, cultural conflicts, and safety concerns are related to engagement (e.g., Gross et al., 2001; Woolfolk & Unger, 2009). The following quotes from interviews with parents show the connections between parents' emotions, their assumptions about practitioners, and their motivation to participate in intervention. The first quote involves an African American mother speaking about her parent educator. The second quote comes from a white parent from rural Appalachia, expressing initial concerns about participating in a university-affiliated group. This quote highlights that cultural concerns are not limited to ethnic minorities.

> "Because [she is] White and because I'm Black ... it's like a certain way that she might do something that I don't do. I don't know what she's talking about. We was not raise like that. I just put up with her. I mean, because you have your way of doing things, and I have mine, we come from two totally different backgrounds." (in Woolfolk & Unger, 2009, p. 193)

> "I was afraid that you were going to push down our throats how we should raise our kids, and I didn't want to hear that." (in Owens, Richerson, Murphy, Jageleweski, & Rossi, 2007, p. 188)

Now, as we return to Crystal and Rena, imagine Crystal feeling similarly to these parents.

- Is it possible that Crystal could feel this way even though she and Rena are both black? What might be the intraracial dynamics between Rena and Crystal?

- How will Rena's insistence that she get Jesse into treatment affect Crystal (affectively and cognitively)?
- How does Crystal's passive refusal to participate in treatment affect Rena (affectively and cognitively)?
- Lorraine believes that rather than processing the facts right now, it may be more useful to focus on Rena's feelings. What do you think of this?

We believe that Rena's emotions affect her ability to see alternative perspectives. Perhaps if Rena regulates her affect, she will gain a greater understanding of the situation and see more ways to intervene.

Core Concept 4: Reflective practice is critical to integrating a diversity-informed approach.

Although Rena is in many situations capable of regulating her emotions by herself, when emotions are especially charged, reflective supervision is crucial. As Pawl (1995) noted, "A family with a child with a difficulty that troubles you particularly and with whom you cannot seem to find your balance—that belongs in supervision" (p. 24).

"Let's Think about This Together"

Lorraine paused. She and Rena had only recently begun working together. She hoped that Rena felt comfortable with her. "I can see how hard you've been trying to engage this family" she began. Rena nodded. "It seems like it's been hard." Rena nodded again. "I'm wondering if it might be helpful to talk about how you're feeling?" Rena seemed apprehensive. Lorraine sensed this. Rena was not sure whether she should talk to Lorraine about her feelings. She wanted Lorraine to think that she was competent. Rena also remembered previous encounters with supervisors. She remembered expressing her anger to her supervisor over the interactions of a day care center with a young African American boy she was treating. She felt he was being racially profiled. Her supervisor, a white male, told her that she would need to control her emotions if she was going to be able to work in this field. He said that he understood that, in her culture, it might be acceptable to display anger in this way, but it was not therapeutic. After that experience, understandably, she hesitated to share her feelings with a supervisor.

- It may be helpful to think about the first core concept and reflect on how Rena's experience is shaping her current interaction with Lorraine.

- It may be helpful to review the second core concept and think about whether Rena and Lorraine share the same assumptions and perspective about the process of supervision. Specifically, is supervision a place where you talk about your own experience and feelings?
- Is it important to focus on the potential role of ethnicity and culture in this interaction in terms of perceptions and safety?

The event that Rena is remembering with her former supervisor can be characterized as a "racial microaggression," defined as a "brief and commonplace daily verbal, behavioral or environmental indignity, whether intentional or unintentional, that communicates hostile, derogatory, or negative racial slights or insults towards people of color (Sue et al., 2007, p. 271). While insensitive supervision can occur in any supervision dyad, comments or judgments that appear to be related to race or stereotypical cultural assumptions may be especially detrimental to ethnic-minority practitioners. Constantine and Sue (2007) interviewed African American supervisees and identified seven microaggression themes this group frequently experienced in supervision. Rena's interaction with her former supervisor touches three of these themes: (1) making stereotypical assumptions about black supervisees; (2) focusing primarily on clinical weakness, and (3) invalidating racial–cultural issues. Rena felt like she was being viewed as a stereotypical "angry black woman"; she felt that her insights about racial profiling were being overlooked, and her competence was continually being questioned. Reflective supervision is meant to provide a safe and supportive context in which the supervisor and supervisee work together to regulate emotions and enhance reflection (Shamoon-Shanok, 2009). The supervisor's comments shattered Rena's sense of safety and interrupted her ability to feel free to reflect not only in that relationship but also in later supervisory relationships, such as that with Lorraine. Although Lorraine seemed different, Rena carried the memory of her past supervisor into this relationship.

Unfortunately, the literature suggests that interactions like this occur frequently (Constantine & Sue, 2007; Hird, Cavalieri, Dulko, Felice, & Ho, 2001; McLeod, 2009). Also common is a failure to integrate a diversity-informed perspective into supervision. The integration of diversity-related factors is new in our field (García Coll & Meyer, 1993). Research suggests that supervisors may have less experience and comfort addressing these factors than supervisees, and many supervisors overestimate the degree to which they focus on them (e.g., Duan & Roehlke, 2001).

"Can We Talk about Feelings and about Race and Culture?"

Lorraine, sensing Rena's apprehensions, decides to check her assumptions about whether Rena feels safe talking about her feelings. "I know we don't know each other well, and I know you mentioned that you had some negative supervision experiences. I wonder if you feel safe talking about your feelings or if it even seems like something that is relevant to supervision. I want to be able to support you."

Rena is hesitant but decides to share a little. "I guess I'm frustrated with Crystal. She has an opportunity to really get some help for Jesse, but she doesn't, and I guess I'm frustrated because I really want to help."

Lorraine remembers Rena saying that she returned to Chicago because she wanted to be a part of the solution to the disparities facing African American communities. She says gently, "I can see how hard you are trying. I remember you saying that you wanted to help families in the black community here, and I wonder how you feel given that it has been so hard to help." Rena is at first surprised that Lorraine has mentioned race, albeit tangentially. She feels like a door has opened. She starts talking about how she wanted to be part of a solution, but now, when she works with clients, she feels shut out, like they don't want her help. She talks about how frustrating it is because she returned to Chicago to be able to gain experience working with poor urban black families. These families are not like the families from the stable, working-class black neighborhood where she grew up. She feels overwhelmed by the multiple challenges Crystal faces and her inability to get through despite sharing the same history as a member of the same racial group. Lorraine and Rena speak about the challenges the families face and those that they as workers face.

"It's interesting," says Lorraine, "you're African American, but you are not from the same economic group as Crystal. She may also see you as part of a system that has traditionally not treated the urban poor well."

Rena pauses and then reflects out loud, "I guess I was so busy trying to get them to come in, and I figured we shared the same cultural background. I never stopped to think about how they see me."

"That makes sense. It seems like you were really focused on trying to help Jesse," said Lorraine.

Rena continues to reflect, "Wow, I think I was so focused on getting Jesse what I thought he needed that I didn't think about Crystal. When she talked about the challenges she faced, I tried to problem-solve to see how we could overcome them, so she could come to treatment, but I don't think I ever really acknowledged her reality. I thought a lot about class issues and the stereotypes she and her son live with every day, but I never brought them up."

Lorraine says, "Perhaps we can think about whether that is something you might do with her in the future."

Rena and Lorraine have begun a process wherein regulating their affect enables them to think flexibly about numerous factors related to Crystal's engagement with services. Research shows that positive affect is associated with increased flexibility in thinking and action (Fredrickson, 2001). Because Rena feels that Lorraine is open to understanding her, she becomes open to thinking about Crystal's perspective; we see parallel process in action. Below are some of the questions on which Rena and Lorraine reflect. Not all of them are related to diversity, but many are. Diversity-related considerations are as relevant and offer the possibility of just as rich and important a dialogue as many other clinical considerations. Moreover, it is important to think about how it might feel if diversity-related lines of inquiry are overlooked.

- How might Crystal's early childhood history of neglect and multiple foster homes affect the way she views the "system" and interpersonal relationships? What does Crystal "need" to feel safe enough to engage with Rena?
- How does Rena's early history affect the way she sees Jesse and Crystal? Rena cared for her younger brother. She also left her old neighborhood and her old friends, many of whom never had the opportunities she had.
- How does Crystal see Rena? Rena comes across as upper-middle class, with clothes straight out of a Banana Republic catalog. Rena speaks in clipped Standard English and works hard to maintain an emotionless expression in Crystal's presence. Reading Comaz-Díaz and Jacobsen's (1991) description of patterns of intraethnic transference (e.g., the traitor) and countertransference (e.g., overidentification, survivor's guilt) may be thought provoking.
- Do the goals of treatment match Crystal's perspective and context? Is it "normal" for her to believe she should participate in her son's treatment when he is having problems in his day care?
- What practical barriers and daily stresses may keep Crystal from engaging (including a potentially violent relationship)?

Research on engagement supports the exploration of practical barriers and contextual factors that may impede a person's involvement in therapy with his or her child (McKay, Pennington, Renan, & McCadam, 2001; Staudt, 2007). Practical barriers may include transportation and cost issues, other responsibilities, objective safety concerns potentially related to domestic and community violence and immigration status, and family stress and mental health issues. For example, Crystal goes to school, and cares for her mother and takes her to medical appointments (other responsibilities); she is reluctant to have evening appointments because it is not safe to return home after dark (objective safety concerns), and she has significant symptoms of depression that interfere with her functioning (mental health issues). Process variables may be equally important, including mistrust of the provider or agency; motivation to change; and beliefs about the problem, its possible solutions, and the relevance of services. Crystal does not trust Rena. She feels forced to participate in Jesse's treatment when she believes that he is "just this way—aggressive" and nothing will change him. Reflective supervision offers Rena a space where she can learn more about her reactions and responses so that she can regulate her emotions and make a better assessment of all of these variables (practical, contextual, interpersonal). In this way, she will be better able to hold Crystal's perspective in mind and develop diversity-informed interventions.

SUMMARY

In a book about young children and trauma, it may seem unusual to write a chapter in which the primary focus is not the young child or the trauma. Jesse, the main target of our intervention, is noticeably absent from the chapter. We have not yet reflected on his experience, although we know it includes exposure domestic violence. Our chapter in an earlier book (Lewis & Ghosh Ippen, 2004) focused on cultural issues in the assessment and treatment of young children who have experienced trauma. In many ways, this chapter should precede that one. It is critical to integrate a diversity-informed approach in all aspects of assessment and treatment, but we often do not have the chance to do this because the families we work with fail to engage or drop out of our interventions in the first few sessions. In order to reduce ethnic and socioeconomic disparities in care, it is crucial to focus our efforts on not only assessment and treatment but also engagement, and we need to understand how diversity-related factors influence caregivers' willingness to engage. Jesse will not decide whether he should get help. Crystal will make the decision; therefore, it is crucial for his growth and development that we support the relationship between them. So we need to understand Crystal's perspective. We need to consider how her experience, her personal family's history, and possible historical trauma to her cultural group have influenced her. We also need to think about how she may view us in light of our external characteristics (e.g., race, age, ethnic group, perceived socioeconomic class).

We chose the somewhat provocative title "They Just Don't Get It" because this phrase carries the charged affect many of us experience when we feel that our efforts to help are being rejected. The phrase places the blame for engagement failures on the caregiver and signals that, in the moment, we may be ignoring contextual and interpersonal diversity-related factors that are contributing to disengagement. Rather than attempting to eliminate this phrase, we suggest that we recognize its importance. It shows us that we have lost perspective and may be viewing the family and the "goodness" of the intervention for the family through the lens of our assumptions. It is important to understand and check our assumptions and to reflect on the family's perspective, but to do so, we may first need to regulate our emotions in the context of a safe relationship. Then, from within this relationship in which we feel understood, we can reflect on the multiple factors—practical, interpersonal, and diversity-related—that may be important to address during the engagement phase of intervention.

Throughout this chapter, interactions between Rena, Crystal, and Lorraine have been described and explored. As an interventionist or supervisor doing this work, one becomes a character in the interaction. We hope that the questions posed throughout the chapter will help the reader begin to reflect on how diversity-related factors and history influence interactions with families. Data from a multisite learning collaborative show that introducing diversity-informed engagement strategies into child mental health agencies resulted in an increase in the number of children who engaged in services, from an average of 63 to 81% (Cavaleri et al., 2006). Both research and experience indicates that as a greater focus on diversity is incorporated into our engagement interventions, the result may be a greater uptake of services.

While the data are promising, it is important to remember that engagement is a process that we can influence but not control. Even if we are mindful of our assumptions and affect, and reflective of the perspective of the families with whom we work, many will not engage in services. It is possible that even with Rena's and Lorraine's best intentions and interventions, Crystal may still choose not to receive services. Perhaps her partner objects to Crystal involving his child in the "system." Maybe Crystal has too many other responsibilities (caring for her mother, who is newly sober and attending school) and cannot find time to participate. It is our hope that even in these circumstances, Rena and Crystal will be able to engage in a dialogue in which the full reality of Crystal's life and Jesse's challenges is appreciated, so that if disengagement occurs, it is respectful and allows a positive connection between Crystal and Rena to be maintained. Crystal's interactions with Rena will influence her future assumptions of infant mental health practitioners, and a positive internal working model of her relationship with Rena may allow her to engage in services at another point in time.

DIRECTIONS FOR THE FUTURE

This chapter represents an important beginning. There is a need for more research and practices that contribute to learning in this area. There is also a need to explore further the different types of barriers to engagement. More detail is needed about strategies that might be used clinically to engage in difficult dialogues about race, ethnicity, socioeconomic status, or discrimination. As an example of an area for future development, the mental health field is learning more about the negative consequences of discrimination on children's mental health. Children's reports of perceived racism have been linked to mental health symptoms (Coker et al., 2009). Research on racial socialization suggests that many ethnic-minority parents of young children are aware of discrimination and talk openly with their preschool-age children about both racial pride and how others may perceive them negatively because of their race (Caughy, O'Campo, Randolph, & Nickerson, 2002). As we begin to understand the importance of this and other diversity-related processes, we need to begin to understand how our interventions address them.

ACKNOWLEDGMENT

The development of this chapter and the core concepts for diversity-informed practice were supported by the A. L. Mailman Family Foundation.

REFERENCES

American Psychological Association, Office of Ethnic Minority Affairs. (2008). A portrait of success and challenge—Progress report: 1997–2005. Washington, DC: Author. Retrieved April 2, 2010, from *www.apa.org/pi/oema/cemrrat_report.html*.

Ammerman, R. T., Stevens, J., Putnam, P. W., Altaye, M., Hulsmann, J. E., Lehmkuhl, H. D., et al. (2006). Predictors of engagement in home visitation. *Journal of Family Violence, 21*(2), 105–115.

Bodenhausen, G. V., Sheppard, L. A., & Kramer, G. P. (1994). Negative affect and social judgment: The differential impact of anger and sadness. *European Journal of Social Psychology, 24,* 45–62.

Caughy, M., O'Campo, P. J., Randolph, S. M., & Nickerson, K. (2002). The influence of racial socialization practices on the cognitive and behavioral competence of African American preschoolers. *Child Development, 73*(5), 1611–1625.

Cavaleri, M. A., Gopalan, G., McKay, M. M., Appel, A., Bannon, W. M., Bigley, M. F., et al. (2006). Impact of a learning collaborative to improve child mental health service use among low-income urban youth and families. *Best Practices in Mental Health, 2*(2), 67–79.

Coker, T. R., Elliott, M. N., Kanouse, D. E., Grunbaum, J. A., Schwbel, D. C., Gilliand, J., et al. (2009). Perceived racial/ethnic discrimination among fifth-grade students and its associations with mental health. *American Journal of Public Health, 99*(5), 878–884.

Comas-Díaz, L., & Jacobsen, F. M. (1991). Ethnocultural transference and countertransference in the therapeutic dyad. *American Journal of Orthopsychiatry, 61*(3), 392–402.

Constantine, M. G., & Sue, D. W. (2007). Perceptions of racial microaggressions among black supervisees in cross-racial dyads. *Journal of Counseling Psychology, 54*(2), 142–153.

DeSteno, D., Dasgupta, N., Bartlett, M.Y., & Cajdrie, A. (2004). Prejudice from thin air: The effect of emotion on automatic intergroup attitutdes. *Psychological Science, 15*(5), 319–324.

Duan, C., & Roehlke, H. (2001). A descriptive "snapshot" of cross-racial supervision in university counseling center internships. *Journal of Multicultural Counseling and Development, 29,* 131–146.

Duggan, A., Windham, A., McFarlane, E., Luddy, L., Rohde, C., Buchbinder, S., et al. (2000). Hawaii's healthy start program of home visiting for at-risk families: Evaluation of family identification, family engagement, and service delivery. *Pediatrics, 105*(1), 250–259.

Dunn, J. R., & Schweitzer, M. E. (2005). Feeling and believing: The influence of emotion on trust. *Journal of Personality and Social Psychology, 88*(5), 736–748.

Fadiman, A. (2008). *Cross-cultural challenges in health care: Lessons from* The Spirit Catches You and You Fall Down. Presented at Medical Humanities Grand Rounds, San Francisco General Hospital, San Francisco.

Farkas, G. (2003). Racial disparities and discrimination in education: What do we know, how do we know it, and what do we need to know? *Teachers College Record, 105,* 1119–1146.

Fernandez, M. A., & Eyberg, S. M. (2009). Predicting treatment and follow-up attrition in parent–child interaction therapy. *Journal of Abnormal Child Psychology, 37,* 431–441.

Fredrickson, B. L. (2001). The role of positive emotions in positive psychology: The broaden-and-build theory of positive emotions. *American Psychologist, 56*(3) 218–226.

García Coll, C., & Meyer, E. C. (1993). The sociocultural context of infant development. In C. H . Zeanah, Jr. (Ed.), *Handbook of infant mental health* (pp. 56–69). New York: Guilford Press.

Ghosh Ippen, C. M. (2009). The sociocultural context of infant mental health: Toward contextually congruent interventions. In C. H. Zeanah, Jr. (Ed.), *Handbook of infant mental health* (3rd ed., pp. 104–119). New York: Guilford Press.

Ghosh Ippen, C. (2011). *Core concepts for enhancing a diversity-informed practice.* Manuscript in preparation.

Gomby, D. S., Culross, P. L., & Behrman, R. E. (1999). Home visiting: Recent program evaluations—analysis and recommendations. *The Future of Children, 9*(1), 4–26.

Gross, D., Julion, W., & Fogg, L. (2001). What motivates participation and dropout among low-income urban families of color in a preventive intervention. *Family Relations, 50,* 246–254.

Hird, J. S., Cavalieri, C. E., Dulko, J. P., Felice, A. A. D., & Ho, T. A . (2001). Visions and realities: Supervisee perspectives of multicultural supervision. *Journal of Multicultural Counseling and Development, 29,* 114–130.

Kazdin, A. E., Stolar, M. J., & Marciano, P. L. (1995). Risk factors for dropping out of treatment among white and black families. *Journal of Family Psychology, 9*(4), 402–417.

Kaniasty, K., & Norris, F. H. (2000). Help-seeking comfort and receiving social support: The role of ethnicity and context of need. *American Journal of Community Psychology, 28*(4), 545–581.

Keltner, D., Ellsworth, P. C., & Edwards, K. (1993). Beyond simple pessimism: Effects of sadness and anger on social perception. *Journal of Personality and Social Psychology, 64*(3), 740–752.

Kummerer, S. E., & Lopez-Reyna, N. A . (2006). The role of Mexican immigrant mothers' beliefs on parental involvement in speech and language therapy. *Communication Disorders Quarterly, 27*(2), 83–94.

Leong, F. T. L., & Lau, A. S. L. (2001). Barriers to providing effective mental health services to Asian Americans. *Mental Health Services Research, 3*(4), 201–214.

Lewis, M. L., & Ghosh Ippen, C. (2004). Rainbow of tears, souls full of hope: Cultural issues related to young children and trauma. In J. D . Osofksy (Ed.), *Young children and trauma: Intervention and treatment* (pp. 11–46). New York: Guilford Press.

Lewis, M. L. (2000). The cultural context of infant mental health: The developmental niche of infant–caregiver relationships. In C. H. Zeanah, Jr. (Ed.), *The handbook of infant mental health* (2nd ed., pp. 91–107). New York: Guilford Press.

McCurdy, K., Gannon, R. A., & Daro, D. (2003). Participation patterns in home-based family support programs: Ethnic variations. *Family Relations, 52,* 3–11.

McGuigan, W. M., Katzev, A. R., & Pratt, C. C. (2003a). Multi-level determinants of mothers' engagement in home visitation services. *Family Relations, 52*(3), 271–278.

McGuigan, W. M., Katzev, A. R., & Pratt, C. C. (2003b). Multi-level determinants of retention in a home-visiting child abuse prevention program. *Child Abuse and Neglect, 27,* 363–380.

McKay, M. M., Pennington, J., Renan, C. J., & McCadam, K. (2001). Understanding urban child mental health service use: Two studies of child, family, and environmental correlates. *Journal of Behavioral Health Services and Research, 28*(4), 1–10.

McLeod, A. L. (2009). *A phenomenological investigation of supervisors' and supervisees' experiences with attention to cultural issues in multicultural supervision.* Doctoral dissertation, Georgia State University, Atlanta, GA.

Miller, L. M., Southam-Gerow, M. A., & Allin, R. B. (2008). Who stays in treatment?: Child and family predictors of youth client retention in a public mental health agency. *Child Youth Care Forum, 37,* 153–170.

Nisbett, R. E., Peng, K., Choi, I., & Norenzayan, A. (2001). Culture and systems of thought: Holistic versus analytic cognition. *Psychological Review, 108*(2), 291–310.

Owens, J. S., Richerson, L., Murphy, C. E., Jageleweski, A., & Rossi, L. (2007). The parent perspective: Informing the cultural sensitivity of parenting programs in rural communities. *Child Youth Care Form, 36,* 179–194.

Pawl, J. (1995). On supervision. In L. Eggbeer & E. Fenichel (Eds.), *Educating and supporting the infant/family work force: Models, methods, and materials* (pp. 21–29). Arlington, VA: Zero to Three Press.

Phelps, E. A., O'Connor, K. J., Cunningham, W. A., Funayama, E. S., Gatenby, J. C., Gore, J. C., et al. (2000). Performance on indirect measures of race evaluation predicts amygdala activation. *Journal of Cognitive Neuroscience, 12*(5), 729–738.

Shamoon-Shanok, R. (2009). What is reflective supervision? In S. S . Heller & L. Gilkerson (Eds.), *A practical guide to reflective supervision* (pp. 7–22). Washington, DC: Zero to Three Press.

Snowden, L. R., & Yamada, A. (2005). Cultural differences in access to care. *Annual Review of Clinical Psychology, 1,* 143–166.

Staudt, M. (2007). Treatment engagement with caregivers of at-risk children: Gaps in research and conceptualization. *Journal of Child and Family Studies, 16,* 183–196.

Sue, D. W., Bingham, R. P., Porché-Burke, L., & Vasquez, M. (1999). The diversification of psychology: A multicultural revolution. *American Psychologist, 54*(12), 1061–1069.

Sue, D. W., Capodilupo, C. M., Torino, G. C., Bucceri, J. M., Holder, A., Nadal, K. L., et al. (2007). Racial microaggressions in every day life: Implications for clinical practice. *American Psychologist, 62*(4), 271–286.

Tiedens, L. Z., & Linton, S. (2001). Judgment under emotional certainty and uncertainty: The effects of specific emotions on information processing. *Journal of Personality and Social Psychology, 81*(6), 973–988.

Trieu, M. (2008). *Ethnic chameleons and the context of identity: A comparative look at the dynamics of intra-national ethnic identity construction for 1.5 and second generation Chinese-Vietnamese and Vietnamese Americans.* Doctoral dissertation, University of Irvine, California.

van Ryn, M., & Fu, S. S. (2003). Paved with good intentions: Do public health and human service providers contribute to racial/ethnic disparities in health? *American Journal of Public Health, 93,* 248–255.

Wagner, M., Spiker, D., Linn, M. I., Gerlach-Downie, S., & Hernandez, F. (2003). Dimensions of parental engagement in home visiting programs: Exploratory study. *Topics in Early Childhood Special Education, 23*(4), 171–187.

Woolfolk, T. N., & Unger, D. G. (2009). Relationships between low-income African American mothers and their home visitors: A parents as teachers program. *Family Relations, 58,* 188–200.

PART II

■ ■ ■ ■

EVALUATION AND TREATMENT MODELS FOR INFANTS AND YOUNG CHILDREN EXPOSED TO TRAUMA

INTRODUCTION TO PART II

Part II reviews best clinical practice in infant mental health, including treatment and evaluation models used to understand and help traumatized infants and young children. Building an effective evidence base for practice and treatment of children and parents or caregivers is crucial. The chapters in this section focus on different practice models for traumatized young children and their families. A well-respected treatment approach, child–parent psychotherapy (CPP) is presented in the first chapter, including adaptations to work with caregivers other than biological parents. CPP, an evidence-based psychotherapy model used with traumatized young children, based on the principle that relationships are central to a young child's healthy emotional and social development, is presented in several of the chapters in this section. CPP was developed with the premise that secure attachment relationships not only help young children organize their responses to stress and trauma but also provide the foundation for the development of resilience. Patricia Van Horn, Lili Gray, Beth Pettinelli, and Natalia Estassi describe the adaptation and use of CPP in cases where children have been removed from their parents' care and placed with relatives. Using sensitive and insightful clinical vignettes, they help the reader understand the implementation of CPP in kinship settings, and describe the strengths and vulnerabilities that are specific to kinship foster care. Expanding our understanding of clinical treatment, Mary Dozier, Johanna Bick, and Kristin Bernard introduce the reader to another helpful and effective treatment modality, the attachment and biobehavioral catch-up (ABC) intervention, designed to address key needs that affect traumatized young children. Working with child–caregiver relationship principles in this attachment-based intervention and treatment for young vulnerable children, the team addresses issues of dysregulation of a young child's emotions and physiology due to the maltreatment and unpredictability of their parents or caregivers. The ABC intervention helps parents recognize their children's problematic coping strategies and encourage new ones, overcome their own issues that interfere with being able to nurture their children, and create an environment that promotes children's biobehavioral regulation. While implementing clinical treatment is crucial, it is also important to carry out research to evaluate the effectiveness of intervention and treatment models. Sheree L. Toth, Jody Todd Manly, and Alisa Hathaway focus on the importance of evaluating relational interventions and treatments for child maltreatment using a developmental psychopathology framework. They include an important discussion of the adverse effects of child maltreatment on stage-salient issues for young children, with an emphasis on attachment organization. Their translational research, which presents results from randomized clinical trials demonstrating the efficacy of CPP for decreasing insecure attachment organization in maltreated infants and young children, is important in substantiating the evidence based for this practice. Toth and her colleagues conclude with recommendations for training and implementation in clinical and community settings to better inform clinical practice. Since relationship-based evaluations set the stage for clinical treatment, in the last chapter in this section, Amy Dickson and Mindy Kronenberg describe ways to carry out evaluations and provide a rationale for the importance of relationship-based evaluations for work with young traumatized children. They describe different methods used in the field of infant mental health to conduct relationship-based evaluations. These authors emphasize that flexibility is needed during the assessment in choosing different interview and observational measures that are sensitive to young traumatized children and their caregivers, and then illustrate the principles of evaluation by presenting a family with a problem that is commonly observed in the field.

CHAPTER 4

■ ■ ■ ■

Child–Parent Psychotherapy with Traumatized Young Children in Kinship Care

Adaptation of an Evidence-Based Intervention

Patricia Van Horn
Lili Gray
Beth Pettinelli
Natalia Estassi

Child–parent psychotherapy (CPP) is a psychotherapy modality for traumatized young children based on the principles that (1) relationships are central to young children's health development, and (2) babies and young children organize their responses to threat and danger around their attachment relationships. Typically developing infants learn to soothe themselves by internalizing the patterns of their earliest caregiving. Early caregiving experiences also teach babies what they can expect from others, and how others see and respond to them. Secure early relationships form the foundation for resilience because babies and toddlers use their caregivers as a secure base from which to explore the world, and to take on the mental and emotional challenges it presents. Thus, secure relationships help young children develop their capacities in three critical domains: (1) self-soothing and emotion regulation, (2) forming sustaining relationships, and (3) cognitive development and problem solving.

When trauma occurs in the lives of infants and very young children, it can be profoundly disruptive of their development in all of these domains because it is so destructive of trust in relationships. Freud (1920/1955) originally proposed the concept that young children rely on their caregivers to provide a protective shield that fends off unbearable levels of stimulation; Bowlby (1969/1982) posited that the baby's expectation of protection and the mother's role in promoting infant survival and generating a sense of security in the baby in circumstances of threat and danger are biologically determined. Following these early theorists, contemporary trauma experts have noted that young children have the developmentally appropriate expectation that those who care for them will sense oncoming danger, appraise the level of risk it presents, and provide protection from injury and from overwhelming fear and terror (Marans & Adelman, 1997; Pynoos, Steinberg, & Piacentini, 1999). When young children experience the overwhelming sights, sounds, and internal sensations that combine in a traumatic experience, their expectation of protection is betrayed. Their trust in their caregivers, the sine qua non of children's healthy development, is at least momentarily shattered.

Janoff-Bulman (1992) described the existential crisis that traumatic life experiences create in adults as their assumptions of benevolence, meaning, and self-worth are shattered. For young children, the shattering of trust in caregivers presents a similar existential crisis because the secure relationship with the caregiver is the source of the child's developing assumptions that the world is a benevolent place, that life has meaning, and that the self is worthy. If young children are to be restored to positive and hopeful developmental trajectories after trauma, then it is essential that the ruptures in their relationships with those who care for them be mended. For this reason, CPP focuses on strengthening the caregiving relationship after trauma as the most economical means of protecting children's development and mental health.

Although generally the child's parents provide essential protections from danger, when the parents' protections fail or parents are themselves the source of risk, surrogate caregivers must take on these protective functions. In this chapter we discuss using CPP in cases where children have been removed from their parents' care and placed with relatives. CPP has been described fully elsewhere (Lieberman & Van Horn 2005, 2008, 2009), so here we briefly describe CPP as it was practiced in the randomized trials that established its efficacy, ending with a brief discussion of the evidence that supports it. We next describe some of the traumatic circumstances that result in infants and young children being placed in foster care, discuss some of the strengths and vulnerabilities specific to kinship foster care, and, using clinical vignettes, show how CPP can be adapted best to serve children in these surrogate caregiving relationships.

TRADITIONAL CHILD–PARENT PSYCHOTHERAPY

Theoretical Underpinnings of CPP

CPP emerged from a tradition of relationship-based therapies developed to address situations in which infants or young children suffered abusive or neglectful caregiving, or in which the parents had suffered traumas in their own early caregiving that they renacted with their child, putting the child's development at risk. These relationship-based treatments have been called by a variety of names, including infant–parent psychotherapy (Fraiberg, 1980; Lieberman, Silverman, & Pawl, 2000), toddler–parent psychotherapy (Lieberman, 1992), and preschooler–parent psychotherapy (Toth, Maughan, Manly, Spagnola, & Cicchetti, 2002), leading Lieberman (2004) to advocate that, to minimize confusion, the term CPP be used to describe them all. All of these relationship-based therapies focus on the intergenerational transmission of trauma and psychopathology, and on translating the parent's and the child's feelings and experiences to one another as a means of achieving enhanced emotional reciprocity in the dyad. Interventions are directed at the parent–child relationship itself, particularly addressing the child's sense of the parent as being unable to provide safety and protection, the parent's distorted negative attributions of the child, and the mutual traumatic expectations that the parent and child have of one another.

CPP (Lieberman & Van Horn, 2005, 2008) is psychodynamic and includes a focus on attachment theory. Because it was developed for use with trauma-specific populations, it has incorporated components common to trauma treatments (Marmar, Foy, Kagan, & Pynoos, 1993), including helping the traumatized individual achieve and maintain regular levels of affective arousal, reestablish trust in bodily sensations and emotional cues, and restore the capacity to respond realistically to threat. CPP uses relationship-focused interventions to help traumatized children and their caregivers cope with traumatic reminders and traumatic expectations, and to help them use play or other media to co-create a coherent narrative of their traumatic experiences. CPP is sufficiently flexible to allow the incorporation of interventions based in behavioral and social learning theories when these are deemed the most effective ways to address the clinical problem at hand. CPP does not, however, strive to accomplish behavior change as an end in itself. It seeks to understand the meaning behind children's and parents' behaviors (particularly when the meaning is based in developmentally salient anxieties or traumatic experiences) and to translate these meanings so that the parent and the child can better understand one another's views of the world and motivations.

Clinical ports of entry are not selected a priori according to theory in CPP, but are selected by the clinician as material presents itself, allowing the clinician to select interventions that he or she believes will most effectively advance the goals of helping the parent and child hold realistic, flexible, and reciprocal views of one another and return the child to a healthy developmental trajectory. CPP clinicians are advised to begin with simple interventions, often based in developmental guidance, but the order of intervention is not dictated.

CPP uses a variety of treatment modalities, including (1) supporting the child's developmental momentum through play, physical contact, and language; (2) offering unstructured, reflective, developmental guidance; (3) modeling appropriate protective behavior in situations where the parent does not respond to threat; (4) interpreting feelings and actions; (5) providing emotional support and empathic communication; and (6) offering crisis intervention, case management, and concrete assistance with problems of daily living. As CPP clinicians weave these modalities into unified treatments, they pay special attention to themes of trauma, both in the present and in the parents' or children's pasts. Clinicians help parents and children understand the impact of the trauma on their beliefs and feelings about one another and about the child's other parent; help them form balanced views of one another and the other parent based on positive memories, as well as traumatic ones; and help them notice and cope with traumatic reminders. CPP clinicians also engage in an active quest for beneficent memories from the parents' care-receiving pasts that may guide and sustain them as they care for their children (Lieberman, Padrón, Van Horn, & Harris, 2004).

The Role of Play

Play holds a special place in CPP. In models of individual child psychotherapy, the child plays in the presence of a trusted therapist who may interpret the play or simply play with the child (Slade, 1994). In CPP, however, traumatized children and their caregivers come together in play. The therapist's role is to facilitate the joint play of parents and children or to support parents as they witness their children's play. If the parents are unable to accept the meaning of their children's play, or become affectively overwhelmed by the play because it is too evocative of their own trauma, CPP clinicians are challenged to make it safe for children to tell their stories and for parents to witness them. In CPP, play becomes a vehicle for restoring children's ability, disrupted by trauma, to maintain a working model of their parents as reliable protectors. In CPP, parents witness and come to understand their children's fears and anxieties as expressed through play, and can both help their children grapple with those fears and offer appropriate reassurance. As children and parents grow more able to play together, children share their concerns and vulnerabilities with their parents; play provides parents with a vehicle to help children examine the distorted expectations created by the trauma, to experiment with different outcomes, and to place the trauma in perspective. The more fully the parent is able to engage in the play, the more the CPP clinician steps aside and allows parent and child to collaborate together.

There are, however, a variety of reasons why parents may be reluctant to engage in play, even after many sessions of treatment. The trauma material may continue to be affectively arousing, or parents may be distressed as they come to understand the full impact that traumatic experiences have had on their children. In either of these cases, parents' strong affect may interfere with their ability to play. In some cultures, parents do not see play as part of their role, and they may never be comfortable playing with their children. Parents may have never learned to play when they were children, or they may find it awkward and embarrassing to behave in a "childish" way in front of the clinician. In these cases, CPP clinicians' central role remains that of translator. They help parents understand and accept their children's experience and feelings; simultaneously, they help children understand their parents' protective impulses and motivations.

Beginning Treatment in CPP

Although CPP is generally a flexible modality, the beginning of a CPP treatment is structured in two distinct ways. First, so that the clinician can form a strong alliance with the parent, he or she should always meet alone with the parent at least once, and more frequently if possible, before the joint parent–child sessions begin. Several purposes are served by these meetings. The clinician should use them to perform a good clinical assessment, with or without the use of formal instruments. At a minimum, the clinician can learn the parent's concerns about the child, the details of the traumatic experience, and the parent's understanding of how the child's functioning changed after the traumatic experience. He or she can also assess the parent's capacity for affect regulation and can offer psychoeducation about the impact of trauma. The clinician can help the parent understand what to expect from CPP, and perhaps most importantly, plan with the parent precisely what the child should be told about why he or she is coming to therapy.

It is critical in the first parent–child session, and thereafter as necessary, that parent and therapist work together, using the same words to tell the child that the trauma is the reason for coming to therapy. If the child is experiencing posttraumatic symptoms or behavioral problems, these can be woven into the explanation for treatment as well. For example, a child may be told,

> "You saw your daddy hit your mom and make her face bleed. You cried and told him to stop. That is so scary for kids, and your mom is worried that you are still scared about what you saw. She says that you

have bad dreams, and sometimes you get so mad that you hit other people. My job is to help your mom help you understand what happened and help you feel better."

In short, the therapist brings the trauma into the room in the first session, and actively looks for hints that the child is playing out themes of the trauma in play. Thereafter, the therapist generally does not guide the child to play specifically about the trauma. CPP's format allows children to bring up trauma material in their own time. For some children, trauma play may emerge in the first session. For others, a period of organizing play may come before active play about the trauma. For still others, trauma material may come and go in play as children work through both the trauma and developmental concerns that may not be trauma related (e.g., exploring the wish for and the fear of increased autonomy). Consistent with the overall goal of supporting a satisfying and reciprocal parent–child relationship, and returning the child to a positive developmental trajectory, CPP encourages the therapist to follow the child's lead in play, and to support the parent in following the child's lead as well.

Although CPP is flexible, like most trauma treatments, it often proceeds in stages. Early CPP sessions may focus on establishing physical and psychological safety for both parent and child. Interventions during this period may include safety planning, help in finding safe housing or legal assistance, and help in stabilizing the child's preschool or day care placement. It may also include psychoeducation about trauma or help both parent and child learn ways to relax and calm themselves when they are emotionally activated by either trauma reminders or the daily stresses of their lives. In later stages of the treatment there is likely to be a greater focus on creating a trauma narrative and undoing the distorted expectations that parents and children may have formed about each other as a result of the trauma.

The Evidence Base for CPP

CPP was not initially developed to treat traumatized children. Before it was adapted to include specific trauma-treatment goals, CPP was demonstrated to be efficacious with high-risk samples, including anxiously attached toddlers of immigrant mothers (Lieberman, Weston, & Pawl, 1991) and toddlers of depressed mothers (Cicchetti, Toth, & Rogosch, 1999). More recently, randomized trials from two different research groups have provided evidence for the efficacy of CPP with traumatized children between the ages of 12 months and 5 years. CPP has been shown to reduce significantly both posttraumatic stress disorder (PTSD) symptoms and behavior problems in preschool children exposed to physical violence between their parents (Lieberman, Van Horn, & Ghosh Ippen, 2005); these improvements have not only persisted for 6 months after the conclusion of treatment, but both children and parents receiving CPP have continued to improve in their functioning during the months after treatment compared to control group parents and children who received case management plus treatment as usual in the community (generally individual treatment for parent, child, or both) (Lieberman, Ghosh Ippen, & Van Horn, 2006). CPP was found efficacious in improving rates of secure attachment in a sample of maltreated toddlers compared to a control group of children who received treatment as usual (see Toth, Manly, & Hathaway, Chapter 6, this volume; Cicchetti, Rogosch, & Toth, 2006; Toth, Rogosch, & Cicchetti, in press). In a study, CPP was found to improve significantly the quality of maltreated preschoolers' representations of their parents compared to a control group of children who received treatment as usual (Toth et al., 2002).

ADAPTING CHILD–PARENT PSYCHOTHERAPY FOR YOUNG CHILDREN IN KINSHIP CARE

It is without doubt that child abuse and neglect, often resulting in the removal of children from their parents and placement in protective custody, is one of the principal sources of trauma in early childhood. Annually there are 3 million reports of child abuse and neglect, with cases substantiated at the rate of 1 million per year (U.S. Department of Health and Human Services Administration on Children, Youth, and Families, 2005). Young children are disproportionately the direct victims of this violence and neglect. During the first year of life, more children are physically abused and die as the result of the abuse than at any other 1-year period (Zeanah & Scheeringa, 1997). Extrapolating data from 40 states reported to the National Center on Child Abuse and Neglect in 1995, the National Research Council and Institute of Medicine (Shonkoff & Phillips, 2000) found that over one-third of victims of substantiated reports to child protection agencies were under age 5. Children under age 5 are also more likely than older children to be present in homes where domestic violence occurs (Fantuzzo, Brouch, Beriama, & Atkins, 1997), and children under 5 are hospitalized and die from drowning and submersion, burning, falls, suffocation, choking, and poisoning more frequently than children in any other age group (Grossman, 2000). Often these injuries are due to intentional acts or negligence by the children's caregivers, and children who survive their injuries are removed from their homes. As will be shown, these young children are disproportionately placed with relatives (Administration for Children and Families, 2005).

Strengths and Limitations of Kinship Care

Kinship care, either formally through the child protection system or less formally in private arrangements between family members, provides a biological family member as a resource for parents who are unable to care safely for their children. Kinship care has some distinct advantages. Children placed with relatives are more likely to be able to maintain cultural linkages and ties to their neighborhoods, siblings, and social networks; they are also more likely to be placed with siblings and to have contact with their birth parents (Chipungu, Everett, Verduik, & Jones, 1998). There is some evidence that kinship care providers are more committed to the children in their care than are traditional foster parents, and are less likely to abuse them (Benedict, Zuravin, Somerfield, & Brandt, 1996). On the other hand, kinship care providers are more frequently beset by both health and mental health problems, and both may be exacerbated by the stress of caring for children (Minkler, Fuller-Thompson, Miller, & Driver, 2000). Kinship foster care providers disproportionately have socioeconomic burdens, ranging from poverty and single-parent status (Cuddeback, 2004) to compromised parenting capacities and home environments (Jones Harden, Clymen, Kriebel, & Lyons, 2004).

Given that child abuse and neglect are so frequently causes of traumatic stress to infants and young children, and that these children are overrepresented in kinship foster care samples, it is important to adapt psychotherapeutic interventions to serve this vulnerable population. Preliminary pilot data demonstrated that CPP, compared to a customary system of care intervention in matched samples of children under age 6, was associated with fewer behavior problems and symptoms of posttraumatic stress (Habib et al., 2008). These findings indicate that although CPP was originally developed and tested on groups of traumatized young children and their biological parents, it may be a promising intervention for children in kinship care. Below we describe adaptations that we believe will make CPP more likely to succeed by taking advantage of the strengths and addressing the vulnerabilities frequently found in families providing kinship care.

Specific Adaptations of CPP for Families in Kinship Care

Although the basic principles underlying CPP still apply, because of the relational complexities inherent in kinship care, adaptations are required when CPP is used with children being cared for by relatives other than their biological parents. These adaptations fall into four basic clusters: (1) dealing with consequences of the fact that kinship caregivers frequently sacrifice their own developmental needs and expectations in order to care for child relatives; (2) working with confounded attachment and caregiving relationships; (3) working with relationship hurts and conflicts that are alive in current family dynamics rather than appearing as "ghosts"; and (4) serving complex family systems when biological parents and kinship providers struggle to co-parent young children. As is in the case examples that follow show, several of these conditions may occur in a single family. The structural adaptation that is needed is often supplemental sessions with the caregiver. CPP clinicians working with kinship care families must keep these additional complexities in mind so that they can fully empathize with the challenges, as well as the gifts, that kinship care presents to children and caregivers.

Dealing with the Caregiver's Phase of Life and Developmental Needs

Relatives in a range of developmental phases in their own lives may undertake the parenting of young children whose biological parents are unable to provide for their day-to-day care. Some caregivers are older siblings, who have not yet begun to formulate their own identities as parents. Others are actively parenting their own children. When they take in the young child of a family member, they find it necessary to postpone or give up entirely their plans to have additional children of their own in order to preserve the financial and emotional resources they need to raise their relatives' children. Perhaps most commonly, kinship providers are the grandparents of the children they undertake to raise. At a phase of life when they believe that childrearing is behind them, they find themselves starting over again and assuming the responsibility of parenting a young child or children. The conflicts that providers experience connected with this "out of phase" parenting may be exacerbated by the fact that they often feel they have no choice but to take in their young relatives, so that the children will not be cared for by strangers and lost to the family.

CASE EXAMPLE 1

Ms. Martin was a 22-year-old African American woman working full time and completing her nursing degree when she agreed to become the guardian of her brother's 5-year-old twins and newborn daughter after he and his wife were killed in an accident. She knew the children well and loved them, and she took on their care with enthusiasm and hope. She quickly found herself feeling unprepared for the challenges she faced. Both twins, who had witnessed the accident in which their parents died, were having nightmares nearly every night. They were aggressive in ways that previously had not been characteristic of them. The baby was withdrawn and unable to sleep. Ms. Martin dropped out of school to care for the children but still felt that she did not have time to give them the attention they needed. She sought help for the children, and CPP was recommended. The

CPP clinician was able to help Ms. Martin find language to talk with the twins about their loss and to support her as she watched them process the accident in play. The clinician also reinforced Ms. Martin's attuned care of her infant niece. As she became accustomed to the patterns of Ms. Martin's care, the baby's symptoms quickly diminished. The older children, although they remained sad and preoccupied by the loss of their parents, became less aggressive and less beset by nightmares as their confidence in their aunt's ability to tolerate and support their feelings increased. Even as the children became less symptomatic, however, Ms. Martin remained angry, overwhelmed, and tearful. The CPP clinician switched the focus of her attention to Ms. Martin, offering to her individual collateral sessions. In these sessions, the clinician empathized with Ms. Martin's plight. She had put her own career goals on hold and set aside her own need to mourn her brother's death and to care for his children. Although she loved the children, she had never thought of herself as a mother, and she doubted her ability to provide adequate care for children who had suffered such overwhelming losses. The CPP clinician helped Ms. Martin work through her fear that she would not be able to care for the children unless she put her own feelings and needs aside. The clinician supported Ms. Martin it talking to the twins about her own feelings of sadness, and helped her understand that her tears, rather than hurt the children, would instead model for them the possibility of feeling sad, then returning to a calmer, happier state. The clinician also helped Ms. Martin process her feelings about having dropped out of school. With support, Ms. Martin was able to find good infant care for the baby and make a plan for resuming her education once the older children started first grade.

CASE EXAMPLE 2

Ms. Lee was the maternal aunt of the mother of Jeremiah and Judith, ages 4 and 2. She had already retired and saved the money she needed to move out of state when she agreed to foster Jeremiah and Judith, who had been removed from their mother's care because she was involved in a violent relationship with a man who had also physically abused both children. Ms. Lee reluctantly agreed to take on the children; no other family member was able or willing to do so, and Ms. Lee believed that the children would be quickly returned to their mother's care. An additional factor, according to Ms. Lee, was that she always had had a close and protective relationship with her niece, taking Judith in from time to time when her parents' physical violence became too frightening. She felt that it was "just natural" that she take in her niece's children when the need arose.

It soon became clear, however, that a speedy return to their mother's care was not likely. She was not willing to leave her violent partner, and the child protection workers were not willing to return the children to a home in which they had been hurt. As Jeremiah and Judith's stay in her home stretched from weeks to months, with no plan to return them in sight, Ms. Lee felt increasing frustration and anger at both her niece and the children. The combination of the children's affective dysregulation, aggression, and sleeping and toileting difficulties, and Ms. Lee's wish to have her dreams for retirement fulfilled created a living situation that felt out of control and emotionally charged for all of them. Ms. Lee was so flooded by her unspoken, and perhaps unconscious, resentments that she initially was unable to engage in child–parent work. When the clinician attempted to engage her in play or other activities with the children, Ms. Lee either ignored her bids or became dismissive and critical of the children. The clinician offered Ms. Lee a series of individual sessions to supplement the child–parent sessions. In these individual sessions, Ms. Lee had space to discuss her anger and resentment. What emerged was her deep wish to proceed with her own retirement plans, anger at her niece for choosing a violent partner over her children, and conflicted feelings of disloyalty and guilt related to her belief that if she followed through with her wishes, she would be abandoning the children, disappointing her niece, and failing in her role as the family matriarch.

Ms. Lee's discussion of her feelings in the collateral sessions had the paradoxical result that she became more supportive of the children, even as she decided she would proceed with her plans to move out of state. In joint sessions, she witnessed the children's play and helped the clinician narrate their story, empathizing first with how wrenching it had been for the children to move to her home, and later, with their pain at witnessing and sustaining violence. Finally, Ms. Lee was able to acknowledge Jeremiah's confusion over his mother's decision to stay with her violent partner even though he had hurt them all, and to acknowledge that she also was confused and angry about that decision. Ultimately Ms. Lee did leave the children and move out of state. As Ms. Lee struggled with this decision in therapy, the therapist, in supervision, worked through her own anger and disappointment at Ms. Lee's unwillingness to provide a permanent home for the children. Supervision provided a nonjudgmental environment in which the therapist could acknowledge how much she had come to care about these children, and how enraged she sometimes felt because Ms. Lee did not want to keep them. The support she received in reflective supervision enabled the therapist to support Ms. Lee, with the result that Ms. Lee was willing at least to wait until a new foster home could be arranged and a thoughtful transition put in place for the children. Ms. Lee made herself available for transition sessions in which the child–parent therapy was transferred to the children's mother, newly separated from her partner. Although the children and their mother experienced sadness and anger at Ms. Lee's decision, with the therapist's support Ms. Lee was able to talk to them about why she felt the need to leave, and her hope that the children and their mother would be able to be together again.

Although these two cases had different outcomes, they have in common the result that both caregivers were able to use CPP to maximize their individual capacities to be empathic and protective of the children in their care. Had the clinician not been able to take into account and empathize with the specific developmental needs of the caregivers, this added measure of protection could not have been attained.

Confounded Attachment and Caregiving Relationships

Kinship care takes place in a complex web of attachment relationships. Children must cope with the loss of their parents and form a new attachment, but in kinship care, that relationship is with a caregiver with whom they have a preexisting but different relationship. Caregivers, particularly grandparents, must shift caregiving impulses from their own children to a grandchild(ren) whose needs for safety and protection may conflict with those of the caregiver's own children.

CASE EXAMPLE 3

Mr. and Mrs. Johnson undertook the care and legal guardianship of their infant granddaughter Maria, when Maria's mother, Annette, was jailed for possessing and selling controlled substances. Annette suffered from bipolar disorder, which she self-medicated using a variety of street drugs. After she was released from jail, Annette went to court to regain custody of Maria, now nearly 3 years old. The court left Maria in her grandparents' custody but granted Annette the right to unsupervised contact with her. Annette was enraged at her parents for opposing her request for custody. She broke into their home and took nearly $200 in cash and many of Maria's clothes and toys. She telephoned many times a week, demanding to speak to Maria, telling Maria that her grandparents did not love her, and "promising" Maria that she could come home to Mommy soon. Annette also vandalized her mother's car in a way that put Mrs. Johnson's and Maria's lives at risk when they next used it. The CPP clinician working with the family spent many hours thinking with the Johnsons about the risk Annette posed to Maria's well-being. They were conflicted, believing that it was in Maria's best interest for them to return to court and request that her contact with her mother be professionally supervised. They were unable to bring themselves to take this protective action, however, because they believed that it would inevitably result in Annette's being arrested and returned to jail. The clinician worked with them over time, exploring their conflicted feelings, until they were ultimately able to request, and receive, a court order for supervised visits. During this period, the clinician used supervision to contain her own anxiety about Maria's safety during unsupervised visits with her mother, and her frustration with what she perceived as the Johnsons' stubborn refusal to protect their very vulnerable young granddaughter.

CASE EXAMPLE 4

Five-year-old Bev spent most days with her maternal grandparents, returning to the home of her mentally ill mother for dinner and to sleep. Her maternal grandmother petitioned for guardianship in order to ensure Bev's safety as her mother's behavior became increasingly bizarre and dissociative, and Bev's contact with her mother was limited to weekends. The grandmother asked for CPP because she noted that when Bev returned from visits, she showed regression in sleep and toileting, disorganized play, tantrums, and tearful clinging. After visits, Bev also alternately "spaced out," becoming lost in her own world and unreachable, and flew into rages in which she sometimes physically attacked her grandmother.

The CPP clinician hypothesized that both Bev and her grandmother had conflicted feelings about Bev's mother. Bev was frightened by her mother's behavior when they were together, but she worried about her and longed for her when they were separated, taking on some of her mother's bizarre and dissociative behaviors as a way of identifying with her and holding her mentally close. Her grandmother felt guilty that she had allowed Bev to spend so much time in the care of her very disturbed mother, angry at her daughter for hurting and frightening Bev, and frustrated that she could not help her daughter. In a CPP session, the clinician talked with Bev about how confusing it was both to love her mom and be frightened of her, and how guilty she might feel for loving her grandmother and feeling so safe in her care. Bev turned to her grandmother and asked her angrily, "Why can't you take care of my mom the way you take care of me? Why can't you fix her? She shouldn't be alone." The grandmother tearfully apologized to Bev for not being able to help her mother, and said that she felt sad because she could not.

In CPP, both Bev and her grandmother struggled with their dual attachments. Bev desparately needed to find parts of her mother that were less disturbed and frightening with which to identify. Her grandmother was sometimes too caught up in her own anger and guilt to help Bev find the positive aspects of her mother. In sessions, the CPP clinician gently asked Bev's grandmother questions about her positive early memories of her daughter, with the result that, ultimately, the grandmother was able to tell Bev stories of her mother that were filled with humor and with a love of exploration and learning. Bev began to identify with these aspects of her mother, remarking that she had a smart mom, and that was why she did so well in kindergarten. She continued to miss her mother and used the CPP sessions as an opportunity to mourn the loss of her mother, to work through her guilt at being in a good and safe home when her mother was not safe, and to deal with the complications of having a grandmother who also functioned as a mommy. Her grandmother was able, with the help of the CPP clinician, to soften her anger toward her own daughter and to let go of some of the guilt she felt at not having been able to protect her.

Generally CPP works to help a caregiver and child strengthen their attachment, and overcome challenges such as trauma that interfere with its security. As we see in the cases described, when CPP is used to help children in kinship care, clinicians must not only attend to the attachment of the caregiver and child in treatment but also their attachments to the relative they share.

Working through the Ghosts in Present Relationships

Fraiberg (1980) described the powerful hold of "ghosts in the nursery" and caregivers' susceptibility to repeating the traumas of their own early caregiving experiences. When kinship caregivers take in the children of relatives, however, they must deal with not only the ghosts from the past but also the realities of relationships in the present. These relationships are likely to be fraught with conflicted feelings and either impoverished or highly aggressive interactions. When children have been removed from their biological parents because of abuse or neglect, kinship caregivers may find it difficult to be open to discussion of the child's experiences or fears. They may be defensive about any play or discussion that implicates their family member in any wrongdoing. Alternatively, they may be so frightened of, or angry with, the family member that they cannot tolerate the child's need to express feelings of longing for a lost parent.

CASE EXAMPLE 5

Mrs. Lambert referred her 4-year-old grandson Michael for CPP when his preschool reported his "out of control" behaviors, which escalated after visits with his parents. Michael had come to live with Mrs. Lambert when he was 3 but, until then, had a chaotic history of witnessing his parents', Mrs. Lambert's son and his wife, drug use and physical violence.

Mrs. Lambert was a stern woman, not prone to physical affection; still, it was clear that Michael responded well to her consistent and firm limits. The therapist spoke with both of them about how good it felt to Michael that his grandma could help him feel safe by not letting him get out of control.

The therapist also helped Mrs. Lambert consider what might be the meaning behind Michael's behaviors, offering psychoeducation about how children can be triggered by changes in routine or visits with their parents. Still, until nearly 2 months into the treatment, Mrs. Lambert denied that Michael's aggression and tantrums were connected to his visits with his parents. Even when she finally made the connection, Mrs. Lambert clearly struggled with conflicted loyalties. She wanted to support her son's and daughter-in-law's efforts toward reunification, and she believed discussing anything that might be negative about the visits with an outsider who was part of the larger "system" betrayed her duty of loyalty to them. Also fueling Mrs. Lambert's silence about Michael's behavioral outbursts after visits was her fear that she could not manage Michael, and her wish to have him out of her home, a wish that might be thwarted if she reported his postvisit regression. The therapist helped Mrs. Lambert explore the many challenges she faced if she acknowledged how troubled Michael was after contacts with his parents. As she became more at ease with her feelings, Mrs. Lambert became more open to the therapist's hypothesis that Michael's behavior was also fueled by internal conflict: He was overwhelmed with both loving and missing his parents, and loving and yearning for closeness with his grandmother. He accepted and responded well to the structure that his grandmother offered, except when he was reminded by visits how much he longed for his parents. As Mrs. Lambert began to understand what motivated Michael's behavior, she was able to free him of the attribution that his behavior was disrespect aimed at her. Mrs. Lambert noted ruefully that she saw her own son in Michael. She saw Michael as disrespectful, she said, because that had been her experience of her own son when he was a little boy. Now she was forced to relive her son's difficult childhood with her grandson, all while deeply desiring both to send Michael back to his father, and to find redemption for her son's difficult childhood in the relationship with her grandson.

In CPP, Mrs. Lambert and Michael each grew in their understanding of their complicated feelings about each other. Ultimately, Mrs. Lambert also grew in her ability to offer Michael the comfort he needed, reassuring him that she understood how much he loved his mother and father, even though they had been frightening sometimes, and even though he was angry with them for not being able to care for him. With the support of the therapist Mrs. Lambert told Michael that she had two kinds of feelings about his dad also: both loving him and being angry at him for not being able to care for his own son.

The Complications of Co-Parenting in Extended Families

CPP clinicians working with kinship families must often adapt the model to take into account the shifting needs of families as biological parents strive to meet their children's needs.

CASE EXAMPLE 6

Kevin, age 6, had lived with his maternal grandparents, Mr. and Mrs. White, for over 2 years. His mother Karen had asked her parents to take Kevin, saying that she could not manage him. Karen and her husband, Kevin's father, were both polysubstance abusers, and their relationship was marked by frequent physical violence, much of which Kevin witnessed. Karen told her mother that Kevin was aggressive and that, at 4, he had never been toilet trained.

Mrs. White also found Kevin challenging. When she brought him for CPP, Mrs. White told the therapist that although Kevin had lived with her for 2 years, he still suffered from encopresis, had difficulty sleeping, and could not concentrate on an activity for more than a few minutes. As a result, he was doing poorly in school. The therapist working with Mrs. White and Kevin experienced him as anxious, hyperactive, and eager to please. He struggled to do everything for himself, rarely asking his grandparents for help or comfort. Mrs. White spoke openly in the sessions about her wish that Karen would ultimately be able to take Kevin back home and care for him. When the therapist gently questioned this wish, Mrs. White acknowledged that her daughter continued to use drugs, and that her life had become even more complicated with the birth of another baby. Mrs. White struggled with the contradictory wishes to send Kevin home to his mother and to take in his baby brother. Kevin's behavior echoed his grandmother's ambivalence. He was sometimes hyperobedient and almost desperate to please her. At other times he had tantrums, refused to eat, and rejected her attempts to help.

In the first 6 months of treatment, the therapist worked toward two goals: exploring Mrs. White's commitment to Kevin, and allowing Kevin to express his complex feelings about all the members of is family. His play themes included worry about his mother and his baby brother, anger at Mrs. White for not being able to care for his whole family, the wish to go home to his mother, and the equally strong wish that he could stay forever with his grandparents. As Mrs. White observed his play, she increasingly saw how important it was to Kevin that he be able to count on her. She told him clearly that she would protect and care for him, that she knew how much he loved his mother, but that his mother was not able to understand and provide the love and safety a boy needed. As Mrs. White's commitment to Kevin became more solid, he was able to relax in her care, feel calmer, and begin to turn to her for help and comfort.

Six months into treatment, as Kevin's symptoms were clearing, his life changed dramatically. Karen, her husband, and her 2-year-old son arrived without warning at the Whites' home. Karen had been arrested for selling drugs; she came to her parents, hoping that they would pay for her to enter a rehabilitation program. Kevin was thrilled to see his mother and brother.

Karen came to a CPP session and told the therapist she was going into rehab, and that she was sure some day she would be able to take Kevin home with her. Kevin's parents moved into a room in the Whites' home. Kevin was torn: Should he continue to sleep in his own bedroom, or should he sleep in the room with his parents and brother? In the CPP sessions, the therapist helped Mrs. White reassure Kevin that his home would always be with her, that she would always care for him, and that she understood how hard it was for him to sleep in his own room when his parents and brother were downstairs.

In the months that followed, Karen relapsed frequently. When she was clean, she actively participated in Kevin's care, helped him with his homework, and took part in the CPP sessions. Kevin became symptomatic again as he experienced uncertainty about who would care for him. The therapist supported Kevin in expressing his fears; Karen reassured Kevin that she loved him but knew he was better off with Mrs. White. When Karen relapsed, she disappeared for days or weeks at a time, living in the streets and sometimes coming home injured. At these times, her inability to care for Kevin was clear to everyone, including Karen. During the CPP sessions, the therapist helped Kevin process his confusion about his mother and understand that his mother's problems were not his fault, and helped Mrs. White overcome her anger and frustration at Karen and focus on Kevin's needs. When Karen returned, the therapist supported Karen in providing what care she could for Kevin, while maintaining the integrity of his primary attachment to Mrs. White.

CONCLUSION

CPP with kinship families has many similarities to CPP with biological families. Play and other media to encourage children's expression of their internal world are at the heart of the sessions. Kinship care providers, just as do biological parents, make use of developmental guidance and emotional support. The changes required to make CPP effective for kinship families are not adaptations to the structure of the sessions or to the theoretical underpinnings of the model. Rather, they take into account the complex and multilayered dynamics that exist in kinship families, and promote attachments that allow children to experience security even in the midst of these complicated relationships.

REFERENCES

Administration for Children and Families. (2005). *National Survey of Child and Adolescent Well-Being: CPS sample component Wave I data analysis report.* Washington, DC: U.S. Department of Health and Human Services.

Benedict, M. I., Zuravin, S., Somerfield, M., & Brandt, D. (1996). The reported health and functioning of children maltreated while in family foster care. *Child Abuse and Neglect, 20,* 561–571.

Bowlby, J. (1982). *Attachment and loss: Vol. 1. Attachment.* New York: Basic Books. (Original work published 1969)

Cicchetti, D., Rogosch, F. A., & Toth, S. L. (2006). Fostering secure attachment in infants in maltreating families through preventive interventions. *Development and Psychopathology, 18,* 623–650.

Cicchetti, D., Toth, S. L., & Rogosch, F. A. (1999). The efficacy of toddler–parent psychotherapy to increase attachment security in offspring of depressed mothers. *Attachment and Human Development 1,* 34–36.

Chipungu, S., Everett, J., Verduik, M., & Jones, J. (1998). *Children placed in foster care with relatives: A multistate study.* Washington, DC: U.S. Department of Health and Human Services.

Cuddeback, G. S. (2004). Kinship family foster care: A methodological and substantive synthesis of research. *Children and Youth Services Review, 26,* 623–639.

Fantuzzo, J. W., Brouch, R., Beriama, A., & Atkins, M. (1997). Domestic violence and children: Prevalence and risk in five major U.S. cities. *Journal of the American Academy of Child and Adolescent Psychiatry, 36,* 116–122.

Fraiberg, S. (1980). *Clinical studies in infant mental health.* New York: Basic Books.

Freud, S. (1955). Beyond the pleasure principle. In J. Strachey (Ed. & Trans.), *The standard edition of the complete psychological works of Sigmund Freud* (Vol. 18). London: Hogarth Press. (Original work published 1920)

Grossman, D. C. (2000). The history of injury control and the epidemiology of child and adolescent injuries. *The Future of Children, 10*(1), 4–22.

Habib, M., Schneider, A., Knoverek, A., Van Horn, P., Hastings, J., Kisiel, C., et al. (2008, November). *Partnerships that work: Applications of trauma-focused interventions for children and adolescents.* Poster presented at International Society for Traumatic Stress Studies, Chicago.

Janoff-Bulman, R. (1992). *Shattered assumptions: Toward a new psychology of trauma.* New York: Free Press.

Jones Harden, B., Clyman, R. B., Kriebel, D. K., & Lyons, M. E. (2004). Kith and kin care: Parental attitudes and resources of foster and relative caregivers. *Children and Youth Services Review, 26,* 657–671.

Lieberman, A. F. (1992). Infant–parent psychotherapy with toddlers. *Development and Psychopathology, 4,* 559–574.

Lieberman, A. F. (2004). Child–parent psychotherapy: A relationship-based approach to the treatment of mental health disorders in infancy and early childhood. In A. J. Sameroff, S. C. McDonough, & K. L. Rosenblum (Eds.), *Treating parent-infant relationship problems* (pp. 97–122). New York: Guilford Press.

Lieberman, A. F., Ghosh Ippen, C., & Van Horn, P. (2006). Child–parent psychotherapy: 6-month follow-up of a randomized controlled trial. *Journal of the American Academy of Child and Adolescent Psychiatry, 45,* 913–918.

Lieberman, A. F., Padrón, E., Van Horn, P., & Harris, W. (2004). Angels in the nursery: The intergenerational transmission of benevolent parental influences. *Infant Mental Health Journal, 26,* 504–520.

Lieberman, A. F., Silverman, R., & Pawl, J. H. (2000). Infant–parent psychotherapy: Core concepts and current approaches. In C. H. Zeanah, Jr. (Ed.), *Handbook of infant mental health* (2nd ed., pp. 472–484). New York: Guilford Press.

Lieberman, A. F., & Van Horn, P. (2005). *"Don't hit my mommy!": A manual for child–parent psychotherapy with young witnesses of family violence.* Washington, DC: Zero to Three Press.

Lieberman, A. F., & Van Horn, P. (2008). *Psychotherapy with infants and young children: Repairing the effects of stress and trauma on early attachment.* New York: Guilford Press.

Lieberman, A. F., & Van Horn, P. (2009). Child–parent psychotherapy: A developmental approach to mental health treatment in infancy and early childhood. In C. H. Zeanah, Jr. (Ed.), *Handbook of infant mental health* (3rd ed., pp. 439–449). New York: Guilford Press.

Lieberman, A. F., Van Horn, P., & Ghosh Ippen, C. (2005). Toward evidence-based treatment: Child–parent psychotherapy with preschoolers exposed to marital violence. *Journal of the American Academy of Child and Adolescent Psychiatry, 44,* 1241–1248.

Lieberman, A. F., Weston, D., & Pawl, J. H. (1991). Preventive intervention and outcome with anxiously attached dyads. *Child Development, 62,* 199–209.

Marans, S., & Adelman, A. (1997). Experiencing violence in a developmental context. In J. D. Osofsky (Ed.), *Children in a violent society* (pp. 202–222). New York: Guilford Press.

Marmar, C., Foy, D., Kagan, B., & Pynoos, R. (1993). An integrated approach for treating posttraumatic stress. *American Psychiatry Press Review of Psychiatry, 12,* 239–272.

Minkler, M., Fuller-Thompson, E., Miller, D., & Driver, D. (2000). Grandparent caregiving and depression. In B. Hayslip & R. Goldberg-Glen (Eds.), *Grandparents raising grandchildren* (pp. 207–220). New York: Springer.

Pynoos, R. S., Steinberg, A. M., & Piacentini, J. C. (1999). A developmental model of childhood traumatic stress and intersection with anxiety disorders. *Biological Psychiatry, 46,* 1542–1554.

Shonkoff, J. P., & Phillips, D. A. (Eds.). (2000). *From neurons to neighborhoods: The science of early childhood development* (Committee on Integrating the Science of Early Childhood Development, Board on Children, Youth, and Families, Commission on Behavioral and Social Sciences and Education). Washington, DC: National Academies Press.

Slade, A. (1994). Making meaning and making believe: Their role in the clinical process. In A. Slade & D. P. Wolfe (Eds.), *Children at play: Clinical and developmental approaches to meaning and representation* (pp. 81–107). New York: Oxford University Press.

Toth, S. L., Maughan, A., Manly, J. T., Spagnola, M., & Cicchetti, D. (2002). The relative efficacy of two interventions in altering maltreated preschool children's representation models: Implications for attachment theory. *Development and Psychopathology, 14,* 877–908.

Toth, S. L., Rogosch, F. A., & Cicchetti, D. (in press). Toddler–parent psychotherapy reorganizes attachment in young offspring of mothers with major depressive disorder. *Journal of Consulting and Clinical Psychology.*

U.S. Department of Health and Human Services Administration on Children, Youth, and Families. (2005). *Child maltreatment, 2003.* Washington, DC: U.S. Government Printing Office.

Zeanah, Jr., C. H., & Scheeringa, M. S. (1997). The experience and effects of violence in infancy. In J. Osofsky (Ed.), *Children in a violent society* (pp. 97–123). New York: Guilford Press.

CHAPTER 5

■ ■ ■ ■

Attachment-Based Treatment for Young, Vulnerable Children

Mary Dozier
Johanna Bick
Kristin Bernard

At birth, human infants are relatively "altricial," or dependent on caregivers for nurturance. The human infant is "prepared" evolutionarily to depend upon a caregiver, and the biological parent is "prepared" evolutionarily to provide care. The infant is dependent on the parent for help with regulating behavior and physiology across a range of systems (Hofer, 2006). For example, the newborn infant's temperature and needs for comfort are best regulated through being held by the caregiver (Christensson et al., 2008), with effects seen when the infant is provided close physical contact by either the mother or the father (Christensson et al., 2008; Erlandsson, Dsilna, Fagersberg, & Christensson, 2007). Typically, parents provide these "co-regulating" functions, with the young child gradually able to take over the functions him- or herself. Neglect and abuse interfere with children's development of these functions, however. When parents neglect their children, they fail to assume this role in helping children develop regulatory capacities. When parents behave in frightening or abusive ways, they may actively undermine children's developing regulatory capabilities (Main & Solomon, 1990).

When children experience maltreatment at the hands of their parents, they have an unsolvable dilemma according to attachment theorists Mary

Main and Erik Hesse (1990); such children are in a position where they must rely upon someone who is frightening to them. In the face of this dilemma, children cope in ways that may have costs socially, emotionally, and physiologically. Maltreated children often develop disorganized attachments to their parents, marked by a breakdown in their strategy for turning to their parents when distressed. Infants placed in foster care are particularly at risk for developing disorganized attachments because they have suffered maltreatment and separation from their biological parents. Infants with disorganized attachments often show behavioral and neuroendocrine dysregulation (Hertsgaard, Gunnar, Farrell, Erickson, & Nachmias, 1995) and face long-term problematic outcomes, including increased aggression toward peers (Lyons-Ruth, 1996; Lyons-Ruth, Alpern, & Repacholi, 1993) and dissociative symptomatology (Carlson, 1998).

In addition to developing disorganized attachments, young children who have been neglected or abused often experience difficulty regulating behaviors, emotions, and physiology (Bernard, Butzin-Dozier, Rittenhouse, & Dozier, 2010; Kim & Cicchetti, 2010; Maughan & Cicchetti, 2002; Pears & Fisher, 2005). Maltreated children are at increased risk for showing behavioral dysregulation in the form of aggressive behavior (Dodge, Pettit, Bates, & Valente, 1995; Keiley, Howe, Dodge, Bates, & Pettit, 2001) and peer rejection (Kim & Cicchetti, 2010). They are also at increased risk for problems regulating emotions (Kim & Cicchetti, 2010), which may underlie some later behavioral and mental health problems. Furthermore, maltreated children are at increased risk for showing dysregulated neuroendocrine systems, such as blunted patterns of cortisol production (Bernard, Butzin-Dozier et al., 2010; Pears & Fisher, 2005). Longer-term problems with internalizing, externalizing, and dissociative symptoms are also associated with early maltreatment (Clemmons, Walsh, DiLillo, & Messman-Moore, 2007; Kim & Cicchetti, 2010; Maughan & Cicchetti, 2002). Taken together, these findings highlight the need for specialized training that helps parents respond to maltreated infants' needs through nurturing care.

THE ATTACHMENT AND BIOBEHAVIORAL CATCH-UP INTERVENTION

We have developed an intervention protocol that helps parents to recognize children's problematic coping strategies and to encourage new ones, to overcome their own issues that get in the way of nurturing their children, and to create an environment that promotes children's biobehavioral regulation (Dozier, Bernard, Bick, & the Infant–Caregiver Lab, 2009).

Randomized clinical trials have demonstrated the effectiveness of the attachment and biobehavioral catch-up (ABC) intervention. For example, in one study, 46 infants in foster care were randomly assigned to receive the ABC intervention or a control intervention that emphasized infants' cognitive and motor development. Foster parents from each group reported on their foster infants' attachment-related behaviors after distress-eliciting scenarios across 3 days. Foster infants in the ABC intervention group were reported to show less avoidance than foster infants in the control intervention group (Dozier, Lindhiem, 2009). In a second study, 120 infants and their neglecting birth parents were randomly assigned to the ABC intervention or a control intervention following involvement with child protective services. At postintervention assessments, fewer children in the ABC intervention group showed disorganized attachments relative to those in the control intervention group (Bernard, Bick, & Dozier, 2010).

In addition to promoting secure attachment behavior among maltreated infants living in either foster care or with their neglecting birth parents, the ABC intervention has been successful in helping foster infants develop more normative cortisol production relative to that of children in a control intervention (Dozier, Peloso, et al., 2006; Dozier, Peloso, Lewis, Laurenceau, & Levine, 2008). Foster children in the ABC intervention group showed lower levels of cortisol upon arrival to the laboratory for a research visit relative to foster children in the control intervention. These lower levels were more similar to cortisol values observed in a low-risk comparison group of children. In terms of diurnal production of cortisol, foster infants in the ABC intervention group had more normative wake-up to bedtime patterns of cortisol than children assigned to the control intervention 1 month after the completion of the programs (Dozier, Peloso, et al., 2006). Furthermore, foster parents of children in the ABC intervention group reported fewer problematic behaviors compared with foster parents of children in the control intervention group. Taken together, these results support the effectiveness of the ABC intervention in helping children develop secure attachment behaviors and improved behavioral and biological regulation.

In this chapter, we first describe research findings that have led to our intervention targets, then the intervention sessions and our approach to intervening with foster and birth parents of children who have experienced early adversity.

RESEARCH FINDINGS REGARDING KEY ISSUES

Issue 1: Children Push Parents Away

The first issue we identified through our research findings was that young children who have experienced early adversity often behave in ways that push parents away (Stovall & Dozier, 2000; Stovall-McClough & Dozier, 2004). More specifically, young children who have experienced adversity often behave as if they do not need their parents (i.e., they behave in avoidant ways), or as if their parents cannot soothe them (i.e., in resistant ways) even when parents are "securogenic" (i.e., when parents' own state of mind with regard to attachment would have predicted that their biological children would develop secure attachments and turn to them when distressed).

These findings emerged in studies in which foster parents completed a checklist and a brief narrative daily for up to 2 months following the foster children's placement in their home. Foster parents were asked to indicate how their children responded when hurt, when frightened, and when separated from them each day. These behaviors were coded for security (whether children sought out parents directly and were soothed), avoidance (whether children turned away from parents), and resistance (whether children fussed and resisted parents). We found that in the first 2 months of their new placement, young foster children often continued to behave in avoidant or resistant ways when hurt or frightened, or following a separation. This was especially true for children placed into foster care after 12 months of age (Stovall & Dozier, 2000).

Although this finding was concerning, it was even more alarming to find that foster parents often responded "in kind" to children's behaviors (Stovall & Dozier, 2000). When children behaved in avoidant ways, foster parents tended to act as if children did not need them; when children behaved in resistant ways, foster parents tended to act angrily in response. Thus, rather than parents taking the lead in the interaction, children were taking the lead. It appeared that children's behaviors initiated a self-perpetuating cycle in which children's underlying needs for nurturance would not be recognized. Our first intervention component was therefore designed to help parents see that their children need nurturance even though children's behavior may not elicit nurturance.

Issue 2: Parents' Own Issues Get in the Way of Providing Nurturance

Among biological parents and children, attachment state of mind is the strongest predictor of attachment security (van IJzendoorn, 1995). "Attachment state of mind" refers to the way in which adults process attachment-related thoughts, memories, and feelings. Parents who are reflective regarding their own attachment-related experiences (termed "autonomous") most frequently have children who are securely attached to them (van IJzendoorn, 1995), presumably because they are open to their children's experiences of distress and able to respond sensitively. In turn, nonautonomous parents who dismiss or devalue the importance of attachment experiences (termed "dismissing"), parents who become incoherent or angrily enmeshed during discussions of their attachment related experiences (termed "preoccupied"), or parents who show a lapse in reasoning when discussing previous traumatic events most frequently have children who develop insecure or disorganized attachments (van IJzendoorn, 1995). Parents with nonautonomous states of mind are less likely to recognize and respond to their children's distress.

Children in foster care especially need parents with autonomous states of mind, who respond sensitively to their distress, if they are to develop organized attachments to new parents (Dozier, Stovall, Albus, & Bates, 2001). When placed with foster parents with nonautonomous states of mind, children are especially likely to form disorganized attachments that place them at increased risk for a host of later problems (Dozier et al., 2001; Fearon, Bakermans-Kranenburg, van IJzendoorn, Lapsley, & Roisman, 2010). We have suggested that sensitive, nurturing care may be especially important for these children because of the early adversity they have experienced. Given that there is not a large enough pool of available foster parents to select only those with autonomous states of mind, and it is not feasible to provide long-term therapy to change state of mind, we have developed an intervention component to help parents behave in nurturing ways even though they may have nonautonomous states of mind. Thus, our second intervention component is designed to help parents "override" their usual ways of responding to children's distress, providing nurturance even though it may not come naturally to them.

Issue 3: Parents Need to Parent in Nonfrightening Ways

Children who have experienced early trauma are particularly susceptible to the effects of frightening behavior (Schuengel, Bakermans-Kranenburg, & van IJzendoorn, 1999). We first noted the need to intervene with regard to frightening behaviors when we adapted our intervention for high-risk birth parents. Parents often view frightening behavior as an effective means of controlling children. As an example, when children touch prohibited objects, some parents yell, smack, and/or threaten children. We have observed this among parents of children who were too young to understand the prohibition or to control their behavior. For example, parents were seen interacting in such ways with children as young as 6 months. Although frightening behaviors are more obvious among birth parents, some foster parents engage in frightening behaviors as well. For example, some foster parents have warned children that they would call their social workers to pick them up if their behavior did not improve. Although not physically threatening, such verbal warnings essentially threaten abandonment. Our intervention helps parents to see how noxious such behaviors can be. Next, parents are helped to recognize their tendency to display frightening behavior that may occur during routine play interactions. They are then helped to develop skills to minimize frightening behavior at these times and to use alternative strategies, beyond the use of frightening behavior.

Issue 4: Children Are Dysregulated Physiologically and Behaviorally

When children experience early adversity, they often become dysregulated behaviorally and biologically. Neuroendocrine functioning generally and the functioning of the HPA (hypothalamus–pituitary–adrenal) axis in particular are often affected in young children who have experienced maltreatment, abuse, or other adversity (Dozier, Manni, et al., 2006; Dozier, Peloso, et al., 2006; Pears & Fisher, 2005). HPA functioning is reflected in the production of cortisol, which is an end product of the HPA axis.

Among nonhuman animal species in which the young form attachments to their mothers, experiences of abuse and separations from parents have been associated with perturbations to the HPA system (e.g., Levine, Johnson, & Gonzalez, 1985; Wiener & Levine, 1983). Depending on the age of the young and the conditions of separations/abuse, effects on HPA axis functioning can be seen even into adulthood (Weiner & Levine, 1983). Similarly, children in foster care and children who are neglected but continue to live with neglecting parents show changes to their HPA axis functioning that may endure in the absence of intervention (Bernard, Butzin-Dozier, et al., 2010; Dozier, Manni, et al., 2006; Dozier, Peloso, et al., 2006; Pears & Fisher, 2005). Dozier, Manni, and colleagues (2006) and Pears and Fisher (2005) found that preschoolers, in comparison to low-risk children, showed a blunted diurnal pattern of cortisol production. Coupled with our work with infants (Dozier, Peloso, et al., 2006), it seems plausible that following early chronic activation of the system as the result of trauma, the system down-regulates, resulting in a blunted pattern (Gunnar & Vazquez, 2001). This is problematic because the child who has experienced trauma may be more poorly equipped to handle social or immune challenges if the HPA axis down-regulates in this fashion.

In addition to biological dysregulation, children who experience early trauma are at risk for becoming behaviorally dysregulated as well. In a study of children placed into foster care, more frequent placements were associated with less well-developed "inhibitory control" (Lewis, Dozier, Ackerman, & Sepulveda-Kozakowski, 2007), which is the ability to inhibit a dominant (prepotent) response. For example, children with stronger inhibitory control are better able to sit at their desks, attend to a boring task, and refrain from jumping up to look out the window relative to children with weaker inhibitory control. Inhibitory control is a key to children's success in school because children with strong inhibitory control are less likely to engage in behaviors that get them in trouble with teachers, are more likely able to attend to academic assignments (and thus progress academically), and are better able to negotiate peer conflicts than children with weak inhibitory control (Blair, 2002). Given that problems with biological and behavioral regulation are seen in young children who have experienced early adversity, we developed an intervention component that targets this issue. Specifically, the intervention helps parents follow their children's lead in play with delight, allowing children a sense of having an effect on their world.

DESIGN OF THE ATTACHMENT AND BIOBEHAVIORAL CATCH-UP INTERVENTION

ABC is a 10-session intervention that targets the four issues identified as critical. The intervention is "manualized," meaning that a manual guides the activities. As described in more detail below, the manual provides a framework but the content must be conversational (i.e., not read), and individualized to the dyad's issues.

Issue 1: Providing Nurturance Even When Children Push Parents Away

This is the first issue we deal with in our intervention, and the easiest. Through videotapes of other children, we help parents see how much more difficult it is to provide nurturance to a child who is avoidant or resistant than to one who is approaching the parent directly for support and is soothed readily. The videos are edited clips of children and parents who had previously participated in research studies in our lab. These families signed release forms giving permission for the videos to be used for this purpose. Using these videos, the case is made that children's behaviors elicit complementary behaviors from parents (with avoidant behaviors eliciting indifference, and resistant behaviors eliciting anger or annoyance). Parents are helped to see that without intervention, interactions between the child and parents may be increasingly driven by the child's behaviors.

Homework after Session 1 helps bring the focus from children's behavior more generally to the specific behaviors of the particular parent's child. Parents are asked to think about how their children behaved with them when distressed during the previous week, and their reactions to these behaviors. Session 2 focuses more than Session 1 on the relationship between parent and child. As described below in more detail, "in-the-moment" feedback is especially useful and important in directing attention to how the issues are playing out in the interactions of this particular parent and child. Through in-the-moment feedback, the trainer points out ways the child is seeking out the parent directly (or not), and ways the parent is providing nurturing care (or not). Care must be taken that parents feel supported (see item 3 on in-the-moment feedback in the section on keys to implementing the intervention).

Issue 2: Providing Nurturance Even When It Does Not Come Naturally to Parents

Whereas the first issue identified is the easiest to address, this second issue is the most difficult. When we first developed the intervention, we planned to address this second component in Sessions 3 and 4. In several iterations of the manual's development, we placed this component later and later in the intervention. This issue is now addressed in Sessions 7 and 8. The reason that this component is introduced so late in the intervention is that parents must have developed real trust in the trainer and a level of openness about their own issues, such that they can do the work required.

The second intervention component is directed at helping parents become aware of how their own issues affect how they respond to their children's needs. Rather than help them work through and resolve these issues fully, the trainers help parents become aware of these issues, so that they can "override" them. Once aware of their own issues, parents can recognize that other behavioral responses to their children's behavior are possible. Thus, we first help parents become aware of their automatic responses (e.g., "I hate to hear my daughter cry, and so I often quickly say, 'you're a big girl—big girls don't cry'"). When parents become aware of their automatic responses (i.e., they have made their automatic responses nonautomatic, or conscious), they can reflect upon how they want to behave (e.g., "I know that I have the inclination to tell her she should not cry, but it's because that's how my mother responded to me. So instead, I'm going to pick her up and hug her because I know that is what she needs"). We help parents see the value of providing nurturing care to the distressed child even though it does not come naturally to them. We conceptualize this as "overriding" parents' natural tendency to respond.

Issue 3: Parents Need to Behave in Nonfrightening Ways

Parents are helped to see how they might have felt overwhelmed and sometimes frightened by their own parents or other attachment figures when they were young. Relatively innocuous examples are first presented, for example, of relatives tickling them or playing a game beyond the point where it was enjoyable. Other scary behaviors that parents can recall are discussed as well. The unsettling effects of some of these behaviors are discussed. Trainers take an empathic approach to help parents realize that they often behave similarly to the ways in which they were parented. For example, trainers explain that, if frightened by their own parents as children, it is understandable that parents might display frightening behavior to their own children.

After the discussion, trainers then ask parents to play with their children in one of several contexts (e.g., with puppets or an assortment of toys that children are often ambivalent about) while monitoring children's reactions for indications that the interaction is intrusive, scary, or unsettling. These interactions are used to demonstrate how easily games that seem innocuous to adults can feel overwhelming to children. Parents are helped to pay very close attention to children's signals. Video feedback helps parents to reflect on their parenting behaviors that may be scary to children at times.

Issue 4: Children Need Help in Developing Regulatory Capabilities

It may be somewhat less apparent than with other intervention components why we chose to intervene as we did with regard to enhancing children's regulatory capabilities. For this component, we borrowed conceptually from interventions that targeted behavioral dysregulation among young infants born prematurely (e.g., Barnard, Morisset, & Spieker, 1993). These interventions focus upon helping parents learn to follow infants' lead as a means of overcoming children's dysregulation that results from compromised neurobiological development. Although we are intervening not with young infants but with older infants and toddlers, the concept is the same.

We help parents learn to follow children's lead through a series of challenging activities. In one session, parents are asked to follow children's lead by playing with blocks and looking at books together. In a second session, parents are asked to follow children's lead while making pudding. These tasks challenge parents because they involve contexts in which parents typically take the lead. Video feedback highlights parents' strengths in letting their children take charge, their delight in their children, and the children's joy in having parents follow their lead.

Session 1: Providing Nurturance to Your Child

The primary objectives of the training are introduced in Session 1. The trainer discusses how vital it is for children to have nurturing relationships with their parents, and to have controllable, interpersonally responsive worlds. Second, the trainer discusses the characteristics of the child and of the parent that may make it difficult to provide nurturance. Attention is drawn to behaviors of the child that make it difficult to see that he or she needs nurturance. In particular, some children do not show their needs for reassurance directly but may instead turn away from parents when distressed or be difficult to soothe. These behaviors are discussed as a result of the child's history of difficult early experiences. The parent is asked to think of how the child responded recently when upset and to consider his or her own reactions to this and to other responses of the child. In addition, the parent is asked to think about his or her usual way of responding to the child, as well as alternative behavioral responses. Finally, the parent is asked to attend to the effects on the child of his or her responding in different ways.

Session 2: Providing Nurturance—What about the Child Makes It Difficult?

During this session, the focus is on helping the parent reinterpret the child's behavior and developing alternative, more nurturing ways to respond. The homework from the week before is reviewed, with careful attention to the child's behavior when distressed and the parent's response. If the child showed secure behaviors, the trainer points out how, clearly, the child showed his or her needs, and discusses what this behavior elicits from the parent. If the child showed avoidant or resistant behaviors, the trainer points out that the task is harder for the parent, and that the parent must see through the child's presentation to his or her underlying neediness. Then, the trainer discusses other behaviors that the child may not have exhibited, and the reactions these behaviors tend to elicit. The feelings engendered by different child behaviors are discussed, and connections are made between the parent's feelings and behaviors. For example, a parent who feels unneeded by the child is likely to behave in a non-nurturing way with the child. Reinterpreting the child's behavior, then, can result in the parent feeling and behaving differently. During the session, the parent is encouraged to see the neediness underlying the child's avoidant and resistant behaviors, and to consider his or her own responses to these behaviors.

Session 3: Following the Child's Lead with Delight

The primary objective of this session is to help the parent feel comfortable following the child's lead in play, while delighting in the child. The trainer discusses with the parent how important it is to allow the child to have a sense of affecting his or her world, and that one of the most important parts of the child's interpersonal world is the parent. Therefore, if the parent is responsive to the child's cues and is delighted, the child begins to develop a sense that the world is predictable. In particular, following the child's lead and allowing the child autonomy allows the child a sense of having an effect on the world.

While being videotaped, parent and child then look at a book with pull-outs on each page. The parent is encouraged to allow the child to take the lead in looking at the book. The parent's role is to follow along and delight in whatever the child is doing. For example, if the child wants to flip through the book quickly, start at the end of the book instead of the beginning, or just focus on one particular pull-out for the entire activity, the parent is encouraged to support and delight in the child. The parent is then asked to play with blocks with the child, again following the child's lead and delighting in him or her. For example, if the child wants to clap the blocks together, stack them, or just throw them in a bucket, the parent is encouraged to follow along. The book is left with the parent and child. The parent is asked to look at the book with the child several times before the next session.

After the activities, the trainer and parent review the video of the interaction. The trainer and parent discuss times when it was difficult for the parent to follow the child's lead. For example, many parents notice that they tend to control the interaction by reading the book to the child and turning the pages rather than letting the child lead. The trainer identifies specific examples of the parent following the child's lead throughout the video feedback and praises these behaviors. In reviewing the video, parents also have opportunities to notice times when they were "leading" that they may have missed during the interaction.

The task of the trainer is to continue to comment on times when the child signals that he or she needs the parent, and times when the parent is responsive to the child's bids for reassurance. In addition, the trainer needs to comment on all those many opportunities the parent has to follow the child's lead and delight in the child.

Session 4: Helping the Child Take Charge

The primary objective of the next several sessions is to help the parent feel comfortable allowing the child to take charge. The trainer reviews with the parent ways in which following the child's lead and taking delight in the child's efforts will help the child feel a sense of his or her own worth.

After seeing a video of a parent and child making pudding, the trainer invites the parent to make a snack with the child. The trainer asks the parent to follow the child's lead as much as possible and to delight in him or her. For example, the parent is encouraged to let the child open the pudding mix, pour the milk, and stir the pudding. The parent is encouraged to give the child any help he or she needs, but to allow the child to be in control as much as possible. Trainers also emphasize that the parent show delight in the child's efforts while making the pudding. The trainer videotapes the interaction. After the interaction, trainer and parent watch the video together and discuss the parent's strengths in interacting with the child. They discuss the difficulty of competing demands (making the snack, keeping the kitchen neat, allowing the child freedom, etc.). The trainer points out the parent's positive behaviors not only when following the child's lead but also when taking delight in the child and what he or she does. The trainer also talks with the parent about times when this may have been hard for the parent. Strategies for helping the parent to follow the child's lead and to delight in the child, even when it is difficult, are discussed.

Session 5: Attending to the Child's Signals

During this session, the parent is helped to "read" the child's signals for engaging and disengaging during an interaction. The parent is urged to see the importance of being sensitively attuned to these signals. The trainer introduces a set of toys (e.g., puppets, snake, spiders, squeaky toys) as a way of illustrating the importance of not being intrusive or overstimulating. The trainer comments on the child's reaction to the toys (e.g., initial tentativeness mixed with curiosity) and the cues that suggest whether the child is frightened or ready to interact with the toys. The child's reaction to these toys and the parent's response to the child are videotaped. When reviewing the interaction together, trainers help the parent become more aware of the child's signals for engagement or disengagement. The trainer helps the parent to notice times when the child may have been showing obvious or subtle signs of being frightened or overwhelmed. The parent is also praised for sensitive responses to the child's signals.

Session 6: Frightening Behavior

This session is designed to help the parent see that he or she needs to protect the child from frightening conditions rather than be the source of that fear. When children are afraid of their parents, it is likely that they cannot use them effectively for support and reassurance. Instead, such children are at increased risk for developing dissociative symptoms (e.g., spacing out) and externalizing problems. The session begins with fairly innocuous examples of frightening behavior and moves to a consideration of more threatening behavior.

Sessions 7 and 8: Providing Nurturance; Recognizing Voices from the Past

Sessions 7 and 8 are the most sensitive sessions because they deal directly with parental issues that may interfere with sensitivity to the child's distress. During these sessions, the parent is asked to consider his or her own contributions to difficulties in providing nurturance. It is critical to handle these issues sensitively so as not to alienate the parent.

The parent is then asked to consider his or her reaction to the child needing him or her. This is discussed in very concrete terms, for example, in the voices from the past that run through his or her head when the child cries. The parent is asked to start making him- or herself aware of the words and feelings running through his or her head, so that the parent can begin to understand and control the influence on his or her parenting.

Session 9: The Importance of Touch

The importance of physical contact for all children, but especially children who have experienced difficult early experiences, is discussed. The parent is asked to consider the kinds of conveniences that have been developed—such as strollers, playpens, child gates, and baby swings—that reduce physical contact. Although not important in and of themselves, these conveniences give us some idea that holding children is not always valued by our society. The parent is asked to think about how his or her child responds to touch, as well as any aversive reactions the parent may have to touch. The parent is asked to relate the most pleasant time he or she has had with this child that involved close physical contact, and a time when the child seemed uncomfortable with the contact. The intervention is tailored to the parent and child depending on their comfort level. For a child who is not comfortable with physical contact, the parent is encouraged to hold, snuggle, and make eye contact regularly with the child, but to follow the child's lead in breaking off contact. For a parent who is not comfortable with physical contact, or who does not value it, the importance of touching this child is stressed. In addition, the parent's own discomfort is dealt with as openly as possible. The trainer introduces several activities (e.g., playing with lotion and stickers, lap games) to encourage the parent to engage in physical touching with the child. Video feedback is used to help the parent recognize strengths in his or her own behavior and the child's responses to the physical contact.

Session 10: The Young Child's Emotions

During this session, the parent is taught the importance of reading the child's emotional expressions, and of helping the child develop comfort in experiencing emotions. The importance of a child experiencing both positive and negative emotions is emphasized. Skills in responding empathically to a child's emotions are developed.

Videos from previous sessions in which the child showed strong negative emotions are shown and discussed. Of particular interest are the parent's feelings about, and reactions to, the child's displays of emotion. The parent is helped to recognize the importance of the child's freedom to feel the emotion and his or her role in helping to organize those feelings so that they are not overwhelming for the child. This is the final session because it is relatively nonthreatening and brings together several previous components of the intervention. Finally, trainer and parent celebrate the parent's accomplishments and progress made throughout the 10-session program.

KEYS TO IMPLEMENTING THE INTERVENTION EFFECTIVELY

Several issues are key to effective implementation.

1. *Adherence to protocol.* First, it is critical that trainers adhere to the protocol. There are many other issues that challenge vulnerable children and families, such as threats of electricity being cut off, children being removed from care, safety and health issues. The lives of vulnerable families are often chaotic, and it may be difficult not to attend to the current crisis. But the intervention will be "hijacked" if parent and trainer do not focus on the targets of the intervention.

2. *Conceptualization of the issues.* Following each session, it is important to conceptualize where the parent is with regard to the issues addressed through this intervention. Attention should be paid to ways in which the parent needs to progress by the end of treatment. For example, some parents may struggle more with providing nurturing care in times of need. Others might respond sensitively to the child's distress but be less comfortable following the child's lead and delighting in the child's efforts. Still other parents may respond in nurturing and sensitive ways but become frightening when disciplining their children. Trainers follow the manual in implementing each session, while tailoring the intervention to focus on the particular needs of the parent. A particularly critical time for tailoring to the parent's needs is Sessions 7 and 8, when parents are encouraged to reflect on "voices from their past" that contribute to their current parenting behaviors.

3. *Use of "in-the-moment" feedback.* To implement the intervention effectively, it is critical to use the interactions observed between the parent and the child. For example, often parents indicate that they are responding to babies' cries, but the trainer observes time after time that this is not occurring. The trainer needs to refer continually to the parent–child interactions during the session as examples of what is being discussed. This is potentially threatening, and it is critical that the trainer do this in a way that feels positive and rewarding for the parent. If the parent comes to see the trainer as a supportive figure, the parent often begins to comment on ways that he or she has missed child signals, or failed to pick the child up. The trainer can comment on times when the parent succeeded, even when it is a rare occur-

rence. For example, the trainer may comment on a 5-second period when the parent responded to the child, even if it occurred during a 2-minute period when the parent missed multiple opportunities to respond. Only the parent who feels supported will be able to do the hard work required.

4. *Where the intervention is implemented.* We prefer to deliver the intervention in families' homes. First, parents have many demands on them in their homes, such as other children, a messy house, and extended family. Although these circumstances may be seen in some interventions as obstacles to effective implementation, we see it as critical to intervene in the context in which parents need to provide care. We do not want a parent to practice nurturing one child in an office setting, for example, if he or she then returns to a house with five children—we fear that it will make the training sterile, and that it will not generalize. Second, we schedule intervention sessions at roughly 1-week intervals. Sometimes parents' lives are so chaotic that it is difficult to make the office visits at regular intervals. Meeting parents in their homes increases the likelihood that visits will occur.

CASE EXAMPLES

Two case examples are provided to illustrate how the intervention is implemented at a practical level.

Case Example 1

Ella was a 36-year-old foster mother to Xavier, a 19-month-old boy. At the beginning of the intervention, the trainer observed that Ella had difficulty responding to Xavier's needs. For example, when Xavier approached Ella after playing alone for about 15 minutes, Ella told him that she was busy talking to the trainer and would play with him later. Later in the same session, Xavier was trying to get onto the couch but lost his balance and fell to the floor. Although not visibly hurt, it was clear that he was alarmed by his fall. Instead of comforting and reassuring Xavier, Ella took his hands and clapped them together quickly, and exclaimed, "What a big boy you are, that didn't hurt. Good clapping!"

Although Ella had a difficult time responding to Xavier during times of need, she showed strengths in following Xavier's lead and expressing delight in his efforts. For example, when Xavier decided to line up puzzle pieces from one end of the table to the other (instead of inserting them into the correct places on the board), Ella responded, "Look how long your line is! Great job!" and followed along. These observations, along with many others, helped the trainer conceptualize Ella's strengths and weaknesses. The subsequent sessions were delivered to emphasize Ella's ease at following Xavier's lead and delighting in his efforts, while also helping Ella to become aware of times when she could be more responsive to his bids for nurturance.

In the first two sessions, Ella and the trainer discussed how children who have responsive parents often turn to their parents in times of need. Later in that session, Ella looked over at Xavier after he whimpered but did not go to him or respond further. To emphasize Ella's responsive behavior (rather than point out her nonresponsiveness), the trainer mentioned how great it was that Ella realized that Xavier needed her at that time. The trainer made other, similar comments whenever possible. A few sessions later, Xavier bumped his knee on the coffee table but did not cry. Ella immediately went over to him and said, "Oh, Xavier, that must have hurt!" and rubbed his knee. Xavier then turned to hug her and said, "hurt!" Through video feedback, the trainer was able to show Ella that her nurturing response helped Xavier turn to her. Soon, Ella was able to recognize times when she responded to Xavier and times when she did not.

By Sessions 7 and 8, the trainer and Ella had formed a trusting, comfortable relationship. Ella was able to admit that she struggled when she felt that Xavier was "too needy." She also described her mother and father coming over to the house and telling her things such as "Don't pick Xavier up right now, he is just going to grow up to be whiny!" By the end of the session, Ella acknowledged that her parents had reacted to her needs for nurturance when she was a child the same way that she reacted to Xavier's needs. The trainer helped Ella realize that, based on her past experiences, it was understandable that responding to Xavier was difficult for her. The trainer emphasized how many times Ella had responded to Xavier sensitively in the past few sessions, and that it really seemed to have a positive effect on Xavier. Finally, the trainer and Ella discussed strategies for overriding Ella's "natural" reaction to ignore Xavier's bids for reassurance. By the end of the 10 sessions, Ella was more comfortable responding to Xavier and did so with consistency.

Case Example 2

Cheronda was the biological mother of a 6-month-old girl, Angel. At the start of the intervention, Cheronda was 17 years old and living at home with her mother and teenage siblings. During a preintervention play assessment, it was clear that Cheronda felt very uncomfortable following Angel's lead in play. Cheronda did not take control and lead the interaction; rather, she sat quietly and did nothing. She even stated, "I don't play with my child." During the 10 minutes of play, the only time that Cheronda interacted with

Angel was when she picked up a rubber duck and squeaked it in Angel's face. The trainer anticipated that sessions emphasizing following the child's lead (Sessions 3 and 4) would be particularly challenging for Cheronda. In addition to Cheronda's own discomfort with following the lead and showing delight, Angel was not seeking out her attention during play (e.g., not turning to her, not holding up toys, not smiling), likely making it even more difficult for Cheronda to respond.

During Sessions 1 and 2, Cheronda held Angel on her lap for most of the visits. She understood that crying was Angel's main way of signaling that she needed her, and Cheronda described specific examples of responding to her distress. More importantly, her behavior in the session matched what she said. For example, Angel woke up from a nap crying at the beginning of Session 2. Cheronda picked her up immediately and patted her back, saying, "Mommy's here, Mommy's here." By repeatedly praising Cheronda's appropriate responses to Angel's distress, the trainer reinforced this behavior and bolstered Cheronda's sense of confidence in her ability to provide comfort. Furthermore, the trainer helped Cheronda understand how this would help Angel learn to trust her and others. Finally, this strengthened the relationship between Cheronda and the trainer. Cheronda felt supported by the trainer preparing her for the hard work that was ahead.

In Session 3, the trainer and Cheronda discussed the importance of also being responsive to Angel when she was not upset, hurt, or frightened. The trainer described how following Angel's lead during play would help Angel feel a sense of control over her world. More importantly, the trainer suggested that having her mother take delight in her efforts would help Angel develop confidence in herself and trust in her mother, both of which were critical to her success as she grew up. Although Cheronda could understand the rationale, she still felt very uncomfortable during the practice activities. When the trainer gave Cheronda a book with pull-out shapes to look at, Cheronda let Angel hold it, turn the pages, and chew on the shapes. However, she sat back quietly and did nothing. The trainer scaffolded the activity by suggesting what Cheronda could do (e.g., pick up a shape after Angel picked one up, comment on what Angel did, smile at Angel when she looked at her). The trainer acknowledged that these behaviors could feel silly but encouraged Cheronda to try them out. Whenever possible, the trainer praised Cheronda's behaviors, pointing out specifically and enthusiastically what she did and how it affected Angel. Through video feedback, the trainer was able to show other clear examples of times that Cheronda followed Angel's lead with delight. Sessions 4 and 5 offered additional opportunities to practice. As Cheronda followed Angel's lead more, Angel started turning to her more, making the effort even more rewarding and reinforcing for Cheronda.

During Sessions 7 and 8, Cheronda and the trainer discussed what got in the way of her ability to follow Angel's lead with delight. Cheronda recalled that she did not receive much attention from her own mother when she was growing up. She noticed herself withholding attention and delight from Angel as well, describing that she sometimes could hear her own mom saying, "She doesn't deserve praise for just playing" and "Just let her do her own thing—she doesn't need you." The trainer helped Cheronda understand that these voices from her past prevented her from being responsive when Angel needed her mother to take delight in her. Cheronda came to see that being aware of these voices would help her override them. Throughout the remaining sessions, the trainer praised Cheronda whenever she showed delight in Angel, reminding her that she was giving what she did not get as she was growing up. During Session 10, the trainer presented several video clips showing changes in how Cheronda responded to Angel during play. Cheronda's face lit up with pride as she watched a video clip of herself taking delight in Angel.

SUMMARY

The ABC intervention was developed to address several key needs of young children who have experienced adversity. Specifically, parents are helped to provide nurturing care even when children do not elicit it, and even when it does not come naturally; to behave in nonfrightening ways; and to provide a responsive, controllable interpersonal environment. The intervention was expected to help children develop secure attachments to parents more readily and to develop better regulatory capabilities. In randomized clinical trials, children in the ABC intervention group have shown more secure attachments and more normative cortisol production than children in a control intervention (Dozier et al., 2008; Dozier, Lindhiem, et al., 2009; Dozier, Peloso, et al., 2006).

Given the exciting findings on the effectiveness of the ABC intervention, we have started disseminating the intervention to other sites. Following a 1-week training, trainees receive a year of supervision from an experienced parent trainer in our laboratory. Supervisors watch videotaped sessions of at least three full cases, and provide weekly feedback via e-mail and videoconferencing. Trainees include social workers, therapists, and researchers. Several dissemination sites are also collecting data on maternal sensitivity, children's attachment security, and children's cortisol regulation. We are hopeful that continued research on the ABC intervention will support its effectiveness across sites. Furthermore, we hope that partnerships between researchers and child welfare agencies will ensure that evidence-based interventions, such as the ABC intervention, are extended to children in need.

ACKNOWLEDGMENTS

Support for this research was provided by National Institute of Mental Health R01 Award Nos. 052135, 074374, and 084135 to Mary Dozier. We acknowledge the support of Delaware Division of Family Services and Philadelphia Department of Human Services; and caseworkers, foster families, birth families, and children at both agencies.

REFERENCES

Barnard, K. E., Morisset, C. E., & Spieker, S. J. (1993). Preventive interventions: Enhancing parent–infant relationship. In C. H. Zeanah, Jr. (Ed.), *Handbook on infant mental health* (pp. 386–401). New York: Guilford Press.

Bernard, K., Bick, J., & Dozier, M. (2010). *Differences in attachment quality among children in attachment and biobehavioral catch-up intervention and a control intervention.* Unpublished manuscript, University of Delaware, Newark.

Bernard, K., Butzin-Dozier, Z., Rittenhouse, J., & Dozier, M. (2010). Young children living with neglecting birth parents show more blunted daytime patterns of cortisol production than children in foster care and comparison children. *Archives of Pediatrics and Adolescent Medicine, 164,* 438–443.

Blair, C. (2002). School readiness: Integrating cognition and emotion in a neurobiological conceptualization of children's functioning at school entry. *American Psychologist, 57,* 111–127.

Carlson, E. A. (1998). A prospective longitudinal study of attachment disorganization/disorientation. *Child Development, 69,* 1107–1128.

Christensson, K., Siles, C., Moreno, L., Belaustequi, A., De La Fuente, P., Lagercrantz, H., et al. (2008). Temperature, metabolic adaptation and crying in healthy full-term newborns cared for skin-to-skin or in a cot. *Acta Paediatrica, 81,* 488–493.

Clemmons, J. C., Walsh, K., DiLillo, D., & Messman-Moore, T. (2007). Unique and combined contributions of multiple child abuse types and abuse severity to adult trauma symptomatology. *Child Maltreatment, 12,* 172–181.

Dodge, K. A., Pettit, G. S., Bates, J. E., & Valente, E. (1995). Social information-processing patterns partially mediate the effect of early physical abuse on later conduct problems. *Journal of Abnormal Psychology, 104,* 632–643.

Dozier, M., Bernard, K., Bick, J., & the Infant-Caregiver Lab. (2009). *Attachment and biobehavioral catch-up.* Unpublished manuscript, University of Delaware, Newark.

Dozier, M., Lindhiem, O., Lewis, E., Bick, J., Bernard, K., & Peloso, E. (2009). Effects of a foster parent training program on children's attachment behaviors: Preliminary evidence from a randomized clinical trial. *Child and Adolescent Social Work Journal, 26,* 321–332.

Dozier, M., Manni, M., Gordon, M. K., Peloso, E., Gunnar, M. R., Stovall-McClough, K., et al. (2006). Foster children's diurnal production of cortisol: An exploratory study. *Child Maltreatment, 11,* 189–197.

Dozier, M., Peloso, E., Lewis, E., Laurenceau, J., & Levine, S. (2008). Effects of an attachment-based intervention on the cortisol production of infants and toddlers in foster care. *Development and Psychopathology, 20,* 845–859.

Dozier, M., Peloso, E., Lindhiem, O., Gordon, M. K., Manni, M., Sepulveda, S., et al. (2006). Preliminary evidence from a randomized clinical trial: Intervention effects on foster children's behavioral and biological regulation. *Journal of Social Issues, 62,* 767–785.

Dozier, M., Stovall, K. C., Albus, K. E., & Bates, B. (2001). Attachment for infants in foster care: The role of parent state of mind. *Child Development, 72,* 1467–1477.

Erlandsson, K., Dsilna, A., Fagerberg, I., & Christensson, K. (2007). Skin-to-skin care with the father after cesarean birth and its effect on newborn crying and prefeeding behavior. *Birth, 34,* 105–114.

Fearon, P., Bakermans-Kranenburg, M., van IJzendoorn, M., Lapsley, A., & Roisman, G. (2010). The significance of insecure attachment and disorganization in the development of children's externalizing behavior: A meta-analytic study. *Child Development, 81*(2), 435–456.

Gunnar, M. R., & Vazquez, D. M. (2001). Low cortisol and a flattening of expected daytime rhythm: Potential indices of risk in human development. *Development and Psychopathology, 13,* 515–538.

Hertsgaard, L., Gunnar, M. R., Farrell, M., Erickson, M. F., & Nachmias, M. (1995). Adrenocortical responses to the Strange Situation in infants with disorganized/disoriented attachment relationships. *Child Development, 66,* 1100–1106.

Hofer, M. A. (2006). Psychobiological roots of early attachment. *Current Directions in Psychological Science, 15,* 84–88.

Keiley, M. K., Howe, T. R., Dodge, K. A., Bates, J. E., & Pettit, G. S. (2001). The timing of child physical maltreatment: A cross-domain growth analysis of impact on adolescent externalizing and internalizing problems. *Development and Psychopathology, 13,* 891–912.

Kim, J., & Cicchetti, D. (2010). Longitudinal pathways linking child maltreatment, emotion regulation, peer relations, and psychopathology. *Journal of Child Psychology and Psychiatry, 51,* 706–716.

Levine, S., Johnson, D. F., & Gonzalez, C. A. (1985). Behavioral and hormonal responses to separation in infant Rhesus monkeys and mothers. *Behavioral Neuroscience, 99,* 399–410.

Lewis, E., Dozier, M., Ackerman, J., & Sepulveda-Kozakowski, S. (2007). The effect of caregiving instability on adopted children's inhibitory control abilities and oppositional behavior. *Developmental Psychology, 43,* 1415–1427.

Lyons-Ruth, K. (1996). Attachment relationships among children with aggressive behavior problems: The role of disorganized early attachment patterns. *Journal of Consulting and Clinical Psychology, 64,* 64–73.

Lyons-Ruth, K., Alpern, L., & Repacholi, B. (1993). Disorganized infant attachment classification and maternal psychosocial problems as predictors of hostile–aggressive behavior in the preschool classroom. *Child Development, 64,* 572–585.

Main, M., & Hesse, E. (1990). Parents' unresolved traumatic experiences are related to infant disorganized attachment status: Is frightened and/or frightening parental behavior the linking mechanism? In M. T. Greenberg, D. Cicchetti, & E. M. Cummings (Eds.), *Attachment in the preschool years: Theory, research and intervention* (pp. 161–182). Chicago: University of Chicago Press.

Main, M., & Solomon, J. (1990). Procedures for identifying infants as disorganized/disoriented during the Ainsworth Strange Situation. In M. T. Greenberg, D. Cicchetti, & E. M. Cummings (Eds.), *Attachment in the preschool years: Theory, research, and intervention* (pp. 121–160). Chicago: University of Chicago Press.

Maughan, A., & Cicchetti, D. (2002). Impact of child maltreatment and interadult violence on children's emotion regulation abilities and socioemotional adjustment. *Child Development, 73,* 1525–1542.

Pears, K., & Fisher, P. A. (2005). Developmental, cognitive, and neuropsychological functioning in preschool-aged foster children: Associations with prior maltreatment and placement history. *Journal of Developmental and Behavioral Pediatrics, 26,* 112–122.

Schuengel, C., Bakermans-Kranenburg, M. J., & van IJzendoorn, M. H. (1999). Frightening maternal behavior linking unresolved loss and disorganized infant attachment. *Journal of Consulting and Clinical Psychology, 67,* 54–63.

Stovall, K. C., & Dozier, M. (2000). The development of attachment in new relationships: Single subject analyses for ten foster infants. *Development and Psychopathology, 12,* 133–156.

Stovall-McClough, K. C., & Dozier, M. (2004). Forming attachments in foster care: Infant attachment behaviors in the first two months of placement. *Development and Psychopathology, 16,* 253–271.

van IJzendoorn, M. (1995). Adult attachment representations, parental responsiveness, and infant attachment: A meta-analysis on the predictive validity of the Adult Attachment Interview. *Psychological Bulletin, 117,* 387–403.

Wiener, S., & Levine, S. (1983). Influence of perinatal malnutrition and early handling on the pituitary–adrenal response to noxious stimuli in adult rats. *Physiology and Behavior, 31,* 285–291.

CHAPTER 6

■ ■ ■ ■

Relational Interventions for Young Children Who Have Been Maltreated

Sheree L. Toth
Jody Todd Manly
Alisa Hathaway

Although not all children who have been maltreated are affected similarly, decades of research have coalesced to show that child maltreatment initiates a cascade of compromised developmental processes, often eventuating in lifelong impairment (Cicchetti & Toth, 2009). Not only are children who have experienced maltreatment likely to exhibit negative socioemotional sequelae and diverse forms of psychopathology, but increasingly research also suggests that these youngsters are at heightened risk for compromised psychophysiological functioning and physical problems (Cicchetti, 2003). In fact, child maltreatment contributes to mortality and morbidity not only during childhood but also into the adult years (Brown et al., 2009; Corso, Edwards, Fang, & Mercy, 2008). In view of the heinous effects of maltreatment on both mental and physical health during childhood and throughout the life course, the provision of interventions that can interrupt this negative developmental cascade are of paramount importance.

In this chapter we discuss the utilization of a developmental psychopathology framework as a conceptual scaffold for the design and evaluation of relational interventions. We next describe the adverse effects of child maltreatment on stage-salient issues during the early years of life, with an emphasis on attachment organization. Principles of child–parent psychotherapy (CPP) are then described. We then discuss translational research and present results from randomized clinical trials that demonstrate the efficacy of CPP for decreasing insecure attachment organizations in infants and young children who have been reared in maltreating families. We provide a clinical vignette to illustrate the implementation of this therapeutic modality, and we conclude by offering recommendations that better inform clinical practice.

A DEVELOPMENTAL PSYCHOPATHOLOGY PERSPECTIVE ON PREVENTION AND INTERVENTION

Since its inception, a major goal of developmental psychopathology has been to bridge research and practice in order to promote positive development, and prevent and ameliorate maladaptive and psychopathological outcomes (Cicchetti, 1990; Cicchetti & Toth, 1992, 2009; Toth, Manly, & Nilsen, 2008). A central parameter of developmental psychopathology involves understanding the interface between normal and atypical functioning and, as such, the discipline is well-positioned to contribute to the development of prevention and intervention strategies. Moreover, by urging attention to risk and psychopathology, the elucidation of mediating and moderating processes that can mitigate against the emergence of maladaptation and psychopathology, and the incorporation of principles of normal development into the design and evaluation of interventions, individuals working within the field of developmental psychopathology have contributed significantly to the design, provision, and evaluation of developmentally informed interventions (Cicchetti & Toth, 2006; Egeland & Erickson, 2004; Lieberman, Weston, & Pawl, 1991). As such, the parameters of developmental psychopathology have fostered the conduct of research with implications for decreasing the burden of mental illness in society.

Substantial research within a developmental psychopathology perspective has been guided by the "organizational perspective," which addresses how development proceeds over time by identifying a progression of reorganizations within and among biological, psychological, and social systems (Werner & Kaplan, 1963). Accordingly, development is conceived as comprising a series of age- and stage-relevant tasks that, although ascendant at certain periods of development, continue to influence the emergence and resolution of subsequent tasks that remain important across the lifespan of the individual (Cicchetti, 1993). Within this framework, the successful resolution of an early-stage-salient task increases the likelihood that subsequent issues also will be resolved successfully (Sroufe & Rutter, 1984). As infants and toddlers are confronted with new demands at transitional periods of development, opportunities for growth and resolution, as well as challenges associated with new vulnerabilities, arise. Development within this model is seen as resulting from dynamic transactions between internal and external factors that can result in competent or maladaptive outcomes over the life course. Such a model imparts hope and the potential for change, and highlights the importance of providing interventions that can prevent or ameliorate negative outcomes, particularly during the early years of life before early-stage-salient issues that are not resolved progressively set in motion a negative cascade of failed developmental attainments.

Although historical experiences and current factors contribute to the developmental course, self-organization also plays an important role in development (Cicchetti & Rogosch, 1997; Cicchetti & Tucker, 1994). Across the course of development, the evolving capacities of individuals and their active choices enable new experiences, both internal (e.g., genetic/ biological) and external (e.g., parenting) to be coordinated in increasingly complex ways. Very early in life, positive self-strivings can impart powerful protective influences, and developmental plasticity can be fostered by both biological and psychological self-organization (Cicchetti, 2002). The presence of self-righting or resilient tendencies (Masten, 2001), even in individuals who have experienced extreme adversity, can be partially attributable to self-organization strivings.

THE SEQUELAE OF CHILD MALTREATMENT

The experience of child abuse and neglect during the early years of life may result in negative consequences in one or more domains of development as children negotiate the stage-salient developmental tasks arising during the infant, toddler, and preschool periods. In the first year of life, babies' regulatory systems that influence arousal, sleeping and waking cycles, modulation of emotions, and responses to environmental cues become more organized both physiologically and in a social context. Caregivers assist infants by responding to physical and emotional needs, and by soothing distress. Because maltreating parents have difficulty consistently meeting their children's needs, abused and neglected infants often struggle to develop physiological regulation mechanisms to help them manage stress and modulate their arousal and emotion regulation (Carlson, Sampson, & Sroufe, 2003). Research on stress hormones among maltreated children has documented the dysregulation of hormonal processes in the hypothalamic–pituitary– adrenal (HPA) systems that direct cognitive, emotional, and behavioral responses to threats (Tarullo & Gunnar, 2006; Van Voorhees & Scarpa, 2004). Chronic activation of stress hormones and responses to trauma also can impact brain development in ways that have an enduring impact on the mastery of other developmental tasks. Caregivers who are able to provide physical and emotional security, and to soothe their children in times of distress provide scaffolding that builds a strong base for the development of skills across cognitive, emotional, self-concept, and behavioral areas. By the end of the first year of life, attachment relationships become a prominent focus, and this relational context can assist children in their emotional and self-development, and in the way they relate to their world and to potential relationship partners. Thus, a key area for prevention and early intervention in child maltreatment focuses on supporting the formation of secure attachment relationships between young children and their primary caregivers.

ATTACHMENT RELATIONSHIPS OF MALTREATED CHILDREN

The development of attachment relationships is a stage-salient developmental issue that is not only centrally important during the first 2 years of life but also continues to play a prominent role throughout the life course. Children who receive sensitive and responsive caregiving in infancy develop trust in these early relationships with primary caregivers that extends to positive expectations about other relationships as children's social worlds expand. Children who have had their needs met consistently learn that nurturing adults to whom they can turn in times of stress are available. Children develop representational models of these relationships that can be applied to appropriate help seeking with teachers and other people later in their lives. Children who are confidently secure in their feelings of protection and safety provided by loving adults also develop more positive concepts of themselves because of experiences demonstrating that they are lovable and worthy of attention. With trust in others and confidence in themselves, they also are able to explore their environments, knowing that their caregivers will provide a secure base to which they can return if they are frightened or stressed.

Research examining different relationship patterns that infants and toddlers exhibit when interacting with their primary caregivers has found that early secure attachment is related to the mastery of many skills as development unfolds. Children who have attachment organizations that are secure are more successful in relationships with peers and teachers (Hamre & Pianta, 2001), more behaviorally and academically competent, and more positive in their views of themselves than are children whose early relationships are insecure (Carlson et al., 2003; Sroufe, Egeland, Carlson, & Collins, 2005). However, children in maltreating families do not experience responsive and sensitive caregiving, and their relationships with their primary care-givers are characterized by inconsistency, unpredictability, and insensitivity. Consequently, children may learn to adapt by avoiding drawing attention to their relationship needs and minimizing their bids for attention, an attach-ment organization referred to as "avoidant." Other children may become clingy and demanding of attention; an attachment organization referred to as "anxious–ambivalent." Children who have experienced more extreme relationship difficulties may be unable to develop an organized response style, and they may exhibit freezing or fear in the presence of their caregiv-ers, extreme withdrawal or passivity, high arousal and aggressive behavior, or an incoherent combination of several patterns, none of which are effec-tive in helping them manage their high level of anxiety (Main, 1999; Sroufe, 2005).

These "disorganized" types of attachment relationships have been found frequently among children who have experienced child maltreat-ment (see Cicchetti & Valentino, 2006). Children who have been neglected have experienced parenting that failed to meet their basic needs for food, medical care, clothing, or shelter, and that has been unresponsive to their emotional needs for comfort and reassurance. Children who have been abused experience harm, often from the parents they depend on for care and protection, leading to particular confusion on when, how, and from whom to seek help and comfort. Often familial relationships for abused and neglected children are inconsistent, sometimes offering nurturance and care, and at other times, when families are under stress associated with poverty, domestic or community violence, substance abuse, parental psy-chopathology, or other challenges, failing to provide the consistent caregiv-ing these infants and toddlers need for healthy development. When parents are unable to ensure children's safety and children are removed from their care, young children experience additional disruption to their relationships at a critical period for their development of interpersonal skills and regula-tion of their emotions.

Studies of maltreated children have shown that a huge preponderance of maltreated children not only exhibit disorganized attachment relationships (Cicchetti & Valentino, 2006), but also that these insecure relationships tend to persist over time (Barnett, Ganiban, & Cicchetti, 1999; Cicchetti & Barnett, 1991). These maladaptive relationship patterns are distinct from child temperament and are associated with the severity of parenting prob-lems (Barnett et al., 1999). In particular, disorganized attachment has been related to caregiver displays of frightening and frightened behavior with the child (Lyons-Ruth, Bronfman, & Parsons, 1999; Main & Hesse, 1990). Maltreated children's experience and expression of fear emerge early, and physiological studies of maltreated children and of those in foster care have provided additional evidence that these children have difficulty regulating their emotions, as evidenced physiologically and psychologically (Dozier, Levine, Stovall, & Eldreth, 2001). However, emerging research suggests that stress hormones in children in foster care can be positively affected through the provision of therapeutic interventions (Fisher, Stoolmiller, & Burraston, 2007).

The high frequency of problematic attachment relationships that endure over time places maltreated children at particular risk for developmental problems, in not only interpersonal relationships but also other domains of functioning. Consistent with an organizational perspective on development, insecure attachment relationships increase the probability of future developmental challenges, placing maltreated children at an extreme disadvantage in mastering subsequent developmental tasks. Although children may be resilient in the face of adversity, maltreated children with disorganized attachments probabilistically are on a pathway that is likely to lead to maladaptive outcomes. Insecure attachment relationships are associated with internalizing and externalizing behavior problems (Lyons-Ruth & Easterbrooks, 1995), difficulty in stress management, dissociative behavior (Ogawa, Sroufe, Weinfield, Carlson, & Egeland, 1997; van IJzendoorn, Schuengel, & Bakersman-Kranenburg, 1999), depressive symptoms (Duggal, Carlson, Sroufe, & Egeland, 2001; Toth & Cicchetti, 1996), and future familial difficulties (Feldman & Downey, 1994; Howes & Cicchetti, 1993; Main & Goldwyn, 1984), including difficulties in parenting into the subsequent generation (Crittenden, Partridge, & Claussen, 1991). Thus, prevention of maltreatment and early intervention with families who have experienced maltreatment is essential to avert future maladaptation and psychopathology, and improving the quality of parent–child attachment relationships has the potential for promoting positive child outcomes across a range of social, emotional, and psychophysiological domains. CPP, an intervention and psychotherapeutic treatment described in depth by Van Horn (Chapter 2, this volume), has been utilized to promote attachment security in children with histories of maltreatment (Cicchetti, Rogosch, & Toth, 2006).

CHILD–PARENT PSYCHOTHERAPY

Child–parent psychotherapy is a nondidactic treatment that allows the therapist and family to learn together, and therapists endeavor to see the world through the family's perspective and understand their beliefs and values. The CPP model of intervention focuses on the child–parent relationship and the impact that parents' representations of their relationship histories exert upon the current caregiving of their children. Sessions include the parent and child together at home or in a setting conducive to promoting interaction and play. Therapists observe dyadic interactions and facilitate improvements in parents' sensitivity to children's emotional needs and responsivity to children's verbal and nonverbal communication, as well as promoting children's development and appropriate expression of their needs and feelings. The goals of the CPP model include: (1) expanding the parent's empathic responsiveness, sensitivity, and attunement to her child; (2) promoting the parent's ability to foster her child's autonomy while negotiating both her own and her child's needs positively; and (3) altering any of the parent's distorted perceptions of her child and any inappropriate parental reactions to the child that stem from the parent's existing representational models of her relationship history. Therapists are trained in stage-salient developmental issues for infants, toddlers, and preschoolers. Discussions of normative development are gently introduced into the dyadic sessions, while encouraging parents to support the developmental gains that their children make over time. This developmental guidance focuses on supportive exploration and recognition of strengths rather than instruction in parenting skills.

In the CPP intervention, the caregiver's relationship with the therapist is considered central to the process of therapeutic change. Therefore, it is important to establish a therapeutic relationship that is framed as a collaborative endeavor between the caregiver and the therapist. This collaboration sets the tone for future therapeutic work, as the caregiver's active role in CPP is needed in order to achieve positive results. The therapeutic relationship is the basis for exploring the parent's history of caregiving and addressing past experiences of trauma, loss, or maltreatment that may exert negative influences on parenting. Because the intervention is not targeted toward an individual, but rather toward the *relationship* that exists between parent and child, CPP utilizes the corrective emotional experience in the context of the therapeutic relationship as a means to improve the parent–child attachment relationship. Within the supportive environment of therapy, sessions with the parent, child, and therapist gradually begin to alter the relationship between the parent and the child. In the course of parent–child interactions, opportunities occur to explore the parent's internal representational world as it relates to their perceptions of and responses to the child. Cultural sensitivity is essential for the success of this model because "intimate relationships are regulated by cultural mores, which dictate if, how, and when feelings can be displayed" (Lieberman & Van Horn, 2005, p. 38). Thus, understanding and exploring cultural factors with the family is essential to empathic and nurturing therapeutic services, and the model has been successfully applied with several different cultural groups.

TRANSLATIONAL RESEARCH

In order to develop and evaluate the efficacy and effectiveness of models of intervention, the importance of translational research has been increasingly highlighted. Translational research involves examining how basic behavioral and biological processes can inform the diagnosis, prevention, treatment, and delivery of services for individuals at risk for, or who have developed, a mental illness (National Advisory Mental Health Council on Behavioral Science Workshop, 2000). The era of translational research is affecting all fields of inquiry in the medical, physical, social, and clinical sciences (Gunnar & Cicchetti, 2009). The impetus to conduct translational research in the behavioral sciences emanated largely from the National Institute of Mental Health (Insel, 2005; Insel & Scolnick, 2006) and was spurred by recognition of the tremendous individual, social, and economic burden associated with mental illness (National Advisory Mental Health Council on Behavioral Science Workshop, 2000). Given the emphasis of developmental psychopathology on understanding the reciprocal interplay between basic and applied research, and between normal and atypical development (Cicchetti & Toth, 2006), the parameters of developmental psychopathology lend themselves to fostering translational research that has implications for society, policymakers, and individuals with mental disorders and their families.

Basic research on the negative effects of child maltreatment on attachment relationships (Cicchetti & Valentino, 2006) highlighted attachment as an important stage-salient issue requiring intervention. Given the relational focus of CPP and its attention to the influences of caregivers' past on their parenting, this modality was identified as an intervention model that could be provided to families where maltreatment had occurred. The efficacy findings from randomized controlled trials (RCTs) demonstrate that insecure attachment can be modified and as children move beyond infancy, interventions that specifically target the attachment relationship may be necessary.

RANDOMIZED CONTROLLED TRIALS OF CHILD–PARENT PSYCHOTHERAPY

CPP has been shown in evaluation studies to be effective in fostering attachment security in children with histories of maltreatment (Cicchetti et al., 2006). CPP has been evaluated with several populations, including Latina immigrant mothers (Lieberman, Ghosh Ippen, & Van Horn, 2006; Lieberman, Van Horn, & Ghosh Ippen, 2005), families involved with Child Protective Services (Cicchetti et al., 2006; Toth, Maughan, Manly, Spagnola, & Cicchetti, 2002), and low-income minority families (Cicchetti et al., 2006; Toth et al., 2002). Family risk characteristics have included domestic violence (Lieberman, Van Horn, & Ozer, 2005; Lieberman et al., 2006), maternal depression (Toth, Rogosch, Manly, & Cicchetti, 2006), and maltreatment (Cicchetti et al., 2006; Toth et al., 2002). To evaluate the most effective approach to improving relationship outcomes for families with reports of maltreatment identified by Child Protective Services, two approaches to intervention were compared. With the common goals of fostering infant attachment security in order to avert maladaptive development, two theoretically distinct intervention modalities were provided. One model, psychoeducational parenting intervention, utilized an ecological perspective and was based on models of maltreatment that highlight parental stress and parenting skills deficits as contributors to maltreatment. Therefore, in this model therapists strived to provide social support and developmentally appropriate parent training in order to reduce stress and social isolation, promote more positive parenting, and decrease child maltreatment. CPP was based on research that highlights the importance of parent–child attachment in fostering positive child development, improving parent–child interaction, and decreasing child maltreatment. CPP involved dyadic mother–infant therapy sessions designed to improve parent–child attachment relationships by modifying the influences of negative maternal representational models on parent–child interaction. Both models of treatment are discussed more fully elsewhere (see Cicchetti et al., 2006).

Interventions were initiated when infants were approximately 12 months old and continued for a period of 1 year. Of particular relevance for the outcome evaluation, assessments of the quality of attachment were conducted at baseline (12 months), at the conclusion of the intervention (24 months), and 1 year postintervention. Both the psychoeducational parenting intervention and CPP treatment conditions were found to be efficacious in fostering increased security of attachment in infants.

A second RCT was conducted with maltreated preschoolers. Again, both models of treatment were provided. A number of modifications to the CPP program were made to ensure that the intervention was developmentally appropriate for older children. While the attachment relationship remained the focus of intervention, developmental concerns related to negotiating goal-corrected partnerships characteristic of attachment relationships during the preschool developmental period were addressed.

In contrast to the benefits of both CPP and psychoeducational parenting intervention in fostering increased attachment security between infants and their mothers (Cicchetti et al., 2006), during the preschool years, only CPP improved children's representations of self and of caregiver (Toth, Cicchetti, Macfie, Maughan, & VanMeenen, 2000). These findings suggest that early in development attachment security may be improved even if an intervention does not target the mother–child relationship directly. However, as development proceeds, and as representational and self-system processes become more consolidated, an intervention designed specifically to address the attachment relational system may be necessary.

In order to demonstrate the principles of CPP, we next present a clinical case that exemplifies the positive outcomes that emerged from the RCTs.

CLINICAL ILLUSTRATION

Mary, a 21-year-old single mother, and her 33-month-old daughter, Jasmine, were referred for CPP services by their case manager through the Department of Human Services. Jasmine was in the care of her maternal aunt and had been in this out-of-home placement since she was 9 months of age. Jasmine had been exposed to her mother's drug activity and usage, as well as experiencing neglectful situations as an infant. On one occasion, police raided Mary's apartment and found explosives. At the point that the referral for services was generated, Mary decided that she was tired of the "drugs" and "running the streets," and she was motivated to work toward achieving her personal goals and having Jasmine returned to her care.

Mary grew up as the fifth of seven children living in a household with her biological mother and stepfather. She described her relationships with her siblings as typical, sometimes even "close-knit." Mary characterized her relationship with her stepfather as extremely tenuous. She depicted him as an alcoholic who was very abusive toward her mother. He was in and out of their home on numerous occasions. Mary highlighted that she was always extremely close to and protective of her mother. Mary claimed that she initially felt scared by the physical and verbal disputes between her mother and stepfather, but those feelings shifted to anger as she became older. Eventually, she began to immerse herself in her parents' fighting, with the intent of protecting her mother. Due to ongoing domestic violence circumstances and poor judgment executed by Mary's mother, who was diagnosed as developmentally delayed, Mary was placed in foster care.

According to Mary, she learned to function quite independently as a teenager. Whenever she needed or wanted something, she was typically told "no" by her parents. This seemed to compound the feelings of hurt and anger she already felt from the household domestic violence. Her first response was to cry, then to lash out. Mary turned to the streets and involvement with drug activity. She utilized drugs to try and combat her feelings, and became involved in selling drugs to have money to obtain material possessions. Involvement in the drug world also brought her a sense of connection and control. For a very long time, Mary was able to hide her addiction from those she loved. Following the birth of Jasmine and attempts to care for her as a single mother, in combination with working and attempting to complete high school, Mary became tremendously overwhelmed. She resorted to involvement with the drug culture, which compromised her ability to make safe decisions as a parent. Mary was incarcerated, and Jasmine was placed in the care of her aunt. Mary responded to her loss in a cyclical manner: drugs, incarceration, recovery, drugs, incarceration, recovery. She noted that there was a defining moment in jail where she felt "tired" of what was occurring in her life: "tired of doing drugs," "tired of running the streets," and "tired of feeling so much hurt and anger."

Based on reports from the referral source and an initial assessment period, whereby the intervening therapist observed the interactions between Mary and Jasmine, the attachment relationship between this mother and daughter dyad was best characterized as insecure–disorganized, with both ambivalent and avoidant features. Information regarding Jasmine's caregiving history, her unorganized responses to separations and reunions with her mother, and her exhibition of feelings of fear, confusion, and anxiety toward her mother informed this attachment relationship formulation. At the initiation of CPP at the age of 33 months, Jasmine had been in a relative's care for most of her life and had participated in supervised visitation with her mother since removal from her care. During visitations, Jasmine frequently "tested" her mother to see if she would follow through with what she said, or attempt to elicit a reaction from her mother. It was evident that her feelings of fear that her mother would leave her for a long period of time and not return for the next scheduled visitation incited difficulty in separating from her mother. Jasmine had formed a mental representation of her mother as an adult who was unable to protect her in dangerous situations, or to meet her needs and be present in a consistent, predictable, and nurturing manner. In turn, Mary appeared unsure of how to interact with, or react to, Jasmine. Mary was unable to formulate an organized and consistent response to her daughter. She was ineffectual and unable to respond to or console her daughter during times when she was emotionally distraught, and she would distance herself from Jasmine when she felt angry or frustrated. She held back on assuming a parental role with Jasmine at times because of her guilty feelings about losing the care of her daughter.

Regular weekly dyadic sessions were held at the center where CPP was offered because visitation in the home was not approved. Transportation was provided for both Mary and Jasmine in order to alleviate this potential barrier to participating in treatment. During the initial assessment period, which took place over 8 weeks, a strong therapeutic alliance was established with Mary. The therapist created a therapeutic context whereby Mary could feel free to engage in honest discussions around her feelings and concerns. In turn, on a few occasions, Mary questioned what she and her daughter were doing within the context of therapy. She wondered whether the therapist was judging her parental capacities and intentions, as others in her past had done. Based on her history, Mary had internalized those with whom she had relationships as judgmental and untrustworthy. Mary indicated emerging trust for the therapist by stating, "You're all right. I like you." The therapist encouraged Mary to discuss the prior relationships in her life and her expectations for others. The therapeutic alliance provided the foundation, offering Mary a corrective relationship experience with someone in whom she could trust, and who would tolerate her various expressions of emotion and her struggles with how to interact effectively with, and become a caregiver to, her daughter.

At the onset of treatment, Mary and the therapist established goals around enhancing the parent–child relationship, improving communication, and helping Mary to understand and support Jasmine's emotional needs. Within sessions, Mary and Jasmine were able to learn about one another as individuals and in their roles as parent and child. They had solely engaged one another for 2 years during visitation times, but they had not been able to spend longer periods of time with each other. Given their limited contact, they had not been afforded the opportunities to learn about each other's personality characteristics or likes and dislikes. Mary attempted to function in a parental role during their visitation, but Jasmine viewed her maternal aunt as the primary caregiver. This was evidenced by Jasmine frequently saying "no" and not observing the boundaries and limits her mother was trying to establish. Jasmine appeared wary or unengaged during their interactions. Mary also displayed some anger and disappointment when she heard her daughter refer to her maternal aunt as "Mom." The therapist created dialogue around these scenarios and feelings within the context of safe, supportive sessions, always being mindful of the emotional status of both Mary and Jasmine.

There were multiple ports of entry (Stern, 1995), or avenues, through which the therapist entered into the parent–child system to actuate change. Mary had identified Jasmine's emotional turmoil and confusion, and agreed that it was necessary to gain an awareness of her daughter's emotional needs and to learn ways to respond to Jasmine's expressions appropriately. One struggle was that Mary did not know what her daughter needed from her, so she required assistance in identifying ways to support Jasmine with nurturance, patience, understanding, and consistency. Another focus of therapy was to label a range of emotions to assist Jasmine in learning appropriately to express her needs verbally. Through support, encouragement, and unconditional positive regard, Mary built up confidence in her maternal role with Jasmine. Additionally, the therapist fostered Mary's and Jasmine's abilities to address and rework their internal working models based on previous experiences and relationship histories.

Throughout the course of intervention, Mary was able to participate in conversations around the trials, tribulations, and major influences from her childhood. Mary stated, "My mom did the best she could," but she did not feel that her physical or emotional needs were met as a child. She felt as if she functioned in a parentified role much of the time, protecting her mother from her stepfather, or from the verbal lashing-out of her other siblings. Mary had no one within her family system to provide guidance or set limits for her; no one to model a nurturing, supportive parental role. She had to create her own life pathway, including figuring out what it meant to function as a parent. Mary's internal working models of relationships were based on inconsistent and unreliable support, which was then filtered through anger and resentment. Not until several months into treatment, with the encouragement of the therapist, and through her own internal strength was Mary able critically to explore the relationship she had with her own mother, including what she felt she had deserved but not received as a child. The therapist also provided support for Mary around addressing the feelings emanating from her childhood and facilitated discussion around how this negative history adversely affected her parenting and her relationship with Jasmine.

Mary was able to access the support offered through her therapist within CPP to identify and discuss the myriad feelings she was experiencing, most significantly, anger and guilt. Her anger stemmed from the lack of guidance and nurturance during her childhood, her parentified role during childhood, and the subsequent domestic violence and addictive behaviors that permeated her life. Her guilt revolved around the decisions she made in Jasmine's first several months of life, eventually resulting in Jasmine's removal from Mary's care. Mary acknowledged wanting a different childhood for Jasmine but had been unable to disengage from the internal working models of her own childhood relationships. The therapist challenged her to conceptualize how she could provide an alternative experience for her daughter, based on her own recollections and what she had learned that Jasmine needed from her.

Mary and Jasmine vacillated between displaying warm, nurturing, predictable interactions to tenuous, antagonistic, inconsistent ones. Through commentary and gentle probing from the therapist around the more difficult interactions shared between the two, Mary was able to reflect on her responses to her daughter and the impact these types of interactions were having on them both, as well as their relationship. As time progressed, and responses to one another became more consistent, their ability to sustain more positive interactions grew. Mary and Jasmine began to develop a goal-corrected partnership whereby they mutually decided upon ways to negotiate uncomfortable or problematic situations that arose. As their time together increased outside the context of therapeutic sessions, Mary and Jasmine were able to utilize session time sharing their joy in being with one another more regularly, in addition to the challenges they experienced around negotiating the rules, boundaries, and roles of their family. Mary began to exude more patience and understanding about Jasmine's emotional expressions of anger, accepting that Jasmine needed to release her feelings before they could be addressed. It was apparent that Jasmine began to view her mother as a secure base, whereby her needs would be met on a regular basis, complemented by nurturing, supportive, predictable responses from Mary. Jasmine appeared ultimately to view her mother as a consistent support and source of security.

This case vignette illustrates the adverse effects of maltreatment on the developmental process and, specifically, the emergence of attachment insecurity. The demonstrated malleability of attachment through implementation of CPP during the early years of life highlights the importance of intervening so as to prevent a negative developmental cascade.

CONCLUSION AND FUTURE RECOMMENDATIONS

Findings on the negative developmental consequences of child maltreatment, in conjunction with research that has demonstrated the efficacy of a number of relational interventions (Chaffin et al., 2004; Cicchetti et al., 2006; Lyons-Ruth, Connell, Grunebaum, & Botein, 1990; Osofsky et al., 2007; Toth et al., 2002), offer a window of hope for children and caregivers who have been traumatized by negative parental pasts that intrude into current parenting contexts. Basic research on the effects of child maltreatment has been integral to informing the design and evaluation of intervention strategies (Toth et al., 2008). Unfortunately, despite the increased availability of evidence-based interventions, such models often are not provided in community and clinical settings. A number of impediments need to be addressed to disseminate more fully evidence-based models of treatment to populations most in need. First, academic researchers who develop and evaluate treatment models need to be committed to ensuring their dissemination. Because RCTs often are very circumscribed in minimizing potential confounds when participants are enrolled, some modifications are likely to be necessary when evidence-based models are exported into community contexts. Although it is critical that the core components of models be retained, and that fidelity to the model be monitored, flexibility also is needed to assure service providers that the intervention is feasible and likely to be effective in their nonacademic venues. Administrators in clinical settings also need to commit to making resources available, so that therapists can be trained on evidence-based models. Both monetary investments and time concessions will be necessary if new, efficacious therapeutic strategies are to be incorporated into community settings. It simply is not possible for therapists to learn new models if they do not receive caseload reductions and dedicated time for supervision of their work. When exporting efficacious models, cultural considerations also must be appreciated to ensure that interventions are likely to be effective with diverse ethnic and racial groups. Increasingly, evidence-based models of treatment have been evaluated with diverse populations, and it is important that this information be communicated to community members to increase their receptivity to adopting the intervention. The important issue of cultural sensitivity in implementing interventions and clinical treatment is elaborated by Ghosh Ippen and Lewis (Chapter 3, this volume). In order to realize fully the potential of breaking the cycle of maltreatment and violence through the provision of intervention, researchers, practitioners, and social policy advocates need to commit themselves to continuing to develop, evaluate, and translate effective interventions into real-world clinical and community contexts.

REFERENCES

Barnett, D., Ganiban, J., & Cicchetti, D. (1999). Maltreatment, negative expressivity, and the development of Type D attachments from 12- to 24-months of age. *Society for Research in Child Development Monograph, 64*, 97–118.

Brown, D. W., Anda, R. F., Tiemeier, H., Felitti, V. J., Edwards, V. J., Croft, J. B., et al. (2009). Adverse childhood experiences and the risk of premature mortality. *American Journal of Preventive Medicine 37*(5), 3749–3797.

Carlson, E. A., Sampson, M. C., & Sroufe, L. A. (2003). Implications of attachment theory and research for developmental–behavioral pediatrics. *Developmental and Behavioral Pediatrics, 24* (5), 364–379.

Chaffin, M., Silovsky, J., Funderbunk, B., Valle, L., Brestan, E., Balachova, T., et al. (2004). Parent–child interaction therapy with physically abusive parents: Efficacy for reducing future abuse reports. *Journal of Consulting and Clinical Psychology, 72*, 500–510.

Cicchetti, D. (1990). Perspectives on the interface between normal and atypical development. *Development and Psychopathology, 2*, 329–333.

Cicchetti, D. (1993). Developmental psychopathology: Reactions, reflections, projections. *Developmental Review, 13*, 471–502.

Cicchetti, D. (2002). The impact of social experience on neurobiological systems: Illustration from a constructivist view of child maltreatment. *Cognitive Development, 17*, 1407–1428.

Cicchetti, D. (2003). Neuroendocrine functioning in maltreated children. In D. Cicchetti & E. F. Walker (Eds.), *Neurodevelopmental mechanisms in psychopathology* (pp. 345–365). New York: Cambridge University Press.

Cicchetti, D., & Barnett, D. (1991). Attachment organization in pre-school-aged maltreated children. *Development and Psychopathology, 3*, 397–411.

Cicchetti, D., & Rogosch, F. A. (1997). The role of self-organization in the promotion of resilience in maltreated children. *Development and Psychopathology, 9*, 799–817.

Cicchetti, D., Rogosch, F. A., & Toth, S. L. (2006). Fostering secure attachment in maltreating families through preventive interventions. *Development and Psychopathology, 18*, 623–650.

Cicchetti, D., & Toth, S. L. (1992). The role of developmental theory in prevention and intervention. *Development and Psychopathology, 4*, 489–493.

Cicchetti, D., & Toth, S. L. (2006). Developmental psychopathology and preventive intervention. In A. Renninger & I. Sigel (Eds.), *Handbook of child psychology* (6th ed., pp. 497–547). New York: Wiley.

Cicchetti, D., & Toth, S. L. (2009). The past achievements and future promises of developmental psychopathology: The coming of age of a discipline. *Journal of Child Psychology and Psychiatry, 50,* 16–25.

Cicchetti, D., & Tucker, D. (1994). Development and self-regulatory structures of the mind. *Development and Psychopathology, 6,* 533–549.

Cicchetti, D., & Valentino, K. (2006). An ecological transactional perspective on child maltreatment: Failure of the average expectable environment and its influence upon child development. In D. Cicchetti & D. J. Cohen (Eds.), *Developmental psychopathology: Vol. 3. Risk, disorder, and adaptation* (2nd ed., pp. 129–201). New York: Wiley.

Corso, P., Edwards, V., Fang, X., & Mercy, J. (2008) Health-related quality of life in adults who experienced maltreatment during childhood. *American Journal of Public Health, 98*(6), 1094–1100.

Crittenden, P. M., Partridge, M. F., & Claussen, A. H. (1991). Family patterns of relationship in normative and dysfunctional families. *Development and Psychopathology, 3,* 491–512.

Dozier, M., Levine, S., Stovall, K., & Eldreth, D. (2001). *Atypical diurnal rhythms of cortisol production: Understanding foster children's neuroendocrine regulation.* Unpublished manuscript, University of Delaware.

Duggal, S., Carlson, E. A., Sroufe, L. A., & Egeland, B. (2001). Depressive symptomatology in childhood and adolescence. *Developmental Psychopathology, 13,* 143–164.

Egeland, B., & Erickson, M. (2004). Lessons from STEEP: Linking theory, research, and practice on the well-being of infants and parents. In A. J. Sameroff, S. C. McDonough, & K. L. Rosenblum (Eds.), *Treating parent–infant relationship problems* (pp. 213–242). New York: Guilford Press.

Feldman, S., & Downey, G. (1994). Rejection sensitivity as a mediator of the impact of childhood exposure to family violence in adult attachment behavior. *Development and Psychopathology, 6,* 231–247.

Fisher, P. A., Stoolmiller, M., Gunnar, M. R., & Burraston, B. O. (2007). Effects of a therapeutic intervention for foster preschoolers on diurnal cortisol activity. *Psychoneuroendocrinology, 32*(8–10), 892–905.

Gunnar, M. R., & Cicchetti, D. (2009). Meeting the challenge of translational research in child psychology. In M. R. Gunnar & D. Cicchetti (Eds.), *Meeting the challenge of translational research in child psychology: Minnesota Symposia on Child Psychology* (Vol. 35, pp. 1–27). New York: Wiley.

Hamre, B. K., & Pianta, R. C. (2001). Early teacher–child relationships and the trajectory of children's school outcomes through eighth grade. *Child Development, 72,* 625–638.

Howes, P. W., & Cicchetti, D. (1993). A family/relational perspective on maltreating families: Parallel processes across systems and social policy implications. In D. Cicchetti & S. L. Toth (Eds.), *Child abuse, child development, and social policy* (pp. 249–300). Norwood, NJ: Ablex.

Insel, T. R. (2005). Developmental psychobiology for public health: A bridge for translational research. *Developmental Psychobiology, 47,* 209–216.

Insel, T. R., & Scholnick, E. M. (2006). Cure therapeutics and strategic prevention: Raising the bar for mental health research. *Molecular Psychiatry, 11,* 11–17.

Lieberman, A. F., Ghosh Ippen, C., & Van Horn, P. (2006). Child–parent psychotherapy: Six-month follow-up of a randomized control trial. *Journal of the American Academy of Child and Adolescent Psychiatry, 45,* 913–918.

Lieberman, A. F., Weston, D. R., & Pawl, J. H. (1991). Preventive intervention and outcome with anxiously attached dyads. *Child Development, 62,* 199–209.

Lieberman, A. F., & Van Horn, P. (2005). *"Don't hit my mommy!": A manual for child–parent pscyhotherapy with young witnesses of family violence.* Washington DC: Zero to Three Press.

Lieberman, A. F., & Van Horn, P. (2008). *Psychotherapy with infants and young children: Repairing the effects of stress and trauma on early attachment.* New York: Guilford Press.

Lieberman, A. F., Van Horn, P., & Ghosh Ippen, C. (2005). Toward evidence-based treatment: Child–parent psychotherapy with preschoolers exposed to marital violence. *Journal of the American Academy of Child and Adolescent Psychiatry, 44,* 1241–1248.

Lieberman, A. F., van Horn, P., & Ozer, E. (2005). Preschooler witnesses of marital violence: Predictors and mediators of child behavior problems. *Development and Psychopathology, 17*(2), 385–396.

Lieberman, A. F., Padrón, E., Van Horn, P., & Harris, W. W. (2005). Angels in the nursery: The intergenerational transmission of benevolent parental influences. *Infant Mental Health Journal, 26,* 504–520.

Lyons-Ruth, K., Bronfman, E., & Parsons, E. (1999). Maternal frightened, frightening, or atypical behavior and disorganized infant attachment patterns. *Monographs of the Society for Research in Child Development, 64*(3), 67–96.

Lyons-Ruth, K., Connell, D. B., Gruenbaum, H. U., & Botein, S. (1990). Infants at social risk: Maternal depression and family support services as mediators of infant development and security of attachment. *Child Development, 61,* 85–98.

Lyons-Ruth, K., & Easterbrooks, A. (1995). Attachment relationships among children with aggressive behavior problems: The role of disorganized/controlling early attachment strategies. *Journal of Consulting and Clinical Psychology, 64,* 64–73.

Masten, A. S. (2001). Ordinary magic: Resilience processes in development. *American Psychologist, 56,* 227–238.

Main, M. (1999). Epilogue: Attachment theory. In J. Cassidy & P. R. Shaver (Eds.), *Handbook of attachment: Theory, research, and clinical applications* (pp. 845–888). New York: Guilford Press.

Main, M., & Goldwyn, R. (1984). Predicting rejecting of her infant from mother's representation of her own experience: Implications for the abused-abusing intergenerational cycle. *Child Abuse and Neglect, 8,* 203–217.

Main, M., & Hesse, P. (1990). Parents' unresolved traumatic experiences are related to infant disorganized attachment status: Is frightened and/or frightening parent behavior the linking mechanism? In M. Greenberg, D. Cicchetti, & E. M. Cummings (Eds.), *Attachment in the preschool years: Theory, research and intervention* (pp. 161–182). Chicago: University of Chicago Press.

National Advisory Mental Health Council on Behavioral Science Workshop. (2000).

Translating behavioral science into action: Report of the National Advisory Mental Health Counsel Behavioral Science Group (NIH Publication No. 00-4699). Bethesda, MD: National Institute of Mental Health.

Ogawa, J. R., Sroufe, L. A., Weinfield, N. S., Carlson, E. A., & Egeland, B. (1997). Development and the fragmented self: A longitudinal study of dissociative symptomatology in a normative sample. *Development and Psychopathology, 9,* 855–879.

Osofsky, J. D., Kronenberg, M., Hammer, J. H., Lederman, J. C., Katz, L., Adams, S., et al. (2007). The development and evaluation of the intervention model for the Florida Infant Mental Health Pilot Program. *Infant Mental Health Journal, 28,* 259–280.

Sroufe, L. A. (2005). Attachment and development: A prospective, longitudinal study from birth to adulthood. *Attachment and Human Development, 7*(4), 349–367.

Sroufe, L. A., & Rutter, M. (1984). The domain of developmental psychopathology. *Child Development, 55,* 17–29.

Sroufe, L. A., Egeland, B., Carlson, E., & Collins, W. A. (2005). *The development of the person: The Minnesota Study of Risk and Adaptation from Birth to Adulthood.* New York: Guilford Press.

Stern, D. N. (1995). *The motherhood constellation: A unified view of parent–infant psychotherapy.* New York: Basic Books.

Tarullo, A. R., & Gunnar, M. R. (2006). Child maltreatment and the developing HPA axis. *Hormones and Behavior, 50,* 632–639.

Toth, S. L., & Cicchetti, D. (1996). Patterns of relatedness and depressive symptomatology in maltreated children. *Journal of Consulting and Clinical Psychology, 64,* 32–41.

Toth, S. L., Cicchetti, D., Macfie, J., Maughan, A., & VanMeenen, K. (2000). Narrative representations of caregivers and self in maltreated preschoolers. *Attachment and Human Development, 2,* 271–305.

Toth, S. L., Cicchetti, D., Macfie, J., Rogosch, F. A., & Maughan, A. (2000). Narrative representations of moral-affiliative and conflictual themes and behavioral problems in maltreated preschoolers. *Journal of Clinical Child Psychology, 29,* 307–318.

Toth, S. L., Manly, J. T., & Nilsen, W. J. (2008). From research to practice: Lessons learned. *Journal of Applied Developmental Psychology, 29,* 317–325.

Toth, S. L., Maughan, A., Manly, J. T., Spagnola, M., & Cicchetti, D. (2002). The relative efficacy of two interventions in altering maltreated preschool children's representational models: Implications for attachment theory. *Development and Psychopathology, 14,* 777–808.

Toth, S., Rogosch, F., Manly, J., & Cicchetti, D. (2006). The efficacy of toddler–parent psychotherapy to reorganize attachment in the young offspring of mothers with major depressive disorder. *Journal of Consulting and Clinical Psychology, 74,* 1006–1016.

van IJzendoorn, M. H., Schuengel, C., & Bakersman-Kranenburg, M. J. (1999). Disorganized attachment in early childhood: Meta-analyses of precursors concomitants, and sequelae. *Development and Psychopathology, 11,* 225–249.

Van Voorhees, E., & Scarpa, A. (2004). The effects of child maltreatment on the hypothalamic–pituitary–adrenal axis. *Trauma, Violence, and Abuse, 5*(4), 333–352.

Werner, H., & Kaplan, B. (1963). *Symbol formation.* New York: Wiley.

CHAPTER 7

■ ■ ■ ■

The Importance of Relationship-Based Evaluations for Traumatized Young Children and Their Caregivers

Amy Dickson
Mindy Kronenberg

The course of a young child's development can be understood best in the context of the child's relationship with a caregiver. John Bowlby, the father of attachment theory, stated that healthy infant development is associated with a consistent relationship with an emotionally available caregiver (Bowlby, 1951, 1982). Infant mental health researchers and clinicians recognize that to optimize young children's development, it is crucial to support and build relationships with their caregivers. As Donald Winnicott, a pediatrician and psychoanalyst, stated, "There is no such thing as a baby" (1964, p. 88), meaning that young children cannot grow and develop on their own; but rather, they thrive in the context of a relationship with a sensitive caregiver.

Given the importance of the caregiver's sensitivity and emotional stability for a young child's development, factors that impact the caregiver's ability to be emotionally present and responsive to the child, or those that affect the child's ability to trust the caregiver, are especially important when assessing a child's functioning. Thus, the experience of trauma, which by definition is associated with actual or threatened physical or psychological harm to the child or another individual (Zero to Three, 2005), as well as feelings of fear and helplessness in the adult caregiver (American Psychiatric Association, 2000), is especially important to consider in order to understand a caregiver–child relationship. A caregiver's ability to help a child cope with trauma is inextricably tied to the caregiver's own trauma history (Lieberman, Padrón, Van Horn, & Harris, 2005). Caregivers who have experienced trauma may feel decreased ability to provide protection for a child. Children who have experienced trauma may feel that adults will not be able to protect them. When both a caregiver and a child have experienced trauma, such as living in a violent environment, they may remind each other of the trauma, so that neither feels safe in the other's presence. Each of these situations places the caregiver–child relationship at risk for disruption, thereby increasing the likelihood that the child's developmental trajectory will be negatively impacted.

Related to evaluation, both attachment theory (Bowlby, 1982; Cassidy & Shaver, 2008; Sroufe, 2005) and trauma research (Lieberman & Knorr, 2007; Osofsky, 1995; Osofsky & Osofsky 2010; Streek-Fischer & van der Kolk, 2000) indicate that a young child's functioning should include an assessment of the child within the context of their primary attachment relationship (Miron, Lewis, & Zeanah, 2009). However, many clinicians continue to assess a young child as they would assess older children or adults, utilizing parent report scales, measures of cognitive development, a brief interview of the young child, or observation of the individual child's play. Current clinical practice guidelines promote evaluations that include both parent and child in order to provide a comprehensive picture of the young child's functioning (American Academy of Child and Adolescent Psychiatry, 2010).

This chapter describes how to conduct a relationship-based evaluation of young children that is consistent with current research and clinical practice in the field of infant mental health (Lieberman & Van Horn, 2008; Mares, Newman, & Warren, 2005; Zero to Three, 2005), and focuses on assessment specifically when the caregiver–child relationship has been impacted by trauma. The following example describes a family with a presenting issue that is commonly observed by clinicians who evaluate and treat children under the age of 5.

> Ms. D, the mother of three children, ages 4, 5, and 7, presented to the clinic with concerns about her 4-year-old son Chaz. She stated that he fights everybody and everything, and that he has been expelled from several day care centers and preschools throughout his young life. She said that Chaz behaves for her, but only her, and that none of her few trusted family or friends will take care of him. Thus, Ms. D does not have time to address her own medical needs, which recently have caused her more physical pain and impaired her mobility. As Ms. D spoke to the clinician, she said she felt exhausted. She said it is difficult being a

single mother and that while the children's father lives in the city, he sees the children inconsistently and only intermittently provides financial support. Unfortunately, he often disappoints the children by promising things and then disappearing. Furthermore, Ms. D reported that her family is not supportive and often relies on her for help with their needs. She said that while she understands many of her son's issues, this understanding does not make it any easier for her to care for him. Chaz often does not sleep through the night, and Ms. D worries that Chaz will hurt himself when he is awake and unsupervised while she is asleep. Ms. D reported that Chaz's behavior is affecting her ability to provide financially for her children because she has trouble maintaining employment since nobody is able to watch her son while she works. She stated that several doctors have described Chaz's behaviors as psychotic and wanted to prescribe numerous medications. However, Ms. D did not feel comfortable with her young son taking these medications and sought a psychological evaluation to find other ways of addressing Chaz's behaviors.

How does a clinician conduct an assessment that provides insight into Chaz's social and emotional functioning, and leads to recommendations to address his disruptive behaviors? In a traditional psychological assessment, the clinician would interview Ms. D and obtain data through parent report and/or psychological tests. However, this type of assessment would not necessarily lead to the fullest understanding of Chaz's behavior. Including observations of the child and caregiver provides information about the relationship and Chaz's ability to use his caregiver to regulate his emotions and behavior. When clinicians are not familiar with the intricacies of relationship-based assessment, they can make the mistake of assuming that assessment of the child and/or parent individually is sufficient to understand how the dyad interacts, or how the child relates to others.

Many young children who are brought to the attention of mental health providers have experienced trauma, even though this may not be the reason for referral. It is always important for clinicians to assess for a trauma history in their clinical intake. The inclusion of a relationship-based evaluation consists of a caregiver interview regarding the background of both caregiver and child, the caregiver's perception of the child, and observations of the caregiver and child together.

EVALUATION MEASURES

Caregiver Interview

Background Interview

A relationship-based assessment of a young child and a caregiver should begin with a comprehensive background interview with the caregiver alone, so that a child with sufficient receptive language capacities is protected from overhearing information that is not developmentally appropriate. During the interview, it is important to obtain information regarding all of the child's primary caregivers. Information about the biological parents' physical and mental health helps the clinician ascertain whether the child's behavior problems are associated with biological factors. However, a clinician who conducts relationship-based assessments recognizes that the caregiver's history and present circumstances impact the caregiver–child relationship, as well as the individual child's functioning. As Selma Fraiberg and colleagues (Fraiberg, Adelson, & Shapiro, 1975) poignantly described, "ghosts," or negative and frightening experiences from the caregiver's childhood, may impact how a caregiver interacts with a child and perceives the child's behaviors. Lieberman and colleagues (2005) emphasized that in addition to asking about a caregiver's history of abuse, neglect, and trauma, it is also important to inquire about the "angels," or positive influences, from the caregiver's past. This information is helpful in working with parents because remembering these experiences may help them protect their child in times of trauma and stress.

Obtaining a trauma history should be part of the interview, or the clinician may utilize a standardized measure, such as the Life Stressors Index—Revised (Wolfe, Kimerling, Brown, Chrestman, & Levin, 1996). While some clinicians may feel that it is intrusive to ask about the caregiver's history, many caregivers report appreciation that a professional values their experiences enough to ask questions about their life history. Most individuals do not spontaneously offer personal information during an interview; however, they generally answer in an honest manner if they are asked direct questions in a nonjudgmental fashion. Thus, it is important that the clinician feel comfortable asking personal questions as part of a routine evaluation and not skip questions on the assumption that they will not be applicable. If asked how the caregiver's history is relevant to the child's behavior, this is an opportunity for the clinician to explain to caregivers that many things impact their young child's functioning, and that by learning more about the child's environment the clinician is better able to address the child's behaviors.

A full trauma history for the child should be obtained during the interview. The clinician can use a measure such as the Trauma Events Screening Inventory—Parent Report Revised (Ghosh Ippen et al., 2002). Questions regarding children's behaviors or trauma symptoms may be obtained during the interview or by using a formalized measure, such as the Trauma Symptom Checklist for Young Children (TSCYC; Briere, 2005). Given that many symptom checklists do not cover the full age range (e.g., the TSCYC is not standardized for children under 36 months of age), many clinicians find informal interview and observations of caregiver and child to be sufficient and do not routinely use standardized paper-and-pencil measures. It is important to note that asking a caregiver about the "trauma" the child has witnessed is likely to result in little information regardless of the educational level of the caregiver. Many caregivers do not equate the frightening experiences in their lives or those of their children as traumas. Thus, a caregiver may deny that the child has experienced trauma but later describe traumatic events, such as the child witnessing the murder of a family member. To obtain accurate information, it is important to ask caregivers specific questions, such as "Has anyone close to your family died in the last few years?" or "Has your child ever seen or heard anything so frightening that he had trouble sleeping, didn't want to leave your side, or showed you that he was very upset?"

It is also essential to achieve an understanding of the context within which the family lives by obtaining information on the family dynamics and family support system, including how in-home and extended family members relate. Information regarding the caregiver's use of community or cultural resources, such as community services and religious involvement, helps the clinician identify sources of strength for the family. Similarly, learning how the family is affected by issues such as poverty, housing stability, access to transportation, community violence, or discrimination helps the clinician understand the barriers the family faces and how the caregiver's and the child's environment impacts their relational functioning. Sensitivity to cultural issues is crucial in building a trusting relationship with caregivers (see Ghosh Ippen & Lewis, Chapter 3, this volume).

Working Model of the Child Interview

The Working Model of the Child Interview (WMCI; Zeanah & Benoit, 1995), a clinically relevant tool that may be used as a supplement to the background interview, has been used for research purposes with children and caregivers who have experienced trauma (Schechter et al., 2005). The WMCI, a semi-structured interview, includes a series of questions and probes that promote a discussion of the caregiver's perception of his or her child. The clinician begins by asking about the caregiver's experiences and thoughts about the child during pregnancy and ends by asking the caregiver to predict what the child will be like as a teenager and as an adult. WMCI questions focus on how the caregiver views the child's personality and behavior, and are geared toward understanding the relationship from the caregiver's perspective. The WMCI may uncover the fact that trauma has impacted the caregiver–child relationship, giving the caregiver an opportunity to discuss his or her perception of the child prior to and after the traumatic event. As the interview is conducted in a relaxed, conversational tone, the caregiver may feel more comfortable sharing stories and anecdotes that help the clinician understand any projections or attributions the caregiver places on the child.

The WMCI is conducted with one caregiver at a time, and the interview focuses on one child at a time. No judgments are made until the entire interview is completed and the overall representations are assessed. It is helpful when caregivers provide consent for the interview to be videotaped, so that it may be reviewed by the clinician. In watching the interview, the clinician can focus on the interviewee's behaviors, body posture, affect, and general demeanor when discussing his or her child. A caregiver whose family or children have experienced a trauma often presents in an altered fashion and may demonstrate incongruent affect, blank stares, trouble remembering information, and emotional dysregulation. For this reason, it is helpful to complete this interview at the beginning of treatment; however, it may be repeated when the caregiver has stabilized. More clinical information is provided if more than one caregiver is interviewed about the child, enabling the clinician to compare and contrast the caregivers' perceptions of the same child. This interview can be coded by those who have been trained to produce one of three classifications: balanced, disengaged, and distorted (Zeanah, Benoit, Barton, & Hirschberg, 1996).

When there has been a trauma, balanced caregivers can discuss how both they and their child have been impacted, and how they supported their child during difficult times. If the caregivers were somehow involved in the trauma, either as a perpetrator or as an adult unable to provide protection, they recognize this and take responsibility. These caregivers do not dramatize or minimize the impact of the trauma on the family. In a disengaged interview, caregivers do not seem to be emotionally connected to the child they are discussing. As expected, these caregivers place little importance on how a trauma may have impacted their child or their role in helping the child cope with trauma. For example, one caregiver whose interview was characterized as disengaged, sat on a couch with her hands in odd positions throughout the interview. The caregiver frequently placed her hands behind her back or over her head. It was only when the blanket on her lap suddenly stirred that the clinician realized the infant was on her lap because she never referenced or touched this child throughout the interview. A distorted interview is often characterized by caregivers' projection or attribution of their own fears, desires, and needs on the child. For example, one mother whose 6-week-old infant reached out in a loving manner to touch her face while she fed him, angrily asked whether the clinician had seen the infant hit her, and went on to state that he would grow up to be violent like his father. These caregivers express little or no recognition of the impact of their behavior on the child and, instead, focus on how the child meets, or does not meet, their needs.

After the first appointment at the clinic during which relevant background information was obtained, Ms. D was asked to return for an appointment without her son, in order to complete a WMCI, so that the clinician could gain a deeper understanding of how Ms. D perceived Chaz and understood his behaviors.

> When administered the WMCI, Ms. D revealed that she was very unhappy to be pregnant with Chaz so soon after the birth of her second child. She felt she could not abort the pregnancy, but she engaged in numerous behaviors in the hope that she would miscarry. For example, she threw herself down the stairs and ingested a variety of different medications. Despite her attempts, Ms. D delivered a premature but healthy infant and had no other birth complications. Ms. D admitted to having postpartum depression during the first few months of Chaz's life; however, she also stated that she had mixed feelings and was happy he survived. She believed that Chaz was a beautiful child, but she also felt very alone with no support.
>
> As the interview progressed, the clinician learned that Chaz was an active, temperamental baby who demanded attention from his mother from infancy. Ms. D also reported that when her son was 1 year of age, an unknown woman burst into their home and attacked her with a knife. All of Ms. D's children witnessed this incident. Her 4-year-old daughter called the police while her 2-year-old son hid, and she held Chaz. When the woman lunged at and eventually stabbed her, Ms. D swung Chaz away in an attempt to protect him, and he landed across the room. When the woman was chased out and the police arrived, Ms. D thought Chaz was dead as he lay motionless on the floor. It is unclear whether he was unconscious or in shock; fortunately, he was not seriously physically injured and survived intact. Ms. D was operated on for her injuries and returned home from the hospital after 1 week. It never occurred to Ms. D that Chaz's behaviors might in any way be connected to this incident, although she began to reflect on this during her interview. She also expressed her reality-based fears of what would happen to her son if his out-of-control behavior did not change, since she was living in a city with a high crime rate, in which male adolescents were continually exposed to violence. Ms. D voiced frustrations and fears for her son, while also expressing love for him and hope for his positive future. She was able to see his strengths despite his many challenging behaviors.

In Ms. D's balanced interview, her conflict about her desire to have her son was revealed, as was the trauma they both had experienced. Ms. D was not fully aware of how this trauma had impacted her child. However, she provided a realistic description of Chaz's behavior, and demonstrated flexibility in accepting his positive and negative behaviors, as well as her simultaneous feelings of love and frustration. During the interview, the clinician does not follow-up with probes about specific incidents, as these questions would derail the caregiver's focus on the child and their relationship. However, the skilled clinician makes note of questions in order to follow-up after the interview has ended.

While it is always important to understand how the caregiver perceives the child, the caregiver report can never replace the clinician's observation of a child during an assessment. If the WMCI is included, it is often clinically interesting to complete the interview before observing the caregiver–child relationship. In this way, the clinician can note whether his or her mental picture of the child and the caregiver–child relationship based on caregiver report is representative of the observational assessment.

Parent/Caregiver–Child Observational Assessment

Observation is one of the most valuable tools for the clinician in determining the quality of a relationship, and an observational component is essential for any comprehensive relationship-based evaluation. Furthermore, in order to obtain an accurate representation of how a child relates to caregivers, it is important that the clinician consider the person-specific nature of interpersonal relationships. Thus, a child may have vastly different ways of interacting with different individuals, and to evaluate fully the child's relationships with multiple caregivers, it is necessary to observe the child with each primary caregiver.

Modified Parent–Child Relationship Assessment

The Modified Parent–Child Relationship Assessment (MPCRA) was developed as an observational measure to research caregiver–child interactions in preschool-age children (Crowell & Feldman, 1988; Crowell & Fleischman, 1993) and is accompanied by a coding system to score the caregiver–child interaction (Crowell, Feldman, & Ginsberg, 1988). The Crowell assessment was originally developed for children between the ages of 2 and 4½ years of age and has been adapted by other clinicians (Osofsky et al., 2007) for use with a broader age range of young children. It has been used with children as young as 6 months, who are able to sit independently, and as old as 5 years.

The Crowell assessment includes free play and structured tasks, as well as a brief separation and reunion. Given that both caregiver and child responses are coded across situations, this relationship-based assessment provides a comprehensive evaluation of the range of behaviors seen in the caregiver–child dyad. The adapted versions of the original Crowell coding system are acceptable to use in clinical practice (Miron et al., 2009). The following description of the MPCRA is based on the adaptation by Amy Dickson, which has been used for both clinical and research purposes. It is utilized in any relationship-based assessment for a child who is under age 6.

ADMINISTRATION

When the MPCRA is used for clinical, forensic, or research purposes, it is important to receive training to administer the assessment in a standardized manner. The following guidelines describe the administration of MPCRA and ensure that the assessment results are a valid representation of caregiver–child relationship functioning.

Setting Up the Room. The environment in which the MPCRA is conducted may impact the manner in which the caregiver and child interact; thus, standardization is encouraged. Ideally, two rooms with a one-way mirror or videotaping equipment are set up, so that the clinician may observe the assessment as it is occurring. The room must be baby-proofed, with all windows locked, outlets covered, and large furniture stabilized. Ideally, the room should be free of distractions, such as extraneous toys or wall art, and the parent should not bring bottles, pacifiers, or other objects that would help to soothe the child. For administration, it is important to have either a cabinet that locks or a container that holds toys, a child-size table and chairs, and a carpet or rug in the middle of the room. The table and carpet signal where the caregiver and child should sit, so that they remain in the view of the clinician. It is helpful to have a mirror or reflective surface on the wall opposite the one-way mirror to catch the caregiver's or child's reflections when they are not facing the camera or clinician.

When there is not an ideal room setup, the evaluation can still be completed with modifications. For example, when there is not a separate observation room, the clinician may hide behind a partition in the room and watch the interaction on videotape. If a partition is not available, the clinician may remain in the room but should indicate to the child and the caregiver that he or she will not be talking or interacting but simply videotaping. Ideally, the assessment should not be conducted in the family's home because that environment is often well out of the control of the clinician; however, if it is the only way to accomplish the evaluation, the clinician should bring the toys to the home and ask that the assessment occur in a room with few other toys or distractions. Televisions and phones would need to be turned off, and other family members would need to be in separate rooms. When these modifications are made, it is important that the clinician note how his or her presence may have altered the behavior of the caregiver or child.

Materials. The MPCRA includes free play, transition, and task-oriented segments that require situation-specific toys. During free play, a large rubber bucket with handles works well to hold toys designed to evoke cooperative play and that are nontraumatic in nature. Free-play materials often include play food and a picnic basket, a soft ball, two telephones, trucks, a doctor's kit, baby dolls, and stuffed animals. Trained clinicians have learned not to include police materials, toy guns, and other toys that are often used in the treatment of young trauma survivors because the clinician is not in the room to assist the caregiver and child in coping with these possible trauma reminders. Furthermore, clinicians do not use well-known characters, such as Disney figures, in the free-play materials, since this may hamper the child's creativity or expression of personal thoughts and feelings.

During the transition from cleanup of free-play toys to structured tasks, blowing bubbles provides an opportunity for a calming, low-stress interaction between caregiver and child. Structured tasks are carefully selected, based on the child's developmental level rather than chronological age. The first two tasks should be at the child's developmental level, and the latter two tasks should be slightly above the child's developmental level, so that they require adult assistance. Table 7.1 is an example of a list of tasks by developmental level.

Preparing to Administer the MPCRA. When scheduling a relationship-based assessment, the clinician tries to schedule the appointment when the child is well rested. The parent is instructed to let the clinician know if the child is not feeling well on the day of the assessment, so that it can be rescheduled when the child is at his or her best. These parameters are followed to ensure that the evaluation provides the best assessment of the child and is not influenced by the child being overtired or overstimulated. When the clinician provides the MPCRA instructions to the parent, the caregiver and child should be separated so that the child is not aware of what is going to occur during the assessment; this is helpful given that a goal of the assessment is to observe how the child utilizes the caregiver to regulate and soothe in a novel environment. It is helpful if the caregiver brings a trusted adult to the evaluation so the second adult can care for child while the clinician instructs the caregiver about the assessment; if the caregiver cannot bring another adult, the clinician should enlist the aid of an assistant to play with the child while the clinician speaks with the caregiver. Prior to beginning the assessment, the clinician should attempt to ensure that the child is ready to begin an uninterrupted evaluation; thus, it is helpful if the child has been fed and has gone to the bathroom or had a diaper change. If the child soils his or her diaper or asks to use the bathroom in the middle of the evaluation, the caregiver is instructed to tend to the child's needs, then immediately reengage in the assessment. If this occurs during the separation portion of the assessment, the caregiver reenters the evaluation room with the child to resume play for a period of time before they separate.

Instructions to Parents. The caregiver is instructed to begin the evaluation by playing with the identified free-play toys with the child as they

TABLE 7.1. Developmentally Ordered, Modified Parent–Child Relationship Assessment Tasks

12 months
- Ball—roll back and forth
- Shape sorter (4 blocks without lid)
- Make a tower (3 soft blocks)
- Nesting cups with 2 cups
- Nesting cups with 3 cups
- Snap beads
- Musical ladybug—push button to play song
- Push-top spinner
- Push toy that will move when pushed down upon

19 months
- Simple wood puzzle with knobs on pieces
- Stacking cups
- Rock-a-stack rings
- Pop-up animals (4 step)
- Jack in the box
- Push-top spinner
- Push toy that will move when pressed upon

22 months
- Place Little People into slots on school bus
- Build a tower with 6 smaller blocks
- Nesting 5 cups
- Jack in the box
- Lego Cookie Monster (easiest version)
- Easy puzzle

31 months
- Shapes puzzle
- 6-piece puzzle
- Plastic shape sorter with lid (6 pieces)
- Colored balls to stack on colored pegs
- Stringing beads
- Match tiles to colored picture cards
- Simplified memory game (few cards)
- Barrel of Monkeys

37 months
- Lego Cookie Monster (small parts, preassembled)
- Stringing beads on a rope—replicate

a model (bead shapes include balls, squares, triangles)
- Animal nesting toy
- Puzzle where specific shapes have to fit into slots
- Spool necklace
- Balancing clown game
- Harder puzzle
- Lace/zip/buckle bear/doll

43 months
- Make a lunch
- Lacing cards
- String beads (3 each of balls, squares, triangles)
- Lego Cookie Monster
- Lace/zip/buckle bear/doll
- Balancing clown game
- Barrel of Monkeys (easy)

48 months
- Replicate a simple Lego design with matching blocks
- Lotto cards
- Harder puzzle—fitting pieces into slots
- Stacking clown
- 10-step stacking/nesting cups
- Build a tower with 10 small blocks
- Cootie game
- Assemble figure 8 train track to match picture
- String beads on a rope to replicate design
- Balancing clown game

60 months
- Replicate Lego structure of 10–15 pieces
- 25- to 30-piece jigsaw puzzle
- Assemble train set (easy task for this age)
- String beads to replicate model with a harder design
- Memory game
- Balancing clown game
- Language or math worksheets

normally would at home, until they hear the appointed signal (e.g., a knock or a sound from the phone) to move to the next segment. The caregiver is then instructed to have the child place the toys back in the container and to help the child as necessary. The caregiver is told that after the child cleans up, they should bring the toy container to the door, so that the clinician may inconspicuously remove the toys from the room. After the cleanup portion is complete, the caregiver is instructed to blow the bubbles and allow the child to pop them, until they are signaled again, at which point they are to engage in three to four ordered tasks. When giving instructions, the clinician should demonstrate each task for the caregiver, even if the task seems easy. The tasks should be labeled so that the caregiver is reminded of their order, and the caregiver is instructed to continue with the same task until the signal to change.

After the last task, the caregiver is instructed to place the toys used during the task segments on the floor so the child can play while the caregiver is out of the room. The caregiver is instructed to bring the bubbles and to leave the room as he or she would normally leave at home. Ideally, when the caregiver leaves the room, the child should not be able to open the door; this may be accomplished by using a child-proof door handle or having an assistant hold the door closed. During the separation, the caregiver joins the clinician behind the one-way mirror to observe the child. The separation generally lasts 3 minutes, even if the child shows signs of mild to moderate distress; however, if the child becomes extremely distressed and does not soothe, or if the clinician knows that separation is a trauma trigger for the child, the caregiver is sent back to the room in less than 3 minutes. For the reunion sequence, the clinician instructs the caregiver to knock on the door, say the child's name, and reenter the room. The time for this portion of the assessment varies because the clinician observes the interaction, ideally, until the child has fully calmed. If the child is not upset, the clinician allows a few minutes for caregiver and child to reengage in play before ending the evaluation. See Table 7.2 for a description of each segment.

Often caregivers have many questions about how to engage with the child during the assessment. Since a goal of the evaluation is to observe as typical an interaction as possible, the clinician deflects questions by stating, "Do what you would normally do if you were at home." It is appropriate for the clinician to provide reassurance, for example, by stating that the toys are cleaned regularly and that the room is baby-proofed. The caregiver is also assured that he or she may ask questions aloud and the clinician will respond.

MPCRA SEGMENT EVALUATION

The MPCRA may be coded using a research scale,[1] the Child–Caregiver Interaction Behavior Rating Scales (Katz, Lederman, & Osofsky, in press),

TABLE 7.2 MPCRA Segment Description

Segment	Time (approximate)	Description
Free play	10 minutes	• Unstructured portion of the assessment. • Utilizes toys designed to evoke cooperative, symbolic play. • Caregiver is instructed to play as they normally play at home.
Cleanup	Untimed	• Child cleans up the toys while the caregiver helps as much as necessary.
Bubble play	Up to 3 minutes	• Bubble play serves as a calming transition between the cleanup and task-oriented portions of the assessment.
Tasks 1 and 2	2–4 minutes	• At the child's developmental level.
Task 3	3–5 minutes	• Slightly above the child's developmental level.
Task 4	3–5 minutes	• Above the child's developmental level to induce some frustration.
Separation	3 minutes (or less)	• Child is alone in the room.
Reunion	Varies	• Caregiver returns and reunites with the child.

or simply to gather clinical information based on informal description and evaluation of adaptive and maladaptive interaction patterns.

When using the MPCRA to assess caregiver–child interaction, both are rated separately on each segment. While some dyads interact positively during free play, others become distressed and dysregulated when they do not have structure to guide their interaction, or vice versa. Aspects of both caregiver's and child's emotional and behavioral responses are observed. Variables include both caregiver's and child's affect (e.g., positive affect, withdrawal, depression, and irritability), caregiver's behaviors (e.g., ability to keep the child safe, ability to structure tasks, intrusiveness, praise, harsh or frightening behaviors), and child's behaviors (e.g., compliance, enthusiasm, and aggression). The following sections describe positive and negative reactions commonly seen among traumatized caregivers and children during each segment of the evaluation.

Free Play. The goal of free play is to allow the clinician to observe how the caregiver and child interact in an unstructured setting. Ideally, the caregiver will have a calm and bright tone of voice, be fully engaged with the child, play with the child in an age-appropriate manner, and follow the child's lead. Sensitive caregivers are observed to expand upon the child's play by noting the child's interest in a toy and using the toy in an age-appropriate manner. It is important to observe whether the child appears relaxed and interested when interacting with the caregiver or demonstrates fear of his or her caregiver. During this segment, it will be apparent whether the caregiver and child are used to playing together or whether they appear awkward in their play. Some caregivers taunt and tease children who are visibly protesting. The types of interactions that are observed during the evaluation likely mirror those that occur in the home. However, it is important that the evaluator remember that both the caregiver's and the child's behaviors are influenced by the artificial nature of the assessment.

When caregivers and children who have experienced trauma are observed, they may either reenact the trauma or avoid play themes that remind them of the traumatic situation. They may engage in traumatic play, which is characterized by repetitive and emotionally restricted or incongruent play regarding the event. Traumatized children may also have restricted affect, freeze during the play, be dysregulated (e.g., tantrums or shutting down during the play), or be hypervigilant (e.g., exaggerated startle responses to environmental stimuli). How the caregiver responds to the child's behaviors is significant when assessing the relationship. For example, some caregivers respond sensitively when the child displays fear of a particular toy, while others use the toy to heighten the child's anxiety.

Cleanup and Transitions. Transitioning between tasks may be particularly difficult for certain children. Those who have little time to play individually with their caregivers are most likely to resist cleaning up the toys because they would like to prolong the interaction. A skilled caregiver notes how the child is feeling and explains that there are more toys and play to come. In a stressed or insensitive caregiver, this may provoke harsh commands and/or consequences with the potential for a power struggle. Bubble play is included in the MPCRA to help calm an anxious child. The child who displays no enjoyment of the bubble play is of concern to the clinician, as this often indicates anxiety, depression, or fearfulness. This segment can also evoke a power struggle because older children may want to blow the bubbles.

Tasks. This segment represents a chance to observe whether the caregiver is aware of the child's capacities and limitations. The clinician notes whether the caregiver helps the child as necessary, while allowing the child to explore the task and succeed on his or her own. Evaluators observe the language the caregiver uses with the child, whether the caregiver is attentive and praises the child, and what conversation occurs during this segment. As the tasks become harder, the clinician observes how the caregiver anticipates and handles the child's frustrations.

Caregivers may display exceptional sensitivity to a child who has been traumatized; they may be even more patient because they understand that their child is struggling and becomes easily upset. Conversely, caregivers may become easily frustrated with their child, who may be visibly frightened and so anxious that they are unable to explore or engage in the tasks. When caregivers are anxious about being evaluated, they may rigidly insist that the child complete the tasks as instructed. Other caregivers appear disengaged when the child is completing the tasks and simply watch without comment or assistance.

Separation and Reunion. In assessing a caregiver–child relationship based on the separation and reunion segment, it is important that the clinician have a working knowledge of young children's developmentally appropriate reactions to separation. After entering focused attachment at approximately 7–9 months (Bowlby, 1982; Prior & Glaser, 2006), many normally developing infants become very upset at the absence of their caregiver; they often cry and move to the door. Older children who attend day care or school are used to the departure of their caregiver, and they may accept this absence with less visible distress. Often the level of distress is mediated by the caregiver's preparation prior to departure. Sensitive caregivers prepare children for their departure and often reassure them that they will return shortly. Some do not leave the room until the child has verbalized his or her understanding. However, less sensitive caregivers distract the child and leave the room without warning. Some tell their children to engage in an activity but do not explain that they are leaving or when they will return. This behavior may be due to the caregivers' own anxiety, their inability to cope with their child's negative affect, or their lack of knowledge regarding child development.

During the separation, sensitive caregivers display appropriate empathy for children's experience. If their child is upset, these caregivers are anxious to return to the room to give comfort. If their child is not distressed, these caregivers often enjoy the observation and may share positive stories about their child with the evaluator. Caregivers who have been negatively impacted by trauma may project their own anxiety onto the child and are anxious to return even when the child is playing adequately. Other caregivers do not appear to be interested in their child's response to the separation, or they laugh at the child's distress.

During the separation, children who have experienced the neglect of being left unattended or with a variety of unknown caregivers, without preparation and without explanation as to how long their primary caregiver will be away, may display heightened anxiety. These children respond acutely to being left alone, and they often react immediately to the absence of their caregiver with extreme distress, displayed by crying loudly and vehemently, running to the door and attempting to leave the room, calling out repeatedly for the caregiver, searching the room for the absent caregiver, or sitting frozenly. Other children appear unmoved by the separation. They may continue to play, though the observant clinician will note that the play is less enthusiastic and relaxed.

When the caregiver returns, some children need to be held, while others are content once the caregiver is in view and simply want the caregiver to sit close to them and reengage in their play. Sensitive caregivers continue to attend to their child until they are suitably calm. Other children display avoidant, ambivalent, or disorganized behaviors upon reunion. Children with avoidant attachment behaviors do not go to the caregiver for comfort or show that they are distressed. They ignore the caregiver when he or she returns and may display this by actively walking away, turning away when picked up, pushing to get down, or avoiding eye contact. Children with ambivalent attachment behaviors go to the caregivers for comfort but cannot use them adequately to soothe. These ambivalent children may tearfully approach the caregiver, then push away, only to return, then push away again while still crying or in distress. Of utmost concern is when the evaluator observes a disorganized response, such as a freezing or head banging. These behaviors are almost exclusively seen in children who have experienced severe abuse and/or neglect (Crittenden, 1992; Main, Hesse, & Kaplan, 2005; Prior & Glaser, 2006).

Caregivers' responses to their child upon reunion may also be impacted by their own experience of trauma. Some caregivers who have experienced trauma may not be able to respond to their child's needs. For example, a formerly emotionally available caregiver may be so distressed seeing the child's negative reaction to the separation that he or she reacts defensively by dismissing the child's emotions and need for comfort or becoming distressed him- or herself and overapologizing to the child. This is especially common if the child's negative response serves as a trauma trigger for the caregiver.

As an example of using description and evaluation on an MPCRA, we focus on the interaction between Ms. D and Chaz.

After Ms. D completed the WMCI, the clinician asked her to return to the office for additional evaluation involving a play interaction with Chaz. During this assessment, Chaz was observed to have age-appropriate motor and language skills, but he was also hyperactive and could not focus on the toys or tasks. He was also hypervigilant and easily startled by the noises he heard outside the windows. Since the clinic was in a large medical complex with three hospitals in close proximity, the frequent sounds of sirens increased Chaz's activity level and anxiety. Ms. D attempted to engage Chaz in play, but her son could not sustain a play theme due to his behavioral and emotional dysregulation. Ms. D initially spoke kindly to Chaz and allowed him to choose the toys; however, she became increasingly frustrated with him and did not know what to do. Her frustration turned to anger, and she became harsh with him. In turn, Chaz was distraught when Ms. D abruptly left the room for the planned separation without preparing him. He yanked on the door, cried for her, and looked lost and scared. When she returned, she was angry at him for his response and for his prior behavior. She did not comfort him; rather, she cleaned up the toys in the room and lectured him on his behavior. He remained unsettled, anxious, and was not able to listen to her.

The MPCRA observation and evaluation revealed that Ms. D had some positive parenting skills, as revealed by her attempts to engage her son despite his hyperactive behavior. The clinician also noted Chaz's strengths in motor and language development. However, the clinician witnessed how Chaz became dysregulated by his environment, upset by the loud sounds of sirens, and how his mother misread his anxiety and reacted harshly toward him as if he were being willfully disobedient. It became apparent that Ms. D could not understand Chaz's mental state and how he understood his world and hers. The observations obtained from this assessment provided additional information that was not revealed in the caregiver interviews, although Ms. D attempted to respond to the clinician's questions in an open and honest manner. Through the MPCRA, the clinician gained clinical information that helped guide treatment planning so that treatment goals included helping Ms. D understand her own emotional responses to Chaz's behavior and to read Chaz's cues accurately and meet his needs.

Adaptations for Young Children: The Face-to-Face Still-Face Paradigm

If Chaz had been under the age of 1 and unable to sit independently, the Still-Face procedure (Mesman, van IJzendoorn, & Bakermans-Kranenburg, 2009; Tronick, 1998; Tronick, Als, Adamson, Wise, & Brazelton, 1978; Weinberg & Tronick, 1996) would have been utilized. The Still-Face paradigm assesses whether caregivers can read and sensitively respond to their infants' (up to 6 months of age) cues. During this procedure, young children are placed in their car seat with the handle locked backward so they are propped upright but the seat cannot rock. All pacifiers, bottles, and toys are removed. The children are loosely strapped in so they cannot slide out of the seat. The seat is placed on a table, and the caregiver is seated in front of his or her child. A mirror is placed behind the child, so the camera can catch both the infant's face and the mirror reflection of the caregiver's face. The same requirements as those in the MPCRA are utilized, in that this procedure is only done when the infant is well-rested, healthy, and not during naptime or if the infant has a dirty diaper. Caregivers are asked to interact with their children as they normally would for a period of 2 minutes. They are then asked to disengage from interaction and look at their child with an expressionless face for 2 minutes. In the final sequence of the procedure, the caregivers again interact with their child. Various researchers have lengthened the time up to 3 minutes and have limited the caregiver's ability to touch the child during the interaction (Miron et al., 2009); adaptations to the procedure allow the clinician to assess how both child and caregiver adapt during longer periods of emotional disengagement, and when the caregiver must find ways to soothe the child other than physical comfort.

Through this procedure, it is possible to learn more about the history of the caregiver–child relationship. If a caregiver historically is emotionally available to the child, it is expected that the child will protest when the caregiver disengages and is no longer emotionally available. In this situation, the child attempts to reengage the caregiver by increased movement, vocalization, and sustained eye contact, and is upset when the caregiver does not reengage. In contrast, a child who has been neglected will not view the caregiver's expressionless face as something different from usual interaction. Children who have been neglected or raised by depressed and emotionally unavailable caregivers express little to no distress during the "still face" portion of the procedure given that this is not an unusual occurrence for them. Children with positive relationships with their caregivers enjoy the face-to-face interaction. There is an ongoing and mutually enjoyable exchange during which the caregiver talks to the child, and the child responds by cooing or physical movement. These healthy dyads maintain eye-to-eye contact and reflect affect back to one another.

Caregivers whose interactions with their children are characterized by lack of sensitivity or synchronicity engage in behavior that is intrusive or disengaged from their children. The interaction lacks a sense of familiarity, comfort, enjoyment, and mutual engagement, and the caregivers may appear not to know how to engage in play with their children. For example, a caregiver who is not sensitive to his or her child's needs may attempt to engage the child in positive interaction by exaggerated facial expression, a loud tone of voice, and intrusion into the child's physical space. Although this caregiver is attempting to engage in a positive interaction, he or she is not able to read his child's cues and does not adjust the interaction style when the child turns away, conveying overstimulation and a need for a more sensitive interaction style. It is possible to tell when a child is not used to prolonged or positive interactions with his or her caregiver because such a child appears to be confused by the interaction. Some caregivers project their own feelings onto the child and complain loudly about the constraints of the assessment, stating that the child is distressed when the child exhibits no visible sign of distress. Traumatized babies may display more aversion toward their caregivers if he or she is a trauma trigger for them. Conversely, they may do well with the caregiver until the still-face portion, then become so distressed that they cannot regulate their emotions after the disruption.

CONCLUSION

When a clinician chooses to work with a young child exposed to trauma, there is often tremendous pressure to delve immediately into the presenting issue and help the family members resolve their anxiety, while addressing and resolving the child's symptomatic behavior. Clinicians who normally thoroughly assess a child and family before drawing conclusions and developing a suitable course of treatment may unconsciously deviate from this wise course of action and find themselves beginning treatment without having conducted a comprehensive assessment due to the pressure to help the family in the midst of crisis. The role of a skilled clinician is to allow family members to express their anxiety fully, attempt to contain that anxiety, and move forward to learn all they can about the child and their environment before starting a course of treatment. As noted, an essential component of an overall evaluation is observing and understanding the child's relationships with primary caregivers.

This chapter utilizes the following framework for comprehensive relationship-based assessments for young, traumatized children: (1) a clinical interview that includes information about the caregiver's and the child's trauma exposure; (2) the WMCI, which allows the clinician insight into how the caregiver perceives the child and the attributions that he or she places on the child's behavior; and (3) a relationship-based observation that provides insight into how the caregiver's and the child's feelings impact their relationship. An evaluation including all of these components allows the clinician the greatest understanding of traumatized young children in their environment. However, as discussed in the chapter, for some evaluations, modifications of the components may be required. Caregiver–child relationships provide a buffer and an opportunity to heal for many children exposed to trauma. Inadequate relationships need to be addressed therapeutically because they can impair the child's development and ability to progress following a trauma. This process of assessing the family by utilizing relationship-based measures is of great therapeutic value as the family begins to feel understood and heard. Caregivers often begin to make their own connections and gain an understanding of their child, and themselves in relation to the child, as they complete the assessment process. They begin to reflect on how the trauma has impacted the family and their support systems, and often begin to understand their child's behaviors in a more informed light. Clinicians will learn of family and child strengths to build on and areas of improvement that need to be addressed for the therapeutic work to be most effective.

NOTE

1. Specialized training is required for research coding for relationship-based assessment. To obtain more information regarding coding for research, contact the authors of this chapter.

REFERENCES

American Academy of Child and Adolescent Psychiatry. (2010). Practice parameter for the assessment and treatment of children and adolescents with posttraumatic stress disorder. *Journal of the American Academy of Child and Adolescent Psychiatry, 49,* 414–430.

American Psychiatric Association. (2000). *Diagnostic and statistical manual of mental disorders* (4th ed., text rev.). Washington, DC: Author.

Bowlby, J. (1951). Maternal care and mental health. *World Health Organization Monograph* (Serial No. 2), pp. 355–533.

Bowlby, J. (1982). *Attachment and loss: Vol. 1. Attachment* (2nd ed.). New York: Basic Books.

Briere, J. (2005). *Trauma Symptom Checklist for Young Children (TSCYC): Professional manual.* Odessa, FL: Psychological Assessment Resources.

Cassidy, J., & Shaver, P. R. (Eds.). (2008). *Handbook of attachment: Theory, research, and clinical applications* (2nd ed.). New York: Guilford Press.

Crittenden, P. M. (1992). Quality of attachment in the preschool years. *Development and Psychopathology, 4,* 209–241.

Crowell, J. A., & Feldman, S. S. (1988). Mothers' internal models of relationships and children's behavioral and developmental status: A study of mother–child interaction. *Child Development, 59,* 1273–1285.

Crowell, J. A., Feldman, S. S., & Ginsberg, N. (1988). Assessment of mother–child interaction in preschoolers with behavior problems. *Journal of the American Academy of Child and Adolescent Psychiatry, 27,* 303–311.

Crowell, J. A., & Fleischman, M. (1993). Use of structured research procedures in clinical assessment of infants. In C. H. Zeanah, Jr. (Ed.), *Handbook of infant mental health* (pp. 210–221). New York: Guilford Press.

Fraiberg, S., Adelson, E., & Shapiro, V. (1975). Ghosts in the nursery: A psychoanalytic approach to the problem of impaired infant–mother relationships. *Journal of the American Academy of Child Psychiatry, 14,* 387–421.

Ghosh Ippen, C., Ford, J., Racusin, R., Acker, M., Bosquet, M., Rogers, K., et al. (2002). *Traumatic Events Screening Inventory—Parent Report Revised.* San Francisco: University of California, San Francisco Early Trauma Network.

Hesse, E., & Main, M. (2006). Frightened, threatening, and dissociative parental behavior in low-risk samples: Description, discussion, and interpretations. *Development and Psychopathology, 18,* 309–343.

Katz, L. F., Lederman, C. S., & Osofsky, J. D. (in press). *Child-centered practices for the courtroom and community: A guide to working effectively with young children and their families in the child welfare system.* Baltimore: Brookes.

Lieberman, A. F., & Knorr, K. (2007). The impact of trauma: A developmental framework for infancy and early childhood. *Psychiatric Annals, 37,* 416–422.

Lieberman, A. F., Padrón, E., Van Horn, P., & Harris, W. W. (2005). Angels in the nursery: The intergenerational transmission of benevolent parental influences. *Infant Mental Health Journal, 26,* 504–520.

Lieberman, A. F., & Van Horn, P. (2008). *Psychotherapy with infants and young children: Repairing the effects of stress and trauma on early attachment.* New York: Guilford Press.

Main, M., Hesse, E., & Kaplan, N. (2005). Predictability of attachment behavior and representational processes at 1, 6, and 19 years of age. In K. E. Grossman, K. Grossman, & E. Waters (Eds.), *Attachment from infancy to adulthood: The major longitudinal studies* (pp. 245–304). New York: Guilford Press.

Mares, S., Newman, L., & Warren, B. (2005). *Clinical skills in infant mental health.* Camberwell, Australia: Acer Press.

Mesman, J., van IJzendoorn, M. H., & Bakermans-Kranenburg, M. J. (2009). The many faces of the Still-Face Paradigm: A review and meta-analysis. *Developmental Review, 29,* 120–162.

Miron, D., Lewis, M. L., & Zeanah, C. H., Jr. (2009). Clinical use of observational procedures in early childhood relationship assessment. In C. H. Zeanah, Jr. (Ed.), *Handbook of infant mental health* (3rd ed., pp. 252–265). New York: Guilford Press.

Osofsky, J. D. (1995). The effects of violence exposure on young children. *American Psychologist, 50,* 782–788.

Osofsky, J. D., Kronenberg, M., Hayes Hammer, J., Lederman, C., Katz, L., Adams, S., et al. (2007). The development and evaluation of the intervention model for the Florida Infant Mental Health Pilot Program. *Infant Mental Health Journal, 28,* 259–280.

Osofsky, J. D., & Osofsky, H. J. (2010). How to understand and help traumatized infants and families. In B. Lester & J. Sparrow (Eds.), *Nurturing children and their families: Building on the legacy of T. Berry Brazelton* (pp. 254–263). New York: Wiley.

Prior, V., & Glaser, D. (2006). *Understanding attachment and attachment disorders: Theory, evidence and practice.* London: Atheneum Press.

Schechter, D. S., Coots, T., Zeanah, C. H., Davies, M., Coates, S. W., Trabka, K. A., et al. (2005). Maternal mental representations of the child in an inner-city clinical sample: Violence-related posttraumatic stress and reflective functioning. *Attachment and Human Development, 7,* 313–331.

Sroufe, L. A. (2005). Attachment and development: A prospective, longitudinal study from birth to adulthood. *Attachment and Human Development, 7,* 349–367.

Streek-Fischer, A., & van der Kolk, B. A. (2000). Down will come baby, cradle and all: Diagnostic and therapeutic implications of chronic trauma on child development. *Australian and New Zealand Journal of Psychiatry, 34,* 903–918.

Tronick, E. Z. (1998). Dyadically expanded states of consciousness and the process of therapeutic change. *Infant Mental Health Journal, 19,* 290–299.

Tronick, E. Z., Als, H., Adamson, L., Wise, S., & Brazelton, T. B. (1978). The infant's response to entrapment between contradictory messages in face to face interaction. *Journal of the American Academy of Child Psychiatry, 17,* 1–13.

Weinberg, M. K., & Tronick, E. Z. (1996). Infant affective reactions to the resump-
tion of maternal interaction after the Still-Face. *Child Development, 67*, 905–
914.

Winnicott, D. W. (1964). *The child, the family, and the outside world.* London:
Penguin.

Wolfe, J., Kimerling, R., Brown, P. J., Chrestman, K. R., & Levin, K. (1996). Psy-
chometric review of the Life Stressor Checklist—Revised. In B. H. Stamm (Ed.),
Measurement of stress, trauma, and adaptation (pp. 198–201). Lutherville,
MD: Sidran Press.

Zeanah, C. H., & Benoit, D. (1995). Clinical applications of a caregiver perception
interview in infant mental health. *Child and Adolescent Psychiatric Clinics of
North America, 4*, 539–554.

Zeanah, C. H., Benoit, D., Barton, M. L., & Hirschberg, L. (1996). *Working Model
Interview of the Child coding manual.* Unpublished manuscript, Louisiana
State University.

Zero to Three. (2005). *Diagnostic Classification of Mental Health and Developmental Disorders of Infancy and Early Childhood, Revised (DC:0–3R).* Washington, DC: Zero to Three Press.

PART III

■ ■ ■ ■

YOUNG CHILDREN FROM MILITARY FAMILIES EXPOSED TO TRAUMA, INCLUDING THE STRESS OF DEPLOYMENT

INTRODUCTION TO PART III

This section of the book introduces a relatively new area of concern related to young children impacted by trauma, that is, stress for children in military families. Classic developmental concerns emerge in this work, particularly problems related to separation and loss; changes in structure and routines; and sudden demands for adjustments by families, caused by deployment and transfers and, of course, the significant effect of injuries, and death. With their commitment to service to their country, military families face changes for which they cannot plan. Furthermore, many military families do not feel comfortable discussing emotions; defenses against feelings are important in coping with the many unpredictable events in their lives. In this context, the three chapters provide different approaches and perspectives on ways to work with military families and some of the difficult situations that may arise. Stephen J. Cozza and Margaret M. Feerick from the Uniformed Services University of the Health Sciences Center present the very difficult issue of addressing the needs of families when a service member is injured in combat. Although little work has been done with young children whose parent experiences this trauma, they build on their extensive clinical knowledge in discussing the many ramifications for young children having a parent injured in combat. They emphasize that these vulnerable young children are likely to face unique and possibly greater challenges than older children, due

137

to their developmental immaturity. Their chapter represents an important perspective for future interventions, clinical work, and research in this area. The issue of deployment and the impact on young children needs much more attention in prevention and intervention strategies. Juliet M. Vogel, Jennifer M. Newman, and the late Sandra J. Kaplan describe their sensitive work with young children in the National Guard and Reserves during a family member's deployment and present a perspective on the challenges posed by deployment for young children and their home-front parents. They illustrate and bring to life their important interventions and clinical work by describing their work with a 4-year-old child and his family during the father's deployment. Dorinda Williams and Lynette Fraga, a Zero to Three team, have taken the lead in developing and implementing the program Coming Together Around Military Families (CTAMF) to work with military communities in raising awareness of the needs of young children in military families, and in supporting professionals, parents, and caregivers in building resilience. CTAMF represents a community-based response to the many changing needs of young children whose parents or caregivers are impacted by deployments, injuries, and trauma resulting from separation and losses. This program provides awareness building, education, and outreach in bases throughout the country. All mental health providers and others who provide interventions need to understand more about the impact of trauma on young children in military families relative to deployment, combat-related injuries, and other adversities in order to build effective prevention, intervention, and clinical treatment programs for these families.

CHAPTER 8

■ ■ ■ ■

The Impact of Parental Combat Injury on Young Military Children

Stephen J. Cozza
Margaret M. Feerick

As of April 2010, over 37,000 service members (U.S. Department of Defense, 2010) have been wounded in ongoing combat operations in Iraq (Operation Iraqi Freedom, OIF) and Afghanistan (Operation Enduring Freedom, OEF). Many military service members are parents of young children, who are impacted by the injury and the events that occur in its immediate aftermath, and over the course of longer-term recovery. While there is a growing literature examining the impact of combat injury on families (e.g., Cohen et al., 2006; Cozza, Chun, & Miller, in press; Cozza, Chun, & Polo, 2005; Cozza et al., 2010), young children likely face unique or possibly greater challenges due to their developmental immaturity. Compared to older children, young children are at special risk when confronted with exposure to stressful and traumatic events (e.g., Heim & Nemeroff, 2001; Lieberman, 2004; Schore, 2001). First, because they are undergoing dramatic physical development, including neurological growth, exposure to stressful situations may jeopardize their typical development. Second, because young children are undergoing rapid changes in their cognitive and emotional capacities, they often lack coping mechanisms available to older individuals, and their relatively immature cognitive and emotional systems exacerbate their responses to stressful life events. Finally, because young children develop within the context of their immediate environment, primarily through interactions with family and other care providers, events that affect these social systems pose a threat to young children's development. In this chapter we examine the impact of combat injury on military families, with specific attention to the needs of children from infancy to 5 years old.

DEMOGRAPHICS OF INJURY IN THE MILITARY COMMUNITY

Wartime injuries may result from a number of causes, such as personal combat experience, in-theater accidents, or miscellaneous causes. Blasts and improvised explosive devices (IEDs) are reported as the most common causes of physical injuries in the current OIF and OEF conflicts (Owens et al., 2008). Combat injuries can include but are not limited to musculoskeletal injuries, spinal cord injuries, disfigurement, amputations, burns, and ocular trauma. Service members may also suffer "invisible" injuries, such as traumatic brain injury (TBI). In addition to moderate or severe forms of TBI, milder TBI may not come to medical attention but may result in symptoms, dysfunction, or sense of ill health (Warden, 2006) that can be particularly disturbing to young children, who can be confused by changes in parental cognitive function or personality, or by new erratic behavior.

Serious physical injuries may also result in comorbid psychiatric problems (Zatzick et al., 2007). Mental health symptoms, moreover, may change over time, resolving or worsening during the first year after hospitalization. In one study, nearly 80% of those combat-injured service members who screened positive for either posttraumatic stress disorder (PTSD) or depression at 7 months postinjury screened negative for both conditions at 1 month (Grieger et al., 2006), suggesting that the population's mental status changes throughout the recovery period. Clinicians, therefore, must be vigilant to the mental health status of both injured service members and family members over time. Such changes are likely to have a profound impact on military families.

U.S. Department of Defense (2009) statistics suggest that nearly half (43%) of U.S. service members have children, and that more than 40% of these children are 5 years old or younger. Military service member parents average two children per family (U.S. Department of Defense, 2009), suggesting that more than 30,000 children have been affected by parental combat injury, with approximately 12,000 of these children being in the age range of birth to 5 years old. In fact, some information suggests that children under the age of 5 years may be overrepresented in families with a combat-injured service member. Our own data (Chun et al., 2009), for example, indicated that 64% of children in a sample of families of hospitalized combat-injured service members were 5 years old and younger, with

31% of all children ($N = 85$) in the 3- to 5-year age group, 13% less than 1 year of age, and 20% between 1 and 2 years of age. This overrepresentation may result from younger service members serving in positions of greater risk while in combat theater.

CHALLENGES FACED BY COMBAT-INJURED FAMILIES AND THE INJURY RECOVERY TRAJECTORY

The effects of wartime injuries on children and families are complex and far-reaching. From the initial distress to longer-term injury adjustment challenges, children and families face a range of difficult emotional and practical problems that evolve, based on the time from the original injury. "Injury recovery trajectory" is a term we have used (e.g., Cozza & Guimond, 2011) to describe how injury recovery is experienced by the wounded service member and his or her family and children from the time of the injury throughout the months and years that follow. It is conceptualized within four phases: acute care, medical stabilization, transition to outpatient care, and long-term rehabilitation and recovery. While the acute care phase focuses on immediate combat theater life-saving and life-sustaining interventions, medical stabilization includes definitive stateside tertiary medical/surgical care. Transition to outpatient care begins prior to discharge as follow-up care and ongoing rehabilitation is planned. During rehabilitation and recovery, the injured service member continues to convalesce from the injury, participates in needed rehabilitation, and settles into a new postinjury life. During this phase, families often must transition to new communities and engage new health care providers (Cozza & Guimond, 2011).

The injury recovery trajectory may involve alternating periods of medical stability and instability. Multiple reconstructive surgeries are common with the severely injured, and continuity of care can be complicated by multiple transitions in care facilities, resulting in changes in family living arrangements, family separations and disruptions, and changes in connections to community resources and support. Since many war-related injuries are extensive, the treatment of patients can be time-consuming and often requires months or years of ongoing care (Cozza & Guimond, 2011).

Each phase of injury recovery poses unique challenges to the family with young children, beginning with notification of the family about the injury. Service member injuries result in a flurry of urgent activity and anxiety, leading to disruption of family roles, sources of care, and instrumental support that are critical to healthy development. Often, immediate information regarding the nature and severity of the injury is limited and sometimes inaccurate, causing further anxiety in families. When the family is notified, young children may witness adults who become extremely distressed, tearful, or emotionally volatile. Raw adult emotional responses can be both confusing and overwhelming to young children, challenging their sense of safety.

Once the family has been notified of the injury, a period of intense activity typically follows, often leading to disruptions in the family's schedule, which can be extremely disorganizing to infants, toddlers, and preschoolers. Spouses commonly join injured service members being treated at military hospitals that are far removed from family homes. Young children may be separated from both parents for unspecified periods of time. They may stay in or near their own homes with other adults, or move to live with relatives in distant places for extended periods of time. In some cases, children may accompany noninjured parents to military hospitals. Like adults, children often benefit from the support offered by others in dealing with stress. Young children are in the process of developing important relationships, and are more dependent upon their caregivers than older children and adolescents. Stressful or traumatic experiences, especially to the extent that they disrupt or challenge these relationships, can have profound effects on young children (e.g., Haine, Wolchik, Sandler, Millsap, & Ayers, 2006). As a result, a young child may experience disruption in attachment, parental loss, separation anxiety, fear of death, anxiety related to hospital visits and/ or exposures to medical procedures, and anxiety related to body damage, as well as sadness or depression.

In our own work (Chun et al., 2009), we have found that a very high proportion of children with a combat-injured parent (approximately 67%) live away from their parents during the injured parent's hospitalization, and many families confront significant changes in living arrangements as a result of the injury (Cozza et al., 2008). In one report, approximately three-fourths of 29 spouses of recently combat-injured service members described spending much less time with their children, and more than one-third anticipated moderate to severe changes in the injured service member's parenting role (Cozza et al., 2008). Not surprisingly, these changes were associated with spouse reports of changes in child behavior and increased emotional problems among these same children (Cozza et al., 2008). We also found that nearly 40% of children experienced moderate to significant behavioral changes following the injury, and that 70% of children experienced moderate to severe emotional difficulties (Cozza et al., 2008). In another set of analyses, children's emotional and behavioral symptoms appeared to be more common among children separated from their parents due to the injury, with young children being especially affected by parental separation (Chun et al., 2009). In a further analysis of these data (Cozza et al., 2010), a significant proportion of families reported high child distress following parental combat injury, and reported distress was significantly more likely to occur among families experiencing high levels of postinjury family disruption.

Later, when injured service members leave the hospital, children and other family members may expect a return to the lives they remember. They may become disappointed with changes that they experience in the family, and younger children may be confused or distressed by the emotional changes they see in their parents. Some data suggest that injured service members become more vulnerable as they transition back to their homes and communities (Grieger et al., 2006). Longer-term consequences of severe combat injury can result in medical retirement from the military service, loss of a cherished military career, and movement from homes in military communities to other locations or back to families of origin. While such transitions may increase access to available resources, particularly when the extended family is supportive, these changes are likely to be stressful for both adults and children. Moves from known communities likely mean loss of friends, changes in schools, and relocations to communities that may have little understanding or appreciation of military culture and the unique challenges that the family has faced.

THE YOUNG CHILD AND THE INJURED MILITARY PARENT

Beyond their developing neurological systems, young children's development is marked by comparative cognitive and emotional immaturity. While developmentally appropriate and typical, these normative developmental skills may impose some limitations in how young children react to the stress of parental injury. Compared with older children, younger children lack the cognitive capabilities that may protect them from traumatic events and may have some limitations that amplify the potential for harm. Young children have limited language skills, restricting their ability to communicate their experiences to others and to understand the language others use in interacting with them around trauma. For example, the emergence of "theory of mind," a child's understanding that the internal states of others may be different from their own, only begins to take shape during early childhood. Until it is formed, a child cannot reliably understand that the behaviors evident in others may be unrelated to him or her. So, when a parent experiences grief or distress, a young child is likely to believe that the parent's emotional state is related to some act or behavior of the child. Young children also use "magical thinking," which is characterized by immature cognitive processes that are vulnerable to emotional distortion. When coupled with children's limited understanding of injury and death (e.g., Cotton & Range, 1990; Kenyon, 2001; Poltorak & Glazer, 2006; Slaughter & Lyons,

2003), magical thinking can lead young children to assign responsibility for events inaccurately to themselves or others based on their own fears or fantasies.

Like their cognitive abilities, children's social and emotional skills are also limited when compared with those of older children and adults. Not only are young children's social and emotional skills undergoing development, they are also transient in nature and prone to broad variation even within the normative range of experience (see, e.g., Carter, Briggs-Gowan, & Davis, 2004). The nature of their early emotional experiences creates a dual challenge to providing effective support to young children experiencing stress or trauma. First, there is the potential for the trauma experience to alter normative development toward more atypical extremes. Second, the fluidity of young children's social and emotional regulatory skills makes it challenging to differentiate potential symptoms from normal variation in development (Carter et al., 2004).

All clinicians benefit from an accurate developmental perspective when considering the responses of children to parental injury. For example, while infants and toddlers (0 to 2 years old) may be assumed to have little cognitive capacity to appreciate their parents' injuries, they respond based on changes in the schedules and routines of their lives, and the physical and emotional availability of important adults, as well as any changes in the emotional tenor (anxiety, interpersonal abruptness, irritability) of their households and caregivers. If the combat injury severely disrupts the capacity of the noninjured parent to care for an infant, the young child may evidence problems in sleeping or eating, develop irritability or emotion regulation problems, or manifest a disturbance of attachment. One of the fundamental achievements of a child's first few years of life is the formation of a secure attachment to one or more adults, typically the child's parents, and most typically the mother (Bowlby, 1969/1982; Thompson, 1998). In addition to the potential for disruption in attachment relationships, when a young child experiences a trauma that also dramatically alters the family, a child previously not at risk may suddenly be at heightened risk (Lieberman, 2004).

Preschool children (3 to 5 years old) have greater awareness of the actual nature of the injury. However, this understanding is likely to be undeveloped and fragile. For example, they may worry that the injury is punishment for something that they or their parent did wrong. Young children's cognitive processes may become even less reality based at times of high anxiety, as typically occurs after a parent's injury (Cozza et al., in press). Not uncommonly, preschoolers who see their seriously injured parents become disorganized and extremely anxious. They may wonder, "If this powerful and important person in my life can be hurt in this way, what could potentially happen to me?" (Cozza et al., in press).

CLINICAL VIGNETTES

It is particularly important to carefully prepare children when dramatic changes in a parent's appearance occur, such as those resulting from facial wounds or serious burns. The following vignette (Cozza et al., in press) describes how one couple successfully helped their young son understand the injury and reengage his father.

> Teddy was a 3½-year-old boy whose father, Bill, had been deployed to Iraq for 6 months when a serious injury resulted from an IED explosion. Bill sustained serious injuries to his face and upper extremities, requiring unilateral facial bandaging and resulting in an inability to use his arms and hands effectively. On the day of Teddy's first visit with his father, his mother spent several minutes explaining the nature of the injuries and what he was likely to see upon entering his father's room, including the presence of facial bandages and his father's hoarse, somewhat unrecognizable voice. Teddy became very excited about the prospect of seeing his father. When they entered the room Teddy became silent and transfixed by his father's appearance. While his mother tried to reassure him, Teddy cautiously approached his father and carefully climbed on Bill's lap when invited. Instinctively, Bill began jostling Teddy between his legs, a game they had played often prior to the deployment. The familiarity of this activity eased Teddy, who immediately relaxed and began talking with Bill in a more natural and comfortable way.[1]

Children may express their anxiety and confusion about parental injury in a variety of ways. Oppositionality, aggression, or tantrums can be misperceived as bad behavior rather than expressions of distress. In the following example, the 3- and 5-year-old sons of a seriously injured Marine were referred for clinical assessment because of uncharacteristic oppositional and aggressive behavior that developed after their father's injury (Cozza et al., in press).

> During the evaluation, each child was asked to "draw a person." They were given no additional directions and were not specifically requested to draw their father. The 3-year-old child initiated his drawing as one would expect, completing the face first, but then proceeded to scribble erratically over and around the face. When asked what the picture represented, the younger brother stated, "This is a man in an explosion." After completing the drawing, the boy became motorically hyperactive and refused to continue to discuss the drawing or his father's injury. He shifted to aggressive play with toy dinosaurs and jungle animals. In contrast, his 5-year-old brother completed his drawing in a very careful and methodical fashion. However, unlike children his age, this boy started the drawing with the figure's feet. He then added three ascend-

ing sections to each leg in the drawing, resulting in two long, discon-
nected legs, side by side. At this point, the 5-year-old boy became visibly anxious and drew a brace between the legs in order to connect the
body. This addition betrayed the older son's anxiety about the body's
instability that needed to be supported by an armature. He completed
the drawing by adding arms, powerful shoulder muscles, and a small
head. After drawing the figure the boy became somewhat sullen and
quiet.

This vignette is not provided to describe psychopathology but as an
example of the numerous psychological challenges with which younger
children must struggle to successfully integrate the cognitive and emotional
experience of serious parental injury. Both children just described benefited
from supportive sessions in which they were able to express their distress
and confusion through creative play. Play was initially disorganized, aggressive, and nonverbal. Over time both boys developed a greater capacity to
talk about their father's injury, revealing fantasies and misperceptions about
what had occurred. They were disturbed about not only what had occurred
but also the disruptions in their lives, including the move from their home
to live with their aunt and uncle in another state. As the boys began more
openly to share their feelings about the injury and its consequences, their
parents were helped to understand better the nature of the "misbehavior"
as a symptom of anxiety and injury-related distress. As a result, the more
aggressive symptoms diminished over time (Cozza et al., in press).

YOUNG CHILDREN IN THE HOSPITAL SETTING

Helping to prepare children to visit a hospitalized parent is essential and
often overlooked in the emotional and logistical upheaval common to combat injury situations. Noninjured parents should initially visit the hospital
without young children, so that they can first integrate the experience themselves (Cozza et al., in press). In preparing a child for hospital visits, adults
can explain what to expect during the visit, describe or show pictures of the
injured parent and hospital setting, teach the vocabulary of the injury, reassure the child that the injured parent is still the same person, and discuss
how the child might feel during the visit. As is recommended with other
traumatic situations with young children, it is important to use accurate language rather than euphemisms to avoid any misunderstandings (Cozza et al.,
in press). Noninjured parents can gauge the appropriate amount of injury-
related information (presence of bandages, casts, amputations, or medical
equipment) and mix into the discussion less anxiety-provoking topics, such
as descriptions of the hospital cafeteria, the kind of food the children can eat

while in the hospital, or the hotel or living quarters. With proper planning, most children will feel comfortable when the time for the visit arrives.

Young children's visits to the hospital should be time-limited and structured to ensure that they are beneficial experiences for them, as well as for their parents. The noninjured parent should take cues from the child, refrain from forcing expressions of affection, and be prepared to leave if the child becomes frightened or bored. Allowing children to bring something for the service member (e.g., a drawing, photo, or flowers) may give them a sense that they are helping their parent feel better (Cozza et al., in press).

Specific plans need to be put in place that allow children to be present and involved in their parent's care, while preparing and protecting them from what they are likely to see in the hospital setting. Due to the presence of many injured service members at military medical centers, children who visit are likely to be exposed not only to their own parent's potentially frightening medical condition but also the burns, amputations, or serious injuries of other injured patients receiving care. When young children first see their injured parent, they may experience a broad range of emotions that can be confusing both to themselves and to the important adults in their lives. Some children may be hesitant, fearful, distressed, or reluctant to show affection to the injured parent. As a result, some injured service members express feelings of hurt or disappointment, which can complicate the parent–child relationship. When this occurs, the uninjured parent or another relative may be overly forceful in pushing children, especially young children, to show affection to the injured.

Hospital staff and family members may place unrealistic behavioral expectations on young children (e.g., expecting preschoolers to sit quietly for extended periods of time). Adults may react to children's loud and boisterous behavior with frustration and unnecessary harshness. Medical centers that provide care to injured service members should ensure that there are appropriate areas for family activities that are "child- and family-friendly." Again, children's presence within the hospital should be time-limited and structured. The immature cognitive capacity of young children can lead to an inability to gauge an accurate sense of time, as illustrated in the following example (Cozza et al., in press).

A 3-year-old boy, whose father had multiple injuries and was prescribed extensive bed rest after an amputation, gave his father's wound a kiss and said, "It's all better now, Dad, let's play." He became confused and frustrated when repeatedly told that his father could not yet play with him. The staff worked with the boy and his parents to establish more circumscribed ways of playing that allowed father and son to enjoy their time together.

As many serious injuries can result in months, if not years, of medical treatment and rehabilitative services, the patience of young children can rapidly dissipate. Professional intervention that assists parents both in understanding these developmental limitations and in creating new means of interaction can be invaluable for the future success of the family.

INTERVENTIONS WITH COMBAT-INJURED FAMILIES WITH YOUNG CHILDREN

To date, there is no research on interventions for children and families of combat-injured service members. An expert panel of professionals recently identified the three most important elements of intervention with this population: (1) reducing individual and family distress; (2) supporting child, parent, and family functioning; and (3) ensuring effective communication among family members, and with other professional and personal contacts outside of the family as related to combat injury experience and recovery (Cozza, 2009). This latter concept has been termed "injury communication" and is discussed below in greater detail. These three principles that serve to guide intervention strategies in families with young children recognize the particular importance of social environments, attachment relationships, and establishing safety and normality in the life of the young child. Interventions will also likely benefit from incorporating the principles of psychological first aid, parent guidance, and family-based interventions. In circumstances where a diagnosable child psychiatric disorder is present, other established interventions—such as individual therapy, trauma-focused therapy (e.g., trauma-focused cognitive-behavioral therapy; Cohen, Mannarino, & Deblinger, 2006), play therapy, child–parent psychotherapy (Lieberman, Ghosh Ippen, & Van Horn, 2006; Lieberman & Van Horn, 2008), or parent–child interaction therapy (Zisser & Eyberg, 2010)—may be indicated, depending on the problems the child is exhibiting; however, these latter treatments are not described in this chapter.

Psychological First Aid

Psychological first aid (PFA) is an evidence-informed intervention for early to midlevel mass trauma recovery (Brymer et al., 2006; Pynoos & Nader, 1988; for a review, see Hobfoll et al., 2007) that is particularly relevant to families with a combat-injured service member. Five key principles of PFA intervention emphasize (1) establishing a sense of safety, (2) promoting calm through distress reduction, (3) building a sense of self- and community efficacy, (4) fostering connectedness, and (5) promoting a sense of hope. These PFA principles can best be implemented with children of the combat injured on three levels: (1) community-based programs (e.g., family assistance programs, parent guidance, and respite programs); (2) family and parentally administered support; and (3) coordinated clinical care for those children considered to be at higher risk or exhibiting symptoms of a disorder. Clinicians can provide consultation to parents, other family members, hospital personnel, and other service providers using PFA.

PFA principles must be applied in a developmentally appropriate manner. For example, maintaining daily routines and physical proximity to a trusted adult are essential in establishing feelings of safety in infants, toddlers, and preschoolers. In addition to needs for safety, preschool children (3 to 5 years old) may have unique requirements for managing distress. Their lack of cognitive capacity to understand the situation fully or to describe their feelings necessitates nonverbal outlets. Young children gain mastery through play, practice, and repetition. Playing with toy hospital equipment or military-related toys can help children become more comfortable with the experiences of their parents. One resource developed specifically for children at this age is the Sesame Workshop's *Talk, Listen, Connect* series of DVDs and print materials (accessible at *www.sesameworkshop.org/initiatives/emotion/tlc*).

Parent Guidance and Consultation in the Hospital Setting

Clinicians can begin assisting families early on by providing guidelines for children's hospital visits, as described earlier. Consultation to hospitals may include recommendations for communicating with children about the injury and the hospital setting (see the section "Guidelines for Effective Injury Communication"), creating appropriate areas for family activities that are "child- and family-friendly," allowing children to be present and involved in their parent's care, protecting young children from unnecessary exposure to other injured service members, and advising parents regarding child visits. Examples of such interventions were described earlier in this chapter.

Interventions with children must be developmentally informed and reflect the unique needs, understanding, and emotional capacity of any particular child.

Guidelines for Effective Injury Communication

Since there is often much confusion and fear associated with injury, combat-injured families face unique challenges that can compromise communication. "Injury communication" refers to the multiple requirements for effective communication about injury-related topics and information both within the family and with others in civilian and military communities (Cozza, 2009; Cozza & Guimond, 2011). Effective injury communication requires open and ongoing discussions about the injury and its consequences between and among multiple parties: the injured service member and spouse, family members (to include children), friends, medical personnel, and other community professionals and service providers. When injury communication is properly conducted, it respects the high emotional valence of injury-related topics, as well as the necessity of using developmentally informed and appropriate language when communicating to children of different ages. Most importantly, effective injury communication changes to meet the needs of a family as the members evolve and change over the course of hospitalization, recovery, and reintegration (Cozza & Guimond, 2011).

Sometimes the noninjured parent or other adults have trouble deciding what is appropriate to tell their young children. Adults often struggle with their own emotional reactions, which may make communication about the injury particularly difficult. Parents may not recognize what is appropriate to pass on to children, particularly young children. As a result, some adults may choose to withhold important information related to serious injuries from children in an attempt to protect them. In these circumstances, clinicians need to be aware that such "secrets" cannot realistically be kept from children. Similarly, just as some parents may provide too little information about the injury, others may share more information than children are able to tolerate, or may frighten them by discussing unknown future consequences. Thus, many adults may need help determining the amount, content, and timing of the facts that they share with their children. Health care professionals should communicate to parents that even young children should be given some explanation, without causing them to become overly worried. This is particularly important to help them understand the actions and emotions of the adults they see around them (Cozza & Guimond, 2011).

The primary aim of the clinician's helpful stance toward the families and children of the injured is to increase adults' awareness of their children's experiences and reactions, and to help them notice and respond appropriately to children's emotional signals. In circumstances when injuries lead to longer-term impairments, personality changes, or cognitive problems in parents, young children need to be provided with simple and clear explanations of the behaviors they see (e.g., "Remember that I told you Daddy's brain was hurt. ... Sometimes he gets angry easily and he says things that he doesn't mean ... but that is not your fault. ... Even though he has trouble being in charge of himself, he still loves you"; see Cozza et al., in press; Cozza & Guimond, 2011).

Family-Based Interventions

Combat injury has the capacity to disrupt family structure and functioning in ways that place young children at particular risk. As such, a family-centered approach is essential to address challenges impacting children, spouses, and service members following combat injury. When the injury is serious, the recovery process is likely to be drawn out, requiring effective care management strategies and interventions that can be implemented across time and tailored to the specific needs of each family. Services should include longitudinal supportive engagement; assistance in identifying and connecting with needed resources; parent guidance; help with family problem solving and goal setting; ongoing risk assessment and, when indicated, referral for clinical intervention. Families are expected to need more help at transition points (after initial notification of spouse injury, traveling to the hospital; after stabilization, moving from the hospital to a rehabilitation site, etc.) (Cozza & Guimond, 2011).

A promising new intervention, FOCUS-CI (Families OverComing Under Stress–Combat Injury) integrates two existing evidence-based treatments: Families OverComing Under Stress (FOCUS) and Early Combined Collaborative Care (ECCC). FOCUS (Saltzman et al., 2009) is a well-respected and evidence-informed preventive intervention program that has been successfully used with military families dealing with the impact of deployment. ECCC (Zatzick et al., 2001) is a shared patient–health care provider treatment approach that promotes long-term care management, active sustained follow-up, and continuity in care delivery sectors. FOCUS-CI has seven core components: (1) family-focused care management; (2) emotion regulation skills; (3) psychoeducation; (4) injury communication; (5) problem solving; (6) goal setting; and (7) injury integration.

A primary goal of FOCUS-CI is to encourage long-term, trusting, and helpful relationships with combat-injured families, so that any family needs are identified and addressed as they develop throughout the injury recovery trajectory. Family strengths are emphasized throughout the intervention, and families are encouraged to engage in innovative, mutually developed activities that allow them to practice new ways of relating to each other and being together. The capacity for the parent–child dyad to reestablish healthy and fun modes of interaction is critical to the future health, happiness, and functioning of the family over time. Honest and open discussions between parents can help injured service member parents to reinterpret and reframe their situations, develop new skills, and develop healthy co-parenting strategies and competencies. Special focus on young children can ensure that parents recognize these children's developmental limitations, are sensitive to their sometimes confusing response patterns, and are capable of addressing their unique needs through guided intervention.

CONCLUSION

With two ongoing military conflicts, the potential for harm to parents in military families is especially high. When injured, not only is the parent affected by the specific short- and long-term consequences of the injury, but so is his or her family, including spouses and children. Young children in particular can be profoundly affected by injury to their parents because they may lack cognitive and emotional maturity and skills to cope that many adults possess. In addition, young children are more reliant upon both the injured and noninjured parent to support their development and meet their needs. A family confronting the combat injuries of a parent may not be able to meet these needs. In addition, the injured family member may require specialized rehabilitative or medical services, often geographically distant from their family. This may dramatically alter the nature of the relationships between the child and his or her parents, other family members, and additional trusting adults. Very little is known about the impact of parental combat injury on young children and how to best support young children during phases of parent recovery. More research and adaptation of evidence-based interventions and treatments are required to recognize these consequences and how best to meet the needs of families and young children when combat injury occurs.

NOTE

1. This vignette and the one that follows were originally provided for Cozza et al. (in press). Used with permission from the Borden Institute.

REFERENCES

Bowlby, J. (1982). *Attachment and loss: Vol. 1. Attachment* (2nd ed.). New York: Basic Books. (Original work published 1969)

Brymer, M., Jacobs, A., Layne, C., Pynoos, R., Ruzek, J., Steinberg, A., et al. (2006). *Psychological first aid (PFA): Field operations guide* (2nd ed.). Available at *www.nctsn.org* and *www.ncptsd.va.gov*.

Carter, A. S., Briggs-Gowan, M. J., & Davis, N. O. (2004). Assessment of young children's social–emotional development and psychopathology: Recent advances and recommendations for practice. *Journal of Child Psychology and Psychiatry, 45,* 109–134.

Chun, R. S., Schneider, B., Guimond, J. M., Arata-Maiers, T. L., Maiers, A., & Cozza, S. J. (2009, October). *Descriptions of emotional and behavioral changes in children following parental combat injury.* Poster presented at the annual meeting of the American Academy of Child and Adolescent Psychiatry, Honolulu, HI.

Cohen, J. A., Mannarino, A. P., & Deblinger, E. (2006). *Treating trauma and traumatic grief in children and adolescents.* New York: Guilford Press.

Cohen, J. A., Mannarino, A. P., Gibson, L.E., Cozza, S. J., Brymer, M. J., & Murray, L. (2006). Interventions for children and adolescents following disasters. In E. C. Ritchie, P. J. Watson, & M. J. Friedman (Eds.), *Interventions following mass violence and disasters: Strategies for mental health practice* (pp. 227–256). New York: Guilford Press.

Cotton, C. R., & Range, L. M. (1990). Children's death concepts: Relationship to cognitive functioning, age, experience with death, fear of death, and hopelessness. *Journal of Clinical Child Psychology, 19*(2), 123–127.

Cozza, S. J. (Ed.). (2009). *Proceedings: Workgroup on intervention with combat injured families.* Bethesda, MD: Center for the Study of Traumatic Stress.

Cozza, S. J., Chun, R. S., & Miller, C. (in press). The children and families of combat injured service members. In E. C. Ritchie (Ed.), *Combat and operational behavioral health.* Washington, DC: Borden Institute.

Cozza, S. J., Chun, R. S., & Polo, J. A. (2005). Military families and children during Operation Iraqi Freedom. *Psychiatric Quarterly, 76,* 371–378.

Cozza, S. J., Chun, R. S., Schneider, B., Fullerton, C. S., Guimond, J. M., & Ursano, R. J. (2008, November). *Assessment of concerns and needs of families following combat Injury: PGA-CI record review analysis.* Poster presented at the 24th annual meeting of the International Society for Traumatic Stress Studies. Chicago.

Cozza, S. J., & Guimond, J. M. (2011). Working with combat-injured families through the recovery trajectory. In S. M. Wadsworth & D. Riggs (Eds.), *Risk and resilience in military families* (pp. 259–278). New York: Springer.

Cozza, S. J., Guimond, J. M., McKibben, J. B. A., Chun, R. S., Arata-Maiers, T. L., Schneider, B., et al. (2010). Combat-injured service members and their famlies: The relationship of child distress and spouse-perceived family distress and disruption. *Journal of Traumatic Stress, 23,* 112–115.

Grieger, T. A., Cozza, S. J., Ursano, R. J., Hoge, C., Martinez, P.E., Engel, C. C., et al. (2006). Posttraumatic stress disorder and depression in battle-injured soldiers. *American Journal of Psychiatry, 163,* 1777–1783; quiz, 1860.

Haine, R. A. Wolchik, S. R., Sandler, I. N., Millsap, R. E., & Ayers, T. S. (2006). Positive parenting as a protective resource for parentally bereaved children. *Death Studies, 30,* 1–28.

Heim, C., & Nemeroff, C. B. (2001). The role of childhood trauma in the neurobiology of mood and anxiety disorders: Preclinical and clinical studies. *Biological Psychiatry, 49,* 1023–1039.

Hobfoll, S. E., Watson, P., Bell, C. C., Bryant, R. A., Brymer, M. J., Friedman, M. J., et al. (2007). Five essential elements of immediate and mid-term mass trauma intervention: Empirical evidence. *Psychiatry, 70,* 283–315; discussion, 316–369.

Kenyon, B. L. (2001). Current research in children's conceptions of death: A critical review. *Omega: Journal of Death and Dying, 43*(1), 63–91.

Lieberman, A. F. (2004). Traumatic stress and quality of attachment: Reality and internalization in disorders of infant mental health. *Infant Mental Health Journal, 25,* 336–351.

Lieberman, A. F., Ghosh Ippen, C., & Van Horn, P. (2006). Child–parent psychotherapy: 6-month follow-up of a randomized controlled trial. *Journal of the Academy of Child and Adolescent Psychiatry, 45,* 913–918.

Lieberman, A. F., & Van Horn, P. (2008). *Psychotherapy with infants and young children: Repairing the effects of stress and trauma on early attachment.* New York: Guilford Press.

Owens, B. D., Kragh, J. F., Jr., Wenke, J. C., Macaitis, J., Wade, C. E., & Holcomb, J. B. (2008). Combat wounds in Operation Iraqi Freedom and Operation Enduring Freedom. *Journal of Trauma, 64,* 295–299.

Poltorak, D. Y., & Glazer, J. P. (2006). The development of children's understanding of death: Cognitive and psychodynamic considerations. *Child and Adolescent Clinics of North America, 15*(3), 567–573.

Pynoos, R. S., & Nader, K. (1988). Psychological first aid and treatment approach to children exposed to community violence: Research implications. *Journal of Traumatic Stress, 1,* 445–473.

Saltzman, W., Lester, P., Pynoos, R., Mogil, C., Green, S., Layne, C., et al. (2009). *FOCUS for military families: Individual family resiliency training manual* (2nd ed.). Los Angeles: Semel Institute for Neuroscience and Human Behavior, University of California at Los Angeles.

Schore, A. N. (2001). The effects of early relational trauma on right brain development, affect regulation, and infant mental health. *Infant Mental Health Journal, 22,* 201–269.

Slaughter, V., & Lyons, M. (2003). Learning about life and death in early childhood. *Cognitive Psychology, 46*(1), 1–30.

Thompson, R. A. (1998). Early sociopersonality development. In W. Damon & N. Eisenberg (Eds.), *Handbook of child psychology:* Vol. 3. *Social, emotional, and personality development* (5th ed., pp. 25–104). New York: Wiley.

U.S. Department of Defense. (2010). Military casualty information. Retrieved April 25, 2010, from *www.defense.gov/news/casualty.pdf.*

U.S. Department of Defense. (2009). Report of the 2nd Quadrennial Quality of Life Review. Retrieved from *cs.mhf.dod.mil/content/dav/mhf/qol-library/pdf/ mhf/qol%20resources/reports/quadrennial%20quality%20of%20life%20 review%202009.pdf.*

Warden, D. (2006). Military TBI during the Iraq and Afghanistan wars. *Journal of Head Trauma Rehabilitation, 21,* 398–402.

Zatrick, D. F., Kang, S. M., Hinton, W. L., Kelly, R. H., Hilty, D. M., Franz, C. E., et al. (2001). Posttraumatic concerns: A patient-centered approach to outcome assessment after traumatic physical injury. *Medical Care, 39*(4), 327–339.

Zisser, A., & Eyberg, S. M. (2010). Parent–child interaction therapy and the treatment of disruptive behavior disorders. In J. R. Weisz & A. E. Kazdin (Eds.), *Evidence-based psychotherapies for children and adolescents* (2nd ed., pp. 179–193). New York: Guilford Press.

CHAPTER 9

■ ■ ■ ■

Working with Young Children of the National Guard and Reserve during a Family Member's Deployment

Juliet M. Vogel
Jennifer M. Newman
Sandra J. Kaplan*

> If the plane had no wings, then my daddy couldn't leave.
> —5-year-old Mark, explaining his drawing of a plane without
> wings during a visit to our center right after his father's
> R&R visit and subsequent return to Iraq

Between September 2001 and April 30, 2009, 1,924,810 service members deployed to Afghanistan and Iraq (Institute of Medicine, 2010). Twenty-eight percent were members of the National Guard and Reserves, together called the Selected Reserves. Both Active Duty and Reserve numbers continue to grow, and many deploy multiple times. Slightly more than 40% of deploying Active Duty and Selected Reserve service members leave children behind (ICF International, n.d.). The Selected Reserve is more heterogeneous than the Active Duty component with regard to age, but 51% are

---

*Sandra J. Kaplan died in July 2010. We want to acknowledge not only her contributions to the writing of this chapter but also her support of the work described and her vision as the founding director of the Rosen Center.

age 30 or younger, compared to 67% of the Active Duty members. Correspondingly, a significant proportion of their children are between ages 0 and 5 years, 21% of the Selected Reservists' children, 41% for the Active Duty component. Young children may also be affected by the deployment of other relatives, such as a grandparent or older sibling, or by the deployment of others close to them. This chapter describes supportive and therapeutic interventions with preschool children of National Guard members and Reservists during the deployment of their parents. In this chapter, we also describe the many challenges that deployment poses for young children of National Guard members and Reservists and their home-front parents. Our team has developed an approach to working with families with young children during deployment; the case of 4-year-old "Tom O'Malley" is used to illustrate this. (Demographic information and other details have been changed to protect the identities of the children and families discussed in this chapter.)

These inventions have been done at the Florence and Robert A. Rosen Center for Family Wellness for Law Enforcement and Military Personnel and Their Families, Department of Psychiatry, North Shore–Long Island Jewish Health System. The Center is located on the boundary of New York City and suburban Nassau County. New York State currently ranks fifth among the states in contributing members to the Reserves and National Guard, and many of them are from the Metropolitan New York City area.

ISSUES FOR YOUNG CHILDREN DEALING WITH DEPLOYMENT

The Challenges

Three issues pose particular challenges for families with young children dealing with deployment. First, even a single deployment of a National Guard or Reservist parent typically involves a series of parent–child separations, which can be difficult for a young child to understand. Second, modern communications allow contact and information flow not possible in prior wars. Although this may help keep the missing parent "in the family circle," the availability of this "real-time" communication for many service members and their families can pose its own challenges and difficulties. Finally, the young child is affected by shifts in family structure, as well as by reactions to the deployment of the home front caregiver(s). The most typical structural change is from a two-parent to a single-parent family, but for many children there is a shift of part or all of the parenting responsibilities to extended family members or others.

A Single Deployment with Phased Separations

Both National Guard members and Reservists have schedules that involve a sequence of separations even around a single deployment. Members of the New York Army National Guard participate in drills one weekend per month. If they live near their unit's location, this involves only limited time away from home. However, National Guard members are also required to participate for 2 weeks per year in training that is often located at a distance from home. Also, service members who train for special roles may have additional training periods away from home.

Currently, for an Army National Guard member, the time away from home for a single deployment is approximately 12 months. It is important in understanding the effect on families that during that period, several "separations and reunions" are part of the process. Army National Guard members typically first go for 2 months to a location within the United States to receive more intensive training. At times, there is a brief reunion after this training, before the service member goes oversees. This can include a brief trip home or a trip by part or all of the family to the location where the service member has been training. In the latter case, this can raise issues about whether to include children. (We have known children who have been upset that they were not included in such trips.) Approximately midway through their time overseas, service members often have an R&R (rest and recuperation) trip, at times visiting the family at home or in a "neutral location." The reunion at the end of the tour of duty marks the end of that deployment. Unless the service member leaves the military, drilling resumes 90 days later, as does the possibility of a future deployment.

KEEPING THE PARENT IN THE FAMILY CIRCLE

Literature dating back to World War II suggests that it helps children after deployment when the missing parent can be "kept in the family circle" during the parent's war-related absence (Hill, 1949). While it is difficult for preverbal infants and toddlers to understand preparations for separation and to keep the service member parent "in the child's family circle" during deployment, we have experienced families that are able to function highly effectively at the latter task. One mother described how she and her husband helped their baby, who was born shortly before the father's deployment, in the following ways: Before deploying, the father made recordings of himself reading baby books. During the deployment, the mother established a daily routine that included time listening to the father's stories and looking at his picture. When this child saw her father during an R&R visit middeployment, she showed no signs of stranger anxiety.

For verbal preschool children, there is more possibility of preparing them using both explanations with words and educational materials. Such materials for preschool children include the *Deployments, Homecomings, Changes* DVD prepared by the Sesame Workshop (2008) Talk, Listen, Connect project, and the book *A Paper Hug* (Skolmoski, 2006). These materials have been shown to be useful for the families we serve; however, they usually do not address fully the child's concerns and potential misunderstandings. It is often important to help preschool children deal with possible misconceptions, including "egocentric" interpretations of events that are often characteristic of preschool children (Piaget & Inhelder, 1969)—such as whether the child's behavior contributed to the parent's departure. The availability of cell phone and computer communication may help but may also lead to new challenges, as we discuss below.

PREPARING FOR THE SERVICE MEMBER'S RETURN

We have seen children benefit from concrete strategies for marking time until a reunion (e.g., removing links from a paper chain). Since precise reunion dates are not typically given, and return dates are subject to change, it is important to not be too specific and to help the child prepare for some uncertainty (e.g., to include some extra links on the paper chain). For some families, a small extension of time has been quite stressful for all members because it meant missing the sharing of an important event, such as a major holiday.

Some young children go through a period of ignoring a returning parent after deployment, much as described in classic works by Bowlby (1972) and Robertson and Robertson (1989), who wrote about children who have had prolonged separations from significant figures. Although this behavior does not always occur, parents can experience relief from understanding that this is a common reaction to separation, not taking it personally, and giving the child time.

COMPLEXITIES OF BRIEF REUNIONS AND REPEATED SEPARATIONS

Brief reunions, such as R&R visits, can be a source of not only anticipation and excitement but also anxiety and apprehension. For some families, the home front parent's concern about an anticipated R&R visit is part of the reason for seeking our assistance. Interventions have included talking with different family members about their expectations of what should happen, helping the home front parent and the children discuss differences in their expectations, and helping the home front parent have preparatory discussions with the service member. In one family, mother and young child had very different expectations about "routine" issues, such as what an appropriate greeting would be in public. Children frequently find the separation after an R&R visit to be difficult. As described at the beginning of the chapter, one 5-year-old drew a plane without wings shortly after his father's R&R visit, explaining to his clinician that if his father's plane had not had wings, the father would not have been able to go away again.

Repeated training out of town prior to deployment also can be confusing for young children, and risk of confusion increases when there has already been an actual deployment. For example, one young child we saw was upset when her father, who was between deployments, was out of town for a 2-week training. It is important to realize that young children may not understand the difference between their father's going to a neighboring state and returning to Afghanistan, as was the case for this 5-year-old. The preschool child has a limited understanding of geography, and phone contact may be similar in both cases.

Challenges of Modern Communication

During deployment, many service members have access to cell phone and computer communication, the latter including e-mail and sometimes Skype, which allows both video and audio communication. This is a major shift from World War II letters, which arrived weeks after being mailed and with pieces sometimes cut out by censors. While the frequency of current communication varies, overall, it has increased since the early phases of Operational Iraqi Freedom and Operation Enduring Freedom (the war in Afghanistan). However, it may still vary depending on the location of the service member and specific service activities at any point in time. Thus, a family with relatively frequent communication may have times when this is not possible. Also, it needs to be recognized that there is a significant time difference, and communication times for phone and Skype contacts typically are based on the service member's schedule rather than convenience for children at home.

In our work, three issues have emerged for young children relating to modern phone and computer communication. First, young children are not known for their "reliability" and ability on demand to talk on the phone (or Skype), and this situation is exacerbated when calls are at times not optimal for young children. Therefore, we have recommended to parents that they might want to prerecord a message from the child or prepare a product (e.g., a drawing) that can be shared by Skype to avoid needing to depend on the child's being communicative at the time of the call. Second, when there has been frequent communication, then a gap, considerable anxiety may result for the home front parent. It may be challenging for the parent to deal with his or her own anxiety, then explain the communication gap in a way that does not "flood" young children. Finally, parents often do not realize that "out of sight" is not "out of earshot" when they are communicating to the other parent or to other adults on the phone. When we discussed this at an educational program for a Family Readiness Group (FRG), one FRG leader gave a pertinent example. She had been careful that her children were not in the room when she called other FRG members to inform them of an injury to a member of the unit. Later, her school-age daughter asked her how the injured service member was doing; it was not clear what her preschool child had heard or understood.

Challenges from Shifts in Family Structure and Family Stress

For two-parent families, there is a shift in structure during deployment to effectively becoming single-parent families. The home front parent is typically told, "Don't worry the warrior," about day-to-day issues that are out of the service member's control. In our program with families during deployment, we sometimes serve as sounding boards for parenting concerns, as well as supports for the home front parent in dealing with new roles and challenges. One parent who had met us at a community event referred herself to our center after an incident in which she was told that her husband was injured, although he subsequently was well enough to return immediately to military operations. She realized that not only was the incident very upsetting to her but also her infant was reacting to her distress and also showing distress.

Common Behavioral and Emotional Issues: The Research

Research on children's reactions to the current deployments is only beginning to be available. Some research from the First Gulf War is relevant. However, older research from the Vietnam War and World War II has limited relevance because of the shifts in demographics of the military. Presently we have an all-volunteer army, including more service members with young children, many service members with multiple deployments, and an increased number of women serving, including some in dual-military couples.

Research from the First Gulf War suggests that the majority of children do not show clinical disorders during a parent's deployment; however, mild increases in both behavior and emotional symptoms are relatively common. Thus, mildly elevated depressive symptoms were found for children between 4 and 17 years with slightly higher risk for younger children (Jensen, Martin, & Watanabe, 1966). Navy service women who were mothers reported higher levels of internalizing symptoms for their young children (80% were between 1 and 3 years old) if the mothers deployed (Kelly et al., 2001) and child care workers also reported higher externalizing symptoms; however, symptoms reached a clinically significant level for only a small proportion of children. (Symptoms were assessed shortly before and after deployment.) Spouses reported that during a parent's deployment, many children between ages 1 and 5 years showed problems such as sadness and demanding attention, and for boys, home discipline issues (Rosen, Teitelbaum, & Westhuis, 1993).

For the current wars, there is emerging evidence of increase in behavioral issues for young children with deployed parents (Barker & Berry, 2009; Chartrand, Frank, White, & Shope, 2008). Children's reponses may be related to a variety of factors, including greater risk of internalizing symptoms when there is depression in the home front parent or a higher number of additional stressors (Jensen et al., 1996). However, a recent study found higher levels of behavioral symptoms compared to peers for 3- to 5-year-olds with a deployed parent even when the researchers controlled for caregiver stress and depression (Chartrand et al., 2008). Greater increase in problems during deployment has been reported for young children whose parents have had multiple deployments (Barker & Berry, 2009).

Resilience factors are important to recognize, including the availability of social supports for the home front parent, the parent's "child sense" and attunement with the young child, and the extent to which schools/day care are also supportive by being not only sympathetic but also effective in dealing with issues that may emerge for the child.

PROGRAM FOR RESILIENCE IN DEPLOYMENT: A CHILD AND FAMILY INTERVENTION

The intervention approach developed in our program addresses challenges to the family, including the young child, from a family member's deployment. The program takes into account the child's developmental needs and individual temperament, the fit between the child's needs and the home front parent or caregiver's needs and concerns, and when needed, issues that may occur in preschool or day care settings.

Community Education and Outreach

The first objective of the program is to partner with support systems provided by the New York National Guard and the Reserves, most frequently the Army Reserves. Our program provides community education when possible to help families to identify common issues and learn about strategies and resources for self-care. These community programs also provide opportunity to address the needs of the children.

Both National Guard and Reserves offer family support services. As of January 2011, the New York National Guard Family Support Program includes (but is not limited to) a network of seven Military Family Assistance Centers (MFACs) and five Airman & Family Readiness Program Managers (A&FRPMs), with one more center soon to be added in the Long Island area. Currently there are two MFACs and one A&FRPM in the New York City/Long Island area. In addition, there are two State Youth Program Coordinators. National Guard programs vary in specifics from state to state, but there are now federal guidelines for "Yellow Ribbon" family educational events throughout the deployment cycle, including family reintegration programs at 30- and 60-days postdeployment. For Reserves, there is considerable variation by service branch, as well as local variation within a branch, in the details of operations of family programs.

During deployment, a central aspect of National Guard and Reserve family support structure is the FRG, a military-sponsored group consisting of family members, military personnel, civilian employees, and volunteers associated with a unit to provide a social network for activities and support, including information dissemination. FRGs vary substantially in level of activity, often as a function of the volunteer leadership as well as the characteristics of the families, including their geographic dispersion. Participants include a range of relationships to service members (e.g., parents, adult siblings, spouses, fiancées), and families vary with respect to ages of children. There is typically much to cover at formal programs. While there may be interest in presentations on needs of children, typically there is limited time to focus on the special needs of any specific age group.

Our program plays a flexible role in supporting National Guard and Reserve Family Program and FRG activities. Most frequently, we provide brief presentations at local events, including FRG meetings, highlighting topics related to family and child resilience. At some events, such as Yellow Ribbon reintegration events, we provide a table of resource materials and are available to answer questions. We have also provided crisis intervention services, at times in support of FRGs, when a crisis has occurred, such as a death of a service member.

At other times, our project provides programs directly for children, including preschool children. One example of our initiative with preschoolers has been at National Guard Yellow Ribbon family events. Typically, the National Guard provides programs for children 6 years and older and for adolescents, but only provides baby-sitting for younger children. The New York National Guard Family Programs has allowed our staff to begin to introduce resilience-building activities for 3- to 5-year-olds at Yellow Ribbon family events in our region with leadership by one of the authors (JN).

In addition to providing information to build resilience, the presence of our staff at community events helps families know about the availability of our services should significant issues develop. Over time, through these relationships, our program has been able to establish a level of trust in our ability to understand and address concerns and the complex issues that may arise.

Clinical Services

Referrals come to community programs such as the Rosen Center at the North Shore–Long Island Jewish Health System in a variety of ways. Some people call after hearing us at community events or reading about our program. Others are referred to us by unit or FRG leaders, National Guard or Reserves Family Programs staff, or other professionals. Still others hear about us from families we have served. All telephone "screens" are done by a clinician, usually the Clinical Director, a social worker who is knowledgeable about deployment issues and also has training on engagement strategies (McKay et al., 2004). These strategies are helpful for engaging a population for whom seeking clinical services may be difficult. We also have found it useful to make adaptations for this specific population. Services begin with an intake/evaluation to determine clinical needs and learn more about which family members to include in sessions.

In work with young children and their families during deployment, three treatment configurations seem to be most helpful: (1) work primarily with the parent about his or her infant, with the child present at some sessions; (2) dyadic parent–child work; and (3) a "child guidance" model of parallel parent and child work, with clear integration of the parent and child work.

For example, in a situation in which a mostly resilient mother of an infant/toddler was facing some major deployment-related stressors, we worked primarily with the mother. We helped her with her own issues, as well as strategies to support her infant. The child's presence at many of the sessions allowed the clinician the opportunity to learn more directly about the child's adjustment.

For older preschool children showing significant externalizing (aggression) and/or anxiety issues, our preferred treatment mode is the second configuration, working with the home front parent and child together, helping them to understand each other, and allowing us to model for and coach the parent in how to deal with the child. This work is based in part on the child–parent psychotherapy model developed by Lieberman and Van Horn (2008). In addition to dyadic sessions, it is typical to include meetings and/or phone consultations with the parent alone. The many demands on the home front parent often make individual meetings difficult to arrange, so for our program the consultation is often by phone.

There are some parent–child dyads in which both the home front parent and the child have significant issues, and the parent needs his or her own regular time with a clinician. In those cases, we use the third configuration, assigning separate clinicians to each member of the dyad but making sure that there is bridging of the work with the parent and child. In these cases, there is close collaboration between the two therapists, including times when both of the therapists, the parent, and the child meet together. At other times the parent may join the child and the child's therapist for a part of a session. Finally, there may be phone consultation by the child's therapist with the parent around specific, child-related issues with which the parent needs help.

The therapeutic modalities we use with young children in military families include play, which is central to our work, integrated with more structured components, including cognitive interventions that directly address ability to express and cope with feelings. Behavioral interventions are used to address disruptive behaviors that frequently are present and cause family and/or school difficulties. In addition, the clinical work with the child and family is supplemented by consultation to the child's preschool when needed. All of these elements were present in the following case.

Case Example: The O'Malley Family[1]

Three phases of work with the O'Malley family are described. Phase I took place prior to deployment, when the parents sought our consultation and support about preparing their four children for their father's imminent deployment with the National Guard. Phase II began about 2 months after deployment, when 4-year-old Tom began to have significant difficulties both at home and in preschool. Tom was seen for about 4 months, until the end of his school year. Four moths later, our team did a brief follow-up intervention, which is described as Phase III.

Phase I: Outreach and Predeployment Consultation

As mentioned earlier, much of our work involves outreach to families at community events. This is where we met Mr. O'Malley. Like many soldiers, he had a strong commitment to serving our country but was worried about how his family would do without him. When we asked what he had told his four children (ages 4–10) so far, he reported having said nothing and not knowing where to start. We invited him to contact us for a consultation at the Rosen Center, which he did.

We conceptualized the first phase of treatment as a time-limited consultation, with later use of our services if needed. It is common that people who come in predeployment have a particular issue of concern. For this family, the primary focus was preparing the children for the father's upcoming deployment. The parents initially came in alone for three sessions. We learned that both parents had questions about how to talk to their children and what type of information would be OK to share with them. Both were also worried about how the children would respond to their dad's absence. Although the family had grown used to his being away for a week of training, they had not experienced an extended absence like that of deployment. The parents identified being more concerned about one of the older children and worried that he would be the most upset, based on some earlier adjustment issues. In fact, they predicted incorrectly which child ultimately would end up most in need of our support. In addition to these issues, as for many other families, the upcoming deployment occurred in the context of other stressors (e.g., illness of a family member).

In all of our work, we balance engagement and "hearing people's stories" with objective assessments that often help to guide treatment. In this case, baseline assessment of general functioning of each child was done, as well a brief battery of self-report measures for each parent. This baseline information has been useful to assess progress, in that the measures can be readministered to see changes over time or when families return subsequently, after later deployment transitions. Also, the self-report measures may provide an opportunity to identify issues that people do not readily bring up. For example, Mr. O'Malley reported that he was having significant sleep trouble, which we were able to address prior to his deployment. In another case, we identified a prior trauma that exacerbated levels of stress for a spouse during her husband's deployment.

During the parent sessions, conversations included information about what to expect with this transition (e.g., discussing the normal adjustments that happen during any life transition and some of the specifics related to deployment), clinicians provided concrete tools to aid the family in communicating about deployment (e.g., the Sesame Street Talk, Listen, Connect program *Deployment and Homecomings* DVD), and family members had a forum to talk openly about stress related to deployment. A good measure of how difficult this time was for this family was learning that the parents put off watching the DVD, finally doing so when it was almost time for Mr. O'Malley's deployment. Mr. O'Malley described having a strong emotional reaction while watching it. It was helpful that the parents saw it before the children so they were better prepared to support the children and their reactions.

The family session occurred after the children had watched the video. This time was used to check whether the children understood what was happening, provide additional psychoeducation for the children at age appropriate levels, talk openly about deployment, and address their questions. Additionally, it gave the children an opportunity to become familiar with the Rosen Center staff in case they needed to come in for future work.

Our program makes it clear to the families that we do not see them as "disordered." Rather, we talk about ways in which they are experiencing a healthy or predictable reaction to a significant stressor. We often consider our work to be supportive, while providing education and encouraging resilience. We work to identify strengths within the families, that is, what they are already doing well, and to find ways to support these positive responses during deployment. We also spend time predicting what might be the hardest time for a loved one to be away. The O'Malley's spoke about what it would be like to not have their dad at upcoming holidays and birthdays. We then discussed ways they could include him in these important events (pictures, letters, Skype).

We had brief phone contact with the parents after this session. By then, deployment time had almost come. Although we discussed reasons that the family might call us again, at this point we said our farewells. Mrs. O'Malley described feeling like "everything would be fine and that it would be unlikely for them to call again."

Phase II: During Deployment—"Tom Is Hitting in Preschool"

Several months after saying good-bye, Mr. O'Malley contacted the Rosen Center—from Iraq—because of concerns he had for the youngest son "Tom," age 4 years. As mentioned earlier, this was not the child the parents predicted might have trouble with the deployment. We learned that Tom was not following rules, appeared angry, and was acting aggressive. During the initial family assessment, it was noted that there were some minor issues in these areas but not at the level currently being described. Mr. O'Malley was concerned that his son was reacting to his deployment and asked about having Tom seen at the Rosen Center. The following day, Mrs. O'Malley called. She reported, "Tom is angry. He has low frustration tolerance at home and at school, he is not listening, and he is hitting and scratching his siblings and peers." She made an appointment to come in with Tom.

Tom was significantly changed from the boy we met prior to his father's deployment. He no longer wore the smile or made the jokes he had previously. Instead, through the use of "feeling faces," he identified his mood as "angry." He answered all questions asked, even about his favorite color, with "no" or "nothing." He also hit both his mother and the clinician without being provoked.

We updated our behavioral questionnaires. Both the mother's behavioral questionnaire responses and teacher report forms were consistent with the mother's reports of angry mood, noncompliance with rules, and aggressive behavior. Although we never assumed that this behavior was solely a result of deployment, we were able to identify that some of the preexisting problem behaviors Tom had exhibited during Phase I were exacerbated soon after his dad left.

We conceptualized that much of Tom's acting out was a stress reaction to his father's departure, as well as to the increased demands on Mrs. O'Malley. (As noted earlier, this is a frequent response for children in Tom's age range.) We wanted a treatment model that would not only help Mrs. O'Malley handle Tom's deployment reactions but also give her support as she faced the stresses of being temporarily a single parent. Additionally, we wanted to help Tom communicate how he was feeling, then help him develop effective coping strategies. Mrs. O'Malley had a hectic schedule, working a full-time job and being the sole caretaker for Tom and three other children, which meant that it was particularly important that she and Tom have the session time together to build communication and support. Based on these reasons, it was determined that a dyadic treatment model would be ideal for Tom and his mother, with additional parent guidance offered via phone periodically. We used a combination of behavioral, cognitive, and play-based interventions.

Work in sessions focused on two issues: (1) developing a "safe" frame, and modeling for Mrs. O'Malley how to deal with Tom's challenging behaviors; and (2) helping Tom with expression of and ability to cope with feelings.

The first focus involved using behavioral techniques for managing problem behaviors (e.g., aggression such as hitting). In-session modeling allowed Mrs. O'Malley to see how to set rules and react when those rules were tested (e.g., using time-out methods). Tom was included in rule setting, which was done weekly at the start of each session. He often chose to dictate the rules (e.g., "stay in the room," "good hands and feet [to self]," "play nicely"). Techniques such as planned ignoring, using a warning system, punishment, and positive praise were discussed and modeled. Also, a "mystery prize box" was introduced from which Tom could earn an item if he displayed good behavior throughout the session. During one session, when Tom motioned that he was going to break a crayon, he was prompted not to do this, and the behavior was then ignored. He was encouraged to continue the in-session activity, but he again motioned his intention to break his crayon. He was prompted by the therapist, "Remember the rule, nice hands and nice feet." Tom then broke the crayon. The therapist directed Tom to a time-out spot. Once a brief time-out was completed, he was able to rejoin the activity, which he did appropriately. Mrs. O'Malley stated that she found it helpful to see how effectively this worked. She also found helpful the modeling of the warning/reminder to Tom of the rule.

These behavioral concepts were translated to the home environment as well, with mother and therapist collaborating on how to do so using in-session and phone contact. Tom's mother reported significant improvement in his behavior at home.

The clinician also made contact with Tom's preschool, where his behavior remained problematic. The school was aware of Mr. O'Malley's deployment and for a while tried not to stress Mrs. O'Malley with negative reports about Tom. Unfortunately, by the time they spoke with Mrs. O'Malley, the problems were well-established. Once Tom's behavior in sessions and at home was under better control, a member of the Rosen team did an observation in the preschool. She identified several issues, including the existence of some high-risk times of day and the frequency with which Tom's acting-out behaviors resulted in negative attention. Based on the observation, Tom's clinician was able to work with the staff to develop a behavioral plan for the school setting. The clinician then maintained regular phone contact with the school, getting periodic updates about progress and helping the school staff modify the behavior plan. With guidance, the school was able to make changes so that attention was given more consistently for Tom's positive behaviors rather than for his negative ones. (This response pattern is common in young children showing externalizing behaviors and needs to be recognized by both parents and child care/preschool programs).

The second focus of treatment, emotional expression and improved coping, involved the use of play and cognitive-behavioral exercises. Tom's play involved acting out themes of nurturance and support. These themes were discussed with Mrs. O'Malley so that she understood how Tom was communicating by utilizing play and how she could engage with him in a supportive way through the play. Tom would typically choose to play with people dolls, assigning one to each person in the room. His character, the young boy, would get physically hurt and need care from his mother's character, "the nurse." The clinician's doll often was not involved in the play, as directed by Tom. The therapist coached Mrs. O'Malley in using supportive language during play (e.g., "I feel sad that you're hurt"; "What can I do to make you feel better?"; and "I'm happy you're feeling better, little boy"). After several sessions, mother and child developed and elaborated on their play routine.

The therapist also helped Tom with emotion identification and expression using concrete cognitive-behavioral tools, such as using feeling faces charts, feeling games, and thermometers. For example, Tom would rate how he felt each day when he arrived and during several points throughout the session. Initially, Tom's routine response was to identify his feelings as "angry" and choose the highest point of a feelings thermometer, where the liquid was spilling over the top. By the end of treatment, he had switched to routinely identifying his feelings in session as "happy" at the highest level.

Other changes by the end of treatment were that Tom's aggressive behaviors had decreased significantly, his angry outbursts were shorter, and his listening had improved in session, at home, and at school. The clinician observed that Mrs. O'Malley was praising Tom for good use of his words (instead of behaviors such as hitting) to express his feelings when angry, and she also was using behavioral strategies to address problem behaviors when they occurred. She reported feeling more in control and less overwhelmed. Tom began to ask questions about his father's deployment instead of avoiding the topic. This included asking how he could know that his father was really in Iraq, not still on the airplane. He and the therapist used the computer to look at a map so that he could better understand where his father was.

This phase of treatment ended with the end of the school year. Tom was going to a summer camp, and Mrs. O'Malley expressed confidence that the summer would go smoothly.

Phase III: Follow-Up Consultation

At the end of the summer, Mrs. O'Malley called to check in. She reported that the summer had gone well. She and the therapist spoke about behavioral issues, which were still present but in much better control, and Tom's mood remained improved.

Two months into the new school year, Mrs. O'Malley called again and came back to the Rosen Center for a consultation. At this point her concerns related to Tom's adjustment to the demands of a new school setting. This started a new phase of assessment and problem solving, including another school observation and behavioral plan. Because of a family move and the children's school schedules, the mother was reluctant to resume treatment with Tom. The therapist did provide continued consultation for the family and for the school, which again was helpful. The therapist also discussed the possibility of a testing referral if problems occurred in the future, particularly after Mr. O'Malley's return. Finally, the therapist provided support for Mrs. O'Malley, who was dealing with the stress on the entire family of a delay in Mr. O'Malley's return.

CONCLUSION

The O'Malleys, like the other families we serve, are a caring and resilient family in which several members, including their youngest, struggled with the challenges and transitions involved with military deployment. Each family member brought both strength and vulnerability to this situation. In the work of our program to provide support to both children and their parents, we bring knowledge of child development and techniques for working with young children and families. We work collaboratively with the families in learning about their unique needs and resources. A main goal is to support the young child, the child's caregiver, and the relationship between them.

Information, support, and consultation are also provided to preschool or child care providers, who typically have little experience with deployment issues, because children with whom we work are often the only ones in their schools dealing with deployment.

We have learned that the outreach and educational work our program provides in the community is as important as the work we do with individual families in the clinical setting. Families appreciate the information and support, and, through these efforts, our program is able to reach many families that do not need or would not seek clinical services. In addition, we believe that the presence of staff from our program at the events for service families helps give families confidence that providers who are not part of the military may actually understand the issues associated with military deployment.

Military deployment continues to affect large numbers of children in our communities. The focus of this chapter has been on the needs of children and their families before and during the deployment. It is evident from current and repeat deployment patterns, and from our work and that of others focusing on issues for young children and families during and after deployment, that provision of support and services for these military families will continue to be important.

ACKNOWLEDGMENTS

We thank the Rosen Center families for their service to our country, for the privilege of working with them, and for what we have learned from them. We also thank Elysa LeBron, LCSW, Clinical Director of the Rosen Center, for her contributions to the work described in this chapter.

NOTE

1. The work with Tom O'Malley was done by Jennifer M. Newman in consultation with Juliet M. Vogel. Elysa LeBron did the intake with this family and collaborated on the intake of Phase II.

REFERENCES

Barker, L. H., & Berry, K. D. (2009). Developmental issues impacting military families with young children during single and multiple deployments. *Military Medicine, 174,* 1033–1040.

Bowlby, J. (1972). *Attachment and loss: Vol. II. Separation: Anxiety and anger.* New York: Basic Books.

Chartrand, M. M., Frank, D. A., White, L. F., & Shope, T.R. (2008). Effects of parents' wartime deployment on the behavior of young children in military families. *Archives of Pediatrics and Adolescent Medicine, 162*(11), 1009–1014.

Hill, R. (1949). *Families under stress: Adjustment to the crisis of war separation and reunion.* New York: Harper.

ICF International. (n.d.). Demographics 2008 profile of the military community. Washington, DC: Office of the Deputy Under Secretary of Defense, Military Community and Family Policy. Retrieved April 11, 2010, from *cs.mhf.dod. mil/content/dav/mhf/qol-library/project%20documents/militaryhomefront/ reports/2008%20demographics.pdf.*

Institute of Medicine. (2010). *Returning home from Iraq and Afghanistan: Preliminary assessment of readjustent needs of veterans, service members, and their families.* Washington, DC: National Academies Press.

Jensen, P. S., Martin, D., & Watanabe, H. (1996). Children's response to parental separation during Operation Desert Storm. *Journal of the American Academy of Child and Adolescent Psychiatry, 35*(4), 433–441.

Kelly, M. L., Hock, E., Smith, K. M., Jarvis, M. S., Bonney, J. F., & Gaffney, M. A. (2001). Internalizing and externalizing behavior of children with enlisted Navy mothers experiencing military-induced separation. *Journal of the American Academy of Child and Adolescent Psychiatry, 40*(4), 464–471.

Lieberman, A., & Van Horn, P. (2008). *Psychotherapy with infants and young children: Repairing the effects of stress and trauma on attachment.* New York: Guilford Press.

McKay, M. M., Hibbert, R., Hoagwood, K., Rodriguez, J., Murray, L., Legerski, J., et al. (2004). Integrating evidence-based engagement interventions into "real world" child mental health settings. *Brief Treatment and Crisis Intervention, 4,* 177–186.

Piaget, J., & Inhelder, B. (1969). *The psychology of the child.* New York: Basic Books.

Robertson, J., & Robertson, J. (1989). *Separation and the very young.* Oxford, UK: Free Association Books.

Rosen, L. N., Teitelbaum, J. M., & Westhuis, D. J. (1993). Children's reactions to the Desert Storm deployment: Initial findings from a survey of Army families. *Military Medicine, 158,* 465–469.

Sesame Workshop. (2008). *Talk, listen, connect: Deployments and homecomings* [DVD]. Available at *www.sesameworkshop.org/initiatives/emotion/tlc.*

Skolmoski, S. (2006). *A paper hug.* Available at *www.apaperhug.com.*

CHAPTER 10

■ ■ ■ ■

Coming Together
Around Military Families

Dorinda Silver Williams
Lynette Fraga

Our purpose in this chapter is to offer a snapshot of Coming Together Around Military Families® (CTAMF®), a community-based response to the diverse, evolving needs of young children whose parents or caregivers have been affected by deployment-related stress, injury, and trauma.

Military families are remarkably strong and resilient, with a long history of navigating stressful circumstances and events in support of the service member's commitment to service and sacrifice. Nonetheless, the deployments to Iraq and Afghanistan, constituting the Global War on Terror (GWOT), have been prolonged and repeated (Shanker, 2008), posing potential challenges for even the healthiest of families. For a portion of military families, deployment-related separation and upheaval have become interwoven with the service member's physical injury (Grieger et al., 2006), psychological injury (Grieger et al., 2006); Kline et al., 2010; Schell & Marshall, 2008), or death (*www.icasualties.org*, 2010), constituting overlays of stress and trauma that may threaten the family's overall state of health and well-being.

The needs and interests of military families are inextricably linked with the needs and interests of their children, who represent a large percentage of the military community. Of the 1,365,571 Active Duty members in 2007, 43.1% had dependent children (Office of the Deputy Secretary Under Defense, 2007). Since September 11, 2001, more than 1 million children have had a parent deployed (Ramirez, 2009). Furthermore, at the time of the 2007 report by the Office of the Deputy Secretary Under Defense, 41% of Active Duty members' dependent children were age 5 and under, with 332,771 children between the ages of 0 and 3.

Recognizing the large numbers of children affected by parental combat deployment, Zero to Three extended its efforts to the military community and committed to raising awareness, sensitivity, and support of interdisciplinary professionals and parents/caregivers around building resilience in military families and their very young children. Through these initial efforts, the foundation to CTAMF was built.

CTAMF, developed to address the needs of babies and toddlers on a community level, aimed at strengthening community and agency responses to children and families affected by deployment-related stress and trauma. We have addressed our goals from many angles and perspectives to inform our interdisciplinary, collaborative approach to the work (Abramson & Mizrahi, 1996; Aronoff & Bailey, 2005; Bronstein, 2002, 2003). Additionally, early childhood stress and trauma were explored through the lens of neurobiology, culture, and strengths-based perspectives. Nonetheless, the CTAMF model holds, at its core, the theoretical underpinnings of attachment theory (Ainsworth, Blehar, Waters, & Wall, 1978; Bowlby, 1988). Underlying training, materials, and activities is the primary goal of facilitating optimal quality of caregiver–child relationships as a means of safeguarding early childhood social–emotional health and resilience in the context of potentially traumatic circumstances. To this end, we have employed multiple mechanisms of change, including awareness building, education, community coordination, and dialogue, all grounded in the concept of early caregiving relationships as potential mediators, or moderators, between stressful or traumatic family circumstances and child outcomes (Belsky & Fearon, 2002; Kim & Cicchetti, 2004; Lieberman & Van Horn, 2008).

CTAMF has expanded rapidly and exponentially, a reflection of both the resonance of the intervention components and the intensive need for support and services stemming from the sociopolitical forces that have impacted the military community for nearly a decade. The rapid growth may also be viewed as evidence of a paradigmatic shift in society's recognition of, and response to, the needs of military families and children, translating into the Department of Defense's significant emotional and financial investment into the emotional health and and well-being of military families affected by deployment.

In this chapter, we trace the origins and evolution of CTAMF as a framework for deconstructing its mechanisms of change, providing opportunity for readers to critique and evaluate the work and perhaps to integrate concepts or components into their own approach to moderating early childhood trauma. We share the CTAMF model as a representation of community strength and resilience in the face of adversity, as well as evidence of the enormous impact a small, modestly funded initiative can make when situated at the intersection of crisis and collaboration.

A PLACE TO BEGIN

The work unfolded against the backdrop of September 11, 2001. In the days following the attack, families with young children, like so many others, were still reeling from the shock and horror of the events that had unfolded on national television. Those events were being played out over and over again on virtually every news channel around the world. Families huddled around the television, trying to make sense of a senseless tragedy. Generations of family members, from the oldest to the youngest, sorted through collective feelings of sorrow, anger, confusion, and helplessness. We were in the midst of a national trauma. As our nation coped with the events surrounding September 11, 2001, our youngest children turned to their parents and caregivers for nurturance and reassurance.

Young children are remarkably adept at social referencing; they scan the emotions of others to assess their environment, using the information as a determinant for their own internal states (Campos & Steinberg, 1981). We witness this emotional pulse taking every day, evident in the countless exchanges between young children and the important adults in their lives. A father is playing with his 1-year-old in the park, heading toward the swing, when a flock of birds suddenly disbands, creating a whirling dervish of dust and wings. "What just happened?" the child wonders, thinking "How do I feel about this commotion? Am I safe? Let me look at Daddy. How is he feeling? He seems OK ... yep, still smiling. I guess I must be OK too." In the aftermath of September 11, 2001, many young children searched the faces of their distressed parents/caregivers, wondering "Am I OK?"

Recognizing how families and children might be affected by the events of September 11, 2001, Zero to Three developed *Little Listeners in an Uncertain World: Coping Strategies for You and Your Child after September 11* (Levine, 2002a), a brochure for parents and caregivers, intended to increase awareness and sensitivity around the child's experience of a stressful or traumatic situation. The title conveyed a core message: Very young children are "listening" to the important adults in their lives. Whether or not they understand the actual words, young children can absorb and internalize the charged emotions of their caregivers, interpreting nonverbal cues to construct their own meaning of a stressful or traumatic family event.

The inextricable link between parent and child emotional states emerged as a pervasive theme within the *Little Listeners* brochures. Very young children's capacities to manage, or regulate, their feelings and behaviors are still developing in the first years of life, and they rely heavily on their primary caregivers to help them modulate their strong and powerful emotions. When a mother is able to attend sensitively to her child's emotions, she creates moments of positive interaction that, over time, translate into optimal, trusting patterns of emotional communication, thereby influencing the child's goal-oriented efforts and development, as well as the growing capacity to manage his or her own emotional states (Siegel, 1999; Tronick, 1989). The caregiver's capacity to support his or her child in managing emotions is predicated on the caregiver's capacity to manage his or her own emotions (Slade, 2006). The *Little Listeners* content was reflective of these principles, encouraging parents/caregivers to attend to their own thoughts and feelings, seeking support as needed, as a fundamental step in promoting their children's emotional health and well-being. The message to parents and caregivers was clear: "The first step in taking care of your child is taking care of yourself" (Levine, 2002a, p. 1).

APPRECIATING THE UNIQUE CIRCUMSTANCES OF MILITARY FAMILIES

For military families there were additional considerations and concerns with which to contend. As they continued to process the shared loss of September 11, 2001, military families were faced with a unique, culturally specific crisis—the possibility of having a loved one deployed. Families knew that their military member could be called on, or in the case of National Guard and Reserve families, activated at any time. In the aftermath of the attack, there was tremendous uncertainty and, for some military families, feelings of anticipatory loss. While military families to varying degrees were accustomed to having their service member deployed overseas, this deployment was different. This was war.

Addressing the unique needs of military families was unchartered territory for Zero to Three, a civilian organization with no formal history of military-specific work and no extensive knowledge of the military culture. Lynette Fraga, then a Senior Program Associate at Zero to Three, had an extensive background serving the military community and was a strong advocate for military families. She had formed a productive working relationship and began to collaborate closely with various personnel at the Department of Defense and the Services. Dr. Fraga, through these working relationships, had also begun exploring the possibility of working collaboratively to address deployment and relocation, family stressors inherent to the military lifestyle. Now, following the events of September 11, 2001, these conversations assumed a newfound urgency.

In an interim, short-term response to the comprehensive needs of the military community, staff at Zero to Three acquired Department of Defense support to adapt the *Little Listeners* brochure, revising the content to reflect deployment-related concerns. The revised brochure, titled *Little Listeners in an Uncertain World: Coping Strategies for You and Your Child during Deployment or When a Crisis Occurs* (Levine, 2002b), captured fundamental concepts that would continue to permeate Zero to Three's efforts around military families. Concerns and strategies relating to caregiver awareness and sensitivity, normalization of emotions and experiences, early childhood behaviors and development, family member anticipatory guidance, the essentiality of maintaining routines, parent–child connectedness, and parental self-care continued to bubble up in trainings and materials, reflecting themes that, though culturally and contextually unique, were universal in respect to the core needs of families and babies under stress. Ultimately, these and similar themes would serve as organizers for the work of Military Projects at Zero to Three, constituting a flexible framework for addressing the needs of families caring for their babies and toddlers against the backdrop of extraordinary events and circumstances.

FORGING NEW RELATIONSHIPS

After the development and dissemination of the *Little Listeners* brochures, Zero to Three explored new ways to respond to the increasingly complex needs of its military constituents. Funding was secured for additional initiatives aimed at building awareness, resources, and collaborative efforts on behalf of military families and their very young children. The first initiative, taking inspiration from the development of the brochures, was informally titled *Little Listeners*. Funded through the McCormick Foundation, the small initiative was developed to serve Ft. Riley, a large Army installation in Manhattan, Kansas, and its surrounding community. Ft. Riley, home of the "Big Red One" (1st Infantry Division), was in the midst of a major upheaval. The increase in operations tempo (OPTEMPO), precipitated by the events of September 11, 2001, was overlaid with the anticipated influx of soldiers from far-flung installations designated for closure. Members of the Ft. Riley community, both on- and off-post, were working at a rapid-fire pace to build up its infrastructure in preparation for the transition. Homes were being constructed, and child care centers were being expanded as quickly as troops were being deployed. Although strengthened in its unity and commitment to mission, the Ft. Riley community was nonetheless under significant stress, creating risk factors for the emotional health and well-being of its families and young children.

The community of professionals working on and around Ft. Riley was already invested in promoting the needs and interests of babies and toddlers; programs and services were plentiful. The primary focus of the new initiative was to support the community in working more collaboratively and efficiently, combining and therefore maximizing resources and energy as a means of promoting coordinated and sustained efforts on behalf of families. A multidisciplinary method was utilized, thereby promoting a comprehensive, holistic approach to addressing the needs of service members' young children. In an effort to adopt a collaborative care model of promotion–prevention, in Phase I a variety of professionals, including early childhood educators, medical personnel, mental health providers, and family support professionals, were convened to ensure that all areas of health and development were addressed. In the first phase of the work, Zero to Three staff played a consultative role, assessing community infant mental heath needs and strengths, providing early childhood materials on a range of topics relevant to the military community, and organizing and facilitating discussion groups and trainings. This approach was part of the evolving multidisciplinary training and consultation framework that would eventually undergird the CTAMF initiative. Zero to Three staff members attached to the Ft. Riley work had their own personal connections to the military community, a potential benefit in initiating trusting professional relationships grounded in understanding and respect for the military culture.

In 2005, Phase II of the McCormick-funded initiative began. Zero to Three staff convened the Little Listeners committee, a long-standing workgroup that comprised early childhood professionals representing agencies both on-post and in the surrounding community. The purpose of the meeting was to create space and opportunity for the staff to conduct an interim community needs assessment, the findings of which would inform the activities of Phase II. Zero to Three staff presented newly developed informational articles related to supporting young children through relocation and deployment. "Thank you, but no thank you," the committee responded politely, but definitively. Parents, they explained, were stressed. Parents in some families were overwhelmed. Parents were being bombarded with information and resources but had little, if any, time to use it. Parents were being stretched, pulled, and twisted in every direction as they balanced the demands of war with the demands of caring for their babies and toddlers. Parents had neither the time nor the inclination to sort through pages and pages of reading. As Zero to Three staff listened and learned, an unspoken question hung in the air: "What now?"

Committee members emphasized the need to provide basic information about the needs of babies and toddlers in a format that was easily accessible to families. Dual-purpose items, such as refrigerator magnets and utility bills, were recommended as opportunities to integrate core messages into existing tasks or resources. A theme was beginning to emerge; in an effort to meet the multiple, conflicting demands of wartime deployment, parents and caregivers were multitasking. In order to help them support their babies, the staff needed to cut through the noise and chaos of parents' daily lives and present the information in a manner that could be "heard" and understood. As the discussion continued, the staff took copious notes, scribbling down comments, suggestions, and insights—gaining increased clarity over the direction of the work.

Upon their return to the office, the Military Projects staff conferred with other staff members at Zero to Three, including members of the Communications Department, in an effort to operationalize some of the thoughts and ideas generated during the Little Listeners panel meeting. These brainstorming sessions translated into a series of focused materials and activities, constituting what might best be described as a minimedia campaign for the Ft. Riley community. The materials included flyers, posters, and photo frame magnets, each of which communicated core messages relating to the needs of babies and toddlers in the context of military-specific stressors. The posters and flyers were disseminated to multiple agencies, on- and off-post, so that professionals working with military families with young children could make the content available and accessible to parents and caregivers. These agencies included child care centers, programs within the family support center, and medical facilities. The flyers were distributed to the main shopping facilities on the installation, including the commissary and the exchange. Articles were developed and distributed, but rather than placing the articles directly into the busy hands of families, efforts were focused on integrating the articles into the larger community landscape by inserting them into publications and resources already being accessed by families. As part of the coordinated effort, Zero to Three staff provided the camera-ready articles to the on-post newspaper; the articles were run as part of an ongoing series focusing on a range of issues related to families and young children. By connecting all of these diverse, visible, and accessible agencies, the media campaign served to expand the collaborative, multidisciplinary theme that had permeated Phase I of the Ft. Riley work. The campaign facilitated a comprehensive effort, addressing the needs and interests of families on multiple levels, and from a range of perspectives. The campaign was titled *Coming Together Around Military Separation: Supporting our Babies and Toddlers*, a reflection of the collaborative intent and focus of the community efforts.

In addition to these materials, a children's book was developed for young children whose parents were deployed. The book was multilayered in its intent, encompassing the following goals: to provide comfort and reassurance to a young child whose parent is away on deployment; to keep the deployed parent and child emotionally connected; to give the parent/caregiver at home the words and encouragement to talk about the deployed parent's absence, thus supporting the child in constructing a meaningful narrative about the deployment experience; to support the child in experiencing and integrating the duality of having a parent who is physically absent, yet "holding" the child in his or her heart and thoughts; to encourage story time and reading as an opportunity for the parent/caregiver at home to engage in nurturing activities and interactions to promote constancy and mutuality in the context of family stress and loss; and to provide reassurance to the deployed parent of his or her emotional presence in the home, thereby fostering opportunity for an optimal reintegration experience.

The authors' goals were grounded in the knowledge that stories can help family members create and internalize shared understandings of difficult events. Through storytelling, the parent is able to support the child in organizing these events, constructing a rich, coherent narrative in which the child can make sense and meaning out of his experiences (May, 2005; Siegel, 1999; Siegel & Hartzell, 2003). Ultimately, the narrative may serve as an emotional road map to guide and sustain parent and child during their long and arduous family journey, facilitating opportunities to foster connectedness, security, attunement, and mutuality in the relationship (May, 2005; Siegel, 1999; Siegel & Hartzell, 2003), even in the context of emotionally strenuous circumstances. In this sense, the story informs the intricate relational choreography of the parent–child dance, providing emotional nourishment that, ultimately, may promote family resilience.

It is likely that, for some families, the idea of talking with young children about the service member's deployment may evoke questions and anxieties:

"What words do I use?"
"What if I say the wrong thing?"
"What kinds of emotions might I stir up in my child?"
"What kinds of emotions might I stir up in myself?"
"My child has finally stopped asking about her daddy. Do I want to get her started all over again?"
"What if he asks questions I don't know how to answer?"

These are legitimate concerns, grounded in the pain and confusion of parenting young children in the context of emotionally charged circumstances. In this respect, the children's book is not a directive for parents to talk about the deployment; rather, it is a supportive tool, available to the parent when, and if, the time feels right to help the child make sense of the service member's absence.

Flyers and posters were also developed and distributed throughout Ft. Riley as part of the early childhood media campaign. These materials offered digestible nuggets of information related to caring for young children in the midst of military-specific stress. The text, though simple and sparse, captured central themes and offered substantive strategies for parents and caregivers. The content was anchored in the experiences of young children, providing developmental context and normalizing early childhood responses to change and stress. Overall, the flyers were inviting and engaging; the "voice" and face of the baby were featured prominently. "Don't even talk to me before I've had my morning milk," warned the sleepy baby, hands covering his face as if to ward off the demands of the day. The message to parents/caregivers followed: "Try to keep routines the same during separations and relocations to help babies and toddlers feel more secure." Each of the seven flyers engaged the reader in a similar way, communicating the child's experience with gentle humor and compassion.

The child's experience of the deployment was associated with the child's internal state. Internal states constitute a wide range of mental experiences, including affect, cognitions, beliefs, wants, and intentions (Fonagy, Gergely, Jurist, & Target, 2004; Slade, 2007). The parent's capacity to consider his or her child's, as well as his or her own internal states, constitutes "reflective functioning," or mentalization, which plays a critical role in supporting early childhood emotional health and development. In recent years, there has been a growing awareness of reflective functioning as an essential instrument in facilitating healthy parent–child representations and, ultimately, in deepening the parent's ability to engage in loving, nurturing interactions with the young child, the understanding of which has translated into new parent–child programs that specifically target reflective functioning as a desired outcome (Slade, 2007). In this respect, the overarching purpose of the flyers and posters was to increase sensitivity to the child's perspective, promoting reflective functioning on the part of the parent/caregiver in relation to military-specific stressors and events.

Through the materials, parents/caregivers were invited into their children's internal world. Indeed, they were encouraged, in a nonthreatening but compelling manner, to think about the child's perception of the events and circumstances affecting the family as a whole, thereby allowing them, as described by Slade (2007), to experience their children as unique and separate individuals, capable of experiencing their own thoughts and feelings.

It is important to emphasize that the tools and strategies utilized in this campaign were on a macro-level, with no direct services provided by Zero to Three. The materials did not address specific family dynamics, apart from the deployment and relocation stressors common to all military families. In this respect, the materials were part of a community-oriented promotion and prevention event. Nonetheless, the materials reflected some of the helpful factors identified in interventions geared toward strengthening the quality of the parent–child relationship, including enhancement of reflective functioning (Slade, 2007), consideration and validation of the parent/caregiver's experience and feelings (Lieberman & Van Horn, 2008), and opportunities to construct a coherent family narrative (May, 2005; Saltzman et al., 2009;

Siegel, 1999). Any situation or event has the potential to impact families in ways that undermine the parent–child relationship, threatening the developmental trajectory of the child (Lieberman & Van Horn, 2008). For the Ft. Riley community, even the healthiest families were experiencing change or loss. For those families with preexisting dynamics that could impair parental care and responsiveness, such as maternal depression, financial difficulties, marital discord, histories of maltreatment, or other contextual risk factors, the military-specific stressors created additional, significant layers of relational risk. The materials were designed to respond to these stressors through the provision of information and resources, within the confines of a macro-level approach. Resource contact information was included on each piece of material, so that families could reach out for help and support as needed. Additionally, professionals were strongly encouraged to utilize the materials in the context of their psychotherapeutic or educational relationships with their parent/caregiver clients. In this respect, the materials could be used as conversation starters or empathy builders, eliciting the thoughts and feelings of both parent and child, and ultimately promoting sessions in which the parent–child relationship could be strengthened in the context of a warm, nurturing, and emotionally safe professional relationship.

EXPANDING OUR REACH

In 2006, Military Projects received funding from the Iraq Afghanistan Deployment Impact Fund (IADIF) administered by the California Community Foundation to expand its efforts to 12 military installations and two medical centers around the country. Additional staff was hired to accommodate the rapid growth and development of the work. The new efforts, referred to as the Coming Together Around Military Families (CTAMF) initiative, rested heavily on its foundational efforts; existing materials were modified and new materials were developed to meet the evolving needs of families. The *Over There* book, which had been soft bound, was reprinted as a board book, more conducive to the exuberant handling of a baby or toddler. Another board book, *I'm Here for You Now,* which had originally been developed for a Zero to Three initiative supporting young children impacted by Hurricane Katrina, was now made available for distribution to the CTAMF sites. The book was filled with reassuring messages, as well as suggestions for caregiver–child interactive activities, as a means of fostering caregiver responsiveness and parent–child engagement in the context of stressful and traumatic circumstances.

New materials included a DVD that depicted the experiences, challenges, strengths, and insights of families experiencing deployment that had babies and toddlers. In addition to providing opportunities for families to see their experiences reflected in the experiences of others, the DVDs included tips and strategies from both parents and professionals. Installations were encouraged to run the DVDs in family-oriented waiting areas, to distribute them directly to families, and to use them as an opportunity to engage with parents/caregivers around the family's deployment experiences. In addition, another children's board book, titled *Home Again,* was developed for the purpose of supporting families through the reintegration experience. The content was reflective of the child's perspective, depicting stories of babies and toddlers experiencing the return of their military parent. The book captured a range of responses in an effort to normalize family members' experiences and reactions, as well as to offer anticipatory guidance to parents and caregivers to help them prepare for the inherent uncertainties of the reunion.

Each of these new and revised materials, including the posters, flyers, magnets, and camera-ready articles from the Ft. Riley campaign, were packaged in an attractive, user-friendly kit box as a means of integrating and consolidating the resources. The kit box, with its sturdy handle, allowed greater flexibility in multidisciplinary use. The therapist, pediatrician, or obstetrician-gynecologist could keep the kit box on the shelf, sharing its contents during office visits; the home visitor could keep the kit in his or her car, sharing its contents during parent–child visits; and the early childhood educator could keep his or her kit in the shared resource cabinet, sharing its contents during a parent pick-up or meeting. A newly developed professional guide, offering a description of the materials and suggestions for use of the materials in a variety of settings, was included in the resource kit.

FOCUS ON TRAUMA

During this period of transition, there was a growing awareness and understanding of the intensity of the issues and challenges affecting military families. The deployments had been going on for years, and there was no indication of a reduction in forces any time soon. The sustained increase in OPTEMPO affected not only the persons deployed but also those who remained behind, working to fill the roles of those who were overseas. For military families, the extended, repeated deployments created a shift in relational dynamics, forming a new set of rules by which to negotiate the phases of deployment. Whereas the family's experience of deployment had typically been characterized as cyclical in nature (Pincus, House, Christenson, & Adler, 2010), it was now, according to some families, assuming the shape and energy of a spiral (National Military Families Association [NMFA], 2006). According to the authors of the NMFA report, a pattern was emerging in which family members were taking their unresolved issues or concerns into the next deployment, never returning to their original pre-deployment state.

During this same year, a study released by Rentz and colleagues (2007) examined the rates of child maltreatment in military families. The data suggested that within the state of Texas, the rate of substantiated maltreatment in military families on or after October 1, 2002, compared to before October 2002, had approximately doubled. According to the authors, the incidence of child maltreatment increased by 28% for every 1% increase in the percentage of Active Duty service members with at least one child, who *departed* to an operational deployment, and by 31% for every 1% increase in the percentage of Active Duty service members, with at least one child, who *returned* from an operational deployment (Rentz et al., 2007). In a study released the following year, Gibbs, Martin, Kupper, and Johnson (2007) found that in the families of enlisted U.S. Army soldiers who had at least one substantiated report of child maltreatment, the rates of maltreatment were consistently higher when the service members were on combat-related deployment.

The emerging research on families and children dovetailed with new studies on the returning service member and the physical and psychological injuries he or she sustained as a result of the GWOT (American Psychological Association Presidential Task Force on Military Deployment Services for Youth, Families, and Service Members, 2007; Hoge, Auchterlonie, & Milliken, 2006; Vasterling et al., 2006). For families whose service member experienced physical injury, emotional injury, and/or traumatic brain injury, reunion occurred against a backdrop of significant loss and adjustment. Many military families experienced the permanent loss of their service member; as of May 2010, approximately 5,464 U.S. military personnel serving in Iraq or Afghanistan were killed (see *www.icasualties.org*). It was evident that as the repeated prolonged combat deployments continued, military families were being exposed to, and impacted by traumatic situations and events, and that the implications for the health and well-being of young children whose parents or caregivers were struggling with these issues demanded attention.

There was, and continues to be, a paucity of research on the effects of parental combat deployment on babies and toddlers (American Psychological Association Presidential Task Force on Military Deployment Services for Youth, Families, and Service Members, 2007; Chartrand & Siegel, 2007). Although there is extant research focusing on the Vietnam War service member, many of the studies were conducted decades after the return of the veteran (Jakupcak et al., 2007) and focused on older or adult children. Nonetheless, these studies offered a glimpse into the lives and interactions of families and children affected by a parent's exposure to combat deployment. Several studies indicated a relationship between paternal combat deployment experience and children's behavioral problems (Glenn et al., 2002; Kulka et al., 1990; Matsakis, 1988; Rosenheck & Fontana, 1998), as well as a negative relationship between severity of maternal combat-related PTSD and parenting satisfaction (Gold et al., 2007).

More recent research focusing specifically on infant/toddler–parent relationships in the context of combat deployment was minimal, forcing the early childhood research community to use data compiled outside of military-specific circumstances. Previous studies had found predictive relationships between maternal PTSD and child behavioral challenges (Lieberman, Van Horn, & Ozer, 2005). However, this research involved mothers and young children exposed to domestic violence, not combat-related trauma. Other findings suggested concerning relationships between maternal depression and children's early dysregulation patterns and competence ratings (Maughan, Cicchetti, Toth, & Rogosch, 2007). Findings from a study by Forman and colleagues (2007) suggested that mothers who experienced and were treated for postpartum depression continued to rate their children lower in attachment security, higher in behavior problems, and more negative in temperament than did mothers without diagnosed depression.

Caution was exercised in extrapolating these findings to the emotional health of the military family impacted by combat deployment stress and trauma. The military population was experiencing its own inimitable circumstances, shaped by culturally unique values, strengths, and resources that potentially could buffer the effects of combat deployment and promote family. Nonetheless, these findings suggested that, as service member parents continued to return with increased levels of psychological distress, including depression and PTSD, it was imperative that helping professionals continue to assess and mitigate potential parent–child relational challenges resulting from the impaired psychological health of the returning parent.

A SHIFT IN APPROACH

In the face of parental injury and death, the Military Projects work was taken to a deeper, more intensive level of response. A new, trauma-oriented component was incorporated into the CTAMF scope of work. Duty to Care: Supporting our Babies and Toddlers During Challenging Times, a 2-day, comprehensive training effort, focused on identifying and addressing the needs of babies and toddlers affected by specific combat deployment stressors, including parent/caregiver emotional distress, psychological injury, physical injury, traumatic brain injury, and death. The training was divided into a series of modules, each of which addressed the social–emotional health of babies and toddlers from a different perspective.

The structure and coordination of the training were consistent with the CTAMF collaborative, community-based approach to military families and their young children. The content was developed and organized to meet the needs of a broad, multidisciplinary audience, representing a wide range of roles and agencies with varying levels of knowledge around early childhood health and development. The intention was to maximize community responsiveness by engaging professionals from multiple ports of entry, ranging from the nurse who chatted with families during well-baby checkups to the early childhood educator who soothed frazzled parents and caregivers during early morning drop-offs. In an effort to strengthen collaborative relationships across military and civilian communities, installation representatives were encouraged to invite early childhood professionals serving military families "outside the gates" to participate as well.

The multidisciplinary approach, though a tremendous strength, was also a significant challenge to the development and facilitation of the trainings. The professional differences served to enrich, as well as to complicate, the training experience. The content needed to be responsive to the diverse needs of an audience that comprised professionals from multiple educational and professional backgrounds, each interacting with military families in a manner consistent with its unique agency role, function, and perspective. Individual learning styles and military cultural diversity needed to be accommodated as well. In order to address these challenges, the content was diversified, encompassing a range of themes and topics reflecting varying levels of complexity, and offering relevance and application to any professional working on behalf military families and their babies and toddlers. The sessions combined a didactic and interactive approach, creating space and opportunity for ongoing dialogue and engagement. Experiential activities accommodated diverse learning styles and provided networking opportunities throughout the 2 days of training. Participants were strongly encouraged to share resources, strategies, and perspectives in an effort to moderate fragmentation of services and to promote opportunities for community collaboration and synergy. Finally, the training sessions were facilitated by consultants who embodied a wide range of backgrounds and expertise. Indeed, the professional composition of the consultant trainers was reflective of the professional diversity of the Duty to Care I audience members. Each training session was facilitated by two consultant trainers and coordinated by a Zero to Three staff member in an effort to optimize multidisciplinary responsiveness. As Zero to Three continued to build its reputation as a trusted, knowledgeable friend and partner to the military community, efforts were made to ensure that at least one member of the training team was immersed in the military culture, whether personally or professionally, at each Duty to Care training event.

Prior to the initial training, a 2-day Train the Trainers session was conducted to maximize facilitator familiarity with, and fidelity to, the training content. Train the Trainers also provided a critical opportunity to foster appreciation for the military community as its own culture, with members holding both individual and culturally shared, values, beliefs, and norms. The facilitators were encouraged to be mindful of their presence on the installations as invited guests, and to communicate respect for the installation leadership and the community as a whole. In this respect, cultural competence played a major role in the efficacy of the training, facilitating a trust and openness that served to enhance participants' responsiveness to the content and dialogue.

The first module of Duty to Care I, titled *Infants and Toddlers: Helping Them to Thrive*, provided core information about the developmental needs of babies and toddlers. It served as a refresher for participants immersed in infant mental health, or as a foundation for participants newly acquainted with the early childhood population. During this session, participants were oriented to the strengths and challenges of the military culture, the stressors of which were introduced as potential overlays of normative parental stress. The intent of this initial session was to expand participants' awareness and sensitivity to early childhood responses to change and parental stress, setting the stage for later discussion of deployment-related family trauma.

The second session, titled Building Healthy Minds, provided basic information about the influence of early childhood interactions and relationships on the developing brain. Areas of focus included neuronal exuberance, brain plasticity and "wiring," and early childhood memory development. This content served as a bridge to the next session, Babies' Brains and Stress, which encouraged participants to consider the invisible line between stress and trauma. The content-laden Babies' Brains and Stress session delved deeply into the neurobiological implications of stress and trauma on early childhood health and development as a means of communicating the exigency of safeguarding the interests of families and their young children in the context of potentially traumatic circumstances. The session ended with an overview of the SERVE approach in response to the needs and interests of military families and their young children. SERVE constituted the following areas of intervention: Supporting the child and family; Expanding the family's understanding of what their child might be experiencing in the context of an appropriate developmental framework; Referring the family to supportive resources; being a Voice for babies by supporting parents in understanding their children's needs and giving their children the words to express themselves during difficult times; and Engaging with families to assess fully their strengths and needs.

The next session, Peeling the Onion, explored specific issues affecting military families in the context of combat deployment. These were deli-

cate, culturally embedded issues. Each was unpacked carefully and sensitively, with the understanding that traumatic circumstances did not necessarily translate into traumatization for the service member or his or her
children (Cozza, 2007); each family, given its individual internal and external resources, would respond differently to any given set of circumstances.
Nonetheless, extended and/or repeated separations, parental physical injury,
parental psychological injury, and parental death constituted significant
stressors that, over time, could erode the coping skills of even the strongest families. Participants were encouraged to dig into their professional
"toolkits," brainstorm, and exchange strategies and resources on behalf
of families experiencing these extraordinary circumstances. In this respect,
participants were acknowledged as the "on the ground" experts they were.
The training offered opportunities for these professionals, already immersed
in the family's struggles, to examine the issues from the child's perspective;
to gain fresh insights and clarity; and to share their expertise, resources, and
"lessons learned" with fellow participants. Ultimately, in spite of the emotional heaviness of the content, the primary intent of the Peeling the Onion
was to instill a sense of hope and efficacy on both an individual and community level in responding to the intensive needs of families and children. This
overarching objective, in fact, underscored the training as a whole.

The final session of the Duty to Care I training, titled Building Resilience
in Ourselves: Awareness and Self-Care, provided a brief overview of compassion fatigue and secondary trauma, the potential by-products of caring
for families and children affected by trauma and loss. Tools and strategies to
promote individual wellness were discussed. The 2-day training ended with
the reminder that professional self-care is as important as parental self-care
in promoting community responsiveness in addressing the needs and interests of babies and toddlers, a theme that would drive the development of the
follow-up training, Duty to Care II: Honoring the Healer.

The Honoring the Healer 1-day training was developed in recognition of the deleterious effects that exposure to clients' traumatic material
can have on the caring professional (Collins & Long, 2003; Figley, 1995).
In fact, professionals who bear witness to children's emotional pain might
be particularly vulnerable to internalizing this distress and, consequently,
having their personal lives disrupted (Fenichel, 1992/2005; Figley, 1995;
Osofsky, 2004). Emotional fatigue can jeopardize the integrity of the helping relationship (Barrett, 2008) and eventually translate into professional
erosion (Osofsky, 2007). The Honoring the Healer training experience represented an opportunity for early childhood professionals to explore the
potential cost of their work and to strategize ways to safeguard their own
emotional health as a means of safeguarding the emotional health of the
families and children they served. In keeping with the theme of the "parallel process," in which the quality of the helping relationship is informed by

the quality of the supervisory relationship (Parlakian & Seibel, 2001), the concept of reflective practice in the infant–family setting—the examination of thoughts, feelings, behaviors, and responses that emerge in the context of intensive interactions and experiences with families and their very young children (Eggbeer, Mann, & Siebel, 2007)—was introduced as a systemic tool to strengthen professional resilience. The 1-day training effort utilized both didactic and experiential approaches, with an emphasis on self-explo-ration, open dialogue, and self-care exercises and activities, including the development of a personal self-care plan as a means of operationalizing each participant's proposed behavioral changes.

Ready Reserve Families

Throughout the work, there has been a growing sensitivity to the unique and complex challenges of the Ready Reserve. As of fiscal year 2007, the Ready Reserve constituted 31% of the total military force. These men and women, consisting of the Selected Reserve, the individual Ready Reserve, and the Inactive National Guard (Office of the Deputy Under Secretary of Defense, 2007), have been called upon heavily during the GWOT. As of late 2009, over 64% of the Reserve force had experienced recent deployments (Baker, 2009). As the families of Reservists have continued to negotiate the stressors of combat deployment, many have been caring for young children. According to the Office of the Deputy Under Secretary of Defense (2007) demographics report, there were 104,505 children of Selected Reserve mem-bers, ages 0–3, in 2007. Of the total number of children of Selected Reserv-ists, 24.7% were between the ages of 0 and 5.

The Selected Reservists and their families are subject to special circum-stances that can exacerbate the inherent stressors of wartime deployment. When the service member is deployed, he or she is first activated, a pro-cess that can engender disruptions within the family household, including changes in insurance and income. Typically, the Ready Reservist is embed-ded within the civilian community, distanced from the multiplicity of ser-vices and resources readily available on installation (American Psychologi-cal Association Presidential Task Force on Military Deployment Services for Youth, Families, and Service Members, 2007; NMFA, 2006). Family members may be left to cope on their own, isolated from military commu-nity members who share the common cultural experience of having a loved one deployed.

The circumstances of the Ready Reservists and their families warrant services that are commensurate with their unique service and sacrifice. Mili-tary Projects staff initially addressed the needs of the Selected Reservists by making content available on the Web, accessible to families who were geographically scattered. As the work progressed, the staff became increasingly intentional in focus, working synergistically and collaboratively with representatives from various state and family agencies to promote sensitivity and responsiveness to the needs of babies and toddlers of Selected Reserve families. An activities guide, titled "Kiddies on Guard," was developed and piloted in 2009. The guide, filled with fun, developmentally appropriate ideas and exercises, was designed for use during existing National Guard family events were taking place around the country. These events provided information, resources, and social networking opportunities for geographically dispersed families whose service member was deployed. Many of the "Kiddies on Guard" activities focused on maintaining parent–child connections through creative projects and correspondence, fostering opportunities for family members to celebrate and chronicle their children's developmental milestones and to communicate their children's growth and development to the deployed parent. In this respect, maintaining parent–child mutuality between the child and caregiver at home, as well as the child and the parent abroad, remained a conceptual cornerstone of the work.

As Military Projects continued to concentrate its efforts on addressing the issues of parental injury, trauma, and loss, the importance of translating these efforts to Selected Reservist families became evident. Additional support was provided by the Department of Defense to bring components of the CTAMF activities, including the Duty to Care I and II training and materials dissemination, to 15 states supporting Joint Family Support Assistance Programs (JFSAP) providing services to National Guard and Reservist families. These efforts lay the groundwork for replication on a larger scale, creating opportunity to expand the reach of the training to professionals and families across many more states and agencies.

In the final phase of the CTAMF initiative, a new set of materials was developed to respond to the needs of families and their young children affected by the complications of combat deployment, including parental physical injury, psychological injury, and death. Although the professional guide was comprehensive in content, delineating considerable information on each of the issues, the "voice" of the professional guide remained conversational and informal in tone. The guide was intended to serve as both a source of information and comfort to the weary professional, weighed down by the heaviness of the issues with which he or she helped families cope. The parent/caregiver brochures reflected the content of the professional guide pared down to the bare essentials, presented in a warm, compassionate tone. Both the professional guide and the parent brochures were filled with charts, titled "In a Child's Words," which explored the meaning of children's behavior in the context of specific situations or events and offered parents/caregivers guidance in responding to their children's behavior and needs. These scenarios addressed a wide range of difficult or traumatic situations, from preparing for deployment to visiting the injured service member in the hospital, to supporting the child during a service member parent's memorial service. While the professional guide encompassed all of these different topics and scenarios, each of the parent brochures was specifically devoted to a single issue, either parental injury or parental death.

Several professionals and family members were interviewed in order to honor and reflect the experiences of those the materials would serve. The materials were infused with the stories, quotes, and strategies of individuals who shared their experiences as an opportunity to help other parents or professionals navigate similar situations and events. A panel of multidisciplinary professionals was enlisted to review the materials throughout the development process, both to maximize quality assurance and to maintain the multidisciplinary, collaborative approach that has been an integral part of the CTAMF work.

NEXT STEPS

As the war persists, so, too, do the demands and challenges imposed on military families. These extraordinary circumstances warrant extraordinary measures that capture the extensiveness and complexity of military families' developing needs. Military Projects staff members continue to build on previous efforts, strengthening and deepening existing, collaborative relationships and expanding the reach and availability of the current training and materials. New partnerships are cultivated as an opportunity to promote innovative ideas and practices, in anticipation of the evolving needs of military families and their young children who have been impacted by parental physical injury, psychological injury, and loss.

Because of the success of the pilot and continued support from the Department of Defense, Military Projects was able to replicate CTAMF on an international scale in 2009, providing training, materials, and consultation to 22 installations and six medical treatment facilities around the world. Additionally, support included the addition of 37 states, with the task of supporting Selected Reservist families, to receive Duty to Care I and II training. The enormous expansion of the work will create the opportunity to reach thousands of families and professionals, facilitating community awareness and collaboration on a massive scale.

The Military Projects staff has, at times, been challenged in its efforts to navigate the unique and complicated landscape of the medical centers. The task of the medical center community is the dual role of supporting both its own "neighborhood" of deploying personnel, and the service member patients and their families who are navigating the intensive circumstances of combat injury and recovery. In this respect, the portal of entry for the CTAMF work has felt like a moving target, and the staff has sometimes struggled to meet its intended mark. In an effort to enhance the integrity of the work, Military Projects has procured the specialized skills of a family physician who understands the professional and cultural needs of the medical community, and can coordinate and facilitate the trainings at a more optimal level. In addition, a new children's book, specifically focused on the needs of young children whose parents have experienced physical or psychological injury, has been drafted. Military Projects staff is exploring funding options to develop and disseminate the book to medical treatment facilities, as well as other installation- and community-based agencies supporting injured service members and their families.

A pilot initiative, sponsored by the Florida BrAIve Fund, is being spearheaded as an additional opportunity to support the medical community. New materials and trainings are being developed to assist installation- and community-based medical practitioners across North Florida in an effort to facilitate awareness and skills building around deployment-related issues and to engage families around these issues in the context of the pediatric/family practice setting.

Knowing What We Do Not Know

It is evident that military personnel are being affected by wartime deployment. In a 2008 RAND study by Schell and Marshall, the authors found that among personnel previously deployed as part of Operation Enduring Freedom or Operation Iraqi Freedom (OEF/OIF), 14% met criteria for probable PTSD, 14% met criteria for probable major depressive disorder (MDD), and 19% met the criteria for having experienced a probable traumatic brain injury (TBI). It is reasonable to assume that a portion of those returning home with visible or invisible injuries are parents of young children. Nonetheless, there remain very limited data regarding the short- and long-term implications of the service member parent's deployment-related psychological distress on babies and toddlers—a gaping hole in today's early childhood trauma literature.

Building Our Knowledge Base

Military families are negotiating affective terrain that heretofore has remained largely unexplored. In order to be fully responsive to the babies and toddlers whose military parents have been deployed, injured, or killed, we must have a strong sense of how these particular issues, within this specific context, play out in the emotional lives of very young children. Additional research is needed to assess risk and resilience in infants and toddlers in the context of extended and multiple deployments, reintegration, varying levels of support and resources, parental physical injury, and parental emotional illness. Longitudinal studies are needed to assess the health and well-being of infants and toddlers over time so that the longer-term implications for young children and their military families impacted by combat deployment are addressed.

Military Projects staff has a responsibility to ensure that the social–emotional needs and concerns that have been raised are now appropriately addressed through the collection and analysis of relevant data. As informed advocates, we have a professional obligation to extend our professional relationship to the scientific community, articulating the research questions that speak directly to the interests of babies and toddlers. In recognition of this responsibility, Military Projects staff has received funding from the IADIF of the California Community Foundation to promote the development of a research agenda that focuses specifically on infant and toddler outcomes, risk factors, and protective factors in the context of military-specific parental stress and trauma. The funding will support the formation of a research panel that comprises early childhood experts, policy experts, trauma experts, bereavement experts, military family support experts, and researchers. These assembled stakeholders will pool their knowledge and expertise to explore the research that exists, identify research gaps, formulate research questions, exchange ideas and resources in support of accumulating the research, and advance a commitment to evaluative research that studies the efficacy of new and existing assessments and treatments in support of babies and toddlers of military families affected by wartime deployment.

The studies that result from the research panel will inform the long-term efforts of Military Projects, ensuring a depth of knowledge commensurate with the complexity of the issues being addressed. It is anticipated that, ultimately, the research agenda will translate into well-informed, early-childhood policies, programs, and services designed to prevent or attenuate the transmission of military combat trauma from one generation to another.

REFERENCES

Abramson, J. S., & Mizrahi, T. (1996). When social workers and physicians collaborate: Positive and negative interdisciplinary experiences. *Social Work, 41*(3), 270–281.

Ainsworth, M. D., Blehar, M. C., Waters, E., & Wall, S. (1978). *Patterns of attachment: Assessed in the strange situation and at home.* Hillsdale, NJ: Erlbaum.

American Psychological Association Presidential Task Force on Military Deployment Services for Youth, Families, and Service Members. (2007, February). The psychological needs of U.S. military service members and their families: A preliminary report. Retrieved January 11, 2010, from *www.apa.org/about/governance/council/policy/military-deployment-services.pdf.*

Aronoff, N. L., & Bailey, D. (2005). Partnered practice: Building on our small group tradition. *Social Work with Groups, 28*(1), 23–37.

Baker, F. W., III. (2009). Forces progress in transition to operational reserve. Arlington, VA: National Guard Bureau. Retrieved January 11, 2010, from *www. ng.mil/news/archives/2009/10/101909-forces.aspx.*

Barrett, M. J. (2008, March). *Ethical boundaries.* Presentation at the Networker Symposium, Washington, DC.

Belsky, J., & Fearon, R. M. P. (2002). Infant–mother attachment security, contextual risk, and early development: A moderational analysis. *Development and Psychopathology, 14*(2), 293–310.

Bowlby, J. (1988). *A secure base: Parent–child attachment and healthy human development.* New York: Basic Books.

Bronstein, L. R. (2002). Index of interdisciplinary collaboration. *Social Work Research, 26*(2), 113–126.

Bronstein, L. R. (2003). A model for interdisciplinary collaboration. *Social Work, 48*(3), 297–306.

Campos, J., & Stenberg, C. (1981). Perception, appraisal, and emotion: The onset of social referencing. In M. E. Lamb & L. R. Sherrod (Eds.), *Infant social cognition: Empirical and theoretical considerations* (pp. 273–314). Hillsdale, NJ: Erlbaum.

Chartrand, M. M., & Siegel, B. (2007). At war in Iraq and Afghanistan: Children in U.S. military families. *Ambulatory Pediatrics, 7*(1), 1–2.

Collins, S., & Long, A. (2003). Working with the psychological effects of trauma: Consequences for mental health-care workers—a literature review. *Journal of Psychiatric and Mental Health Nursing, 10,* 417–424.

Cozza, S. J. (2007, April). *Children of combat veterans.* Presentation at the Coming Together Around Military Families® Consultant Orientation, Washington, DC.

Eggbeer, L., Mann, T.L., & Seibel, N. (2007). Reflective supervision: Past, present, and future. *Zero to Three, 28*(2), 5–9.

Fenichel, E. (Ed.). (2005). *Learning through supervision and mentorship to support the development of infants, toddlers and their families: A sourcebook.* Arlington, VA: Zero to Three. (Original work published 1992)

Figley, C. R. (1995). Compassion fatigue as secondary traumatic stress disorder: An overview. In C. R. Figley (Ed.), *Compassion fatigue: Coping with secondary traumatic stress disorder in those who treat the traumatized* (pp. 1–20). New York: Brunner/Mazel.

Fonagy, P., Gergely, G., Jurist, E. L., & Target, M. (2004). *Affect regulation, mentalization, and the development of the self.* London: Karnac.

Forman, D. R., O'Hara, M. W., Stuart, S., Gorman, L. L., Larsen, K. E., & Coy, K. C. (2007). Effective treatment for postpartum depression is not sufficient to improve the developing mother–child relationship. *Development and Psychopathology, 19,* 585–602.

Gibbs, D. A., Martin, S. L., Kupper, L. L., & Johnson, R. E. (2007). Child maltreatment in enlisted soldiers' families during combat-related deployments. *Journal of the American Medical Association, 298*(5), 528–535.

Glenn, D. M., Beckham, J. C., Feldman, M. E., Kirby, A. C., Hertzberg, M. A., &

Moore, S. D. (2002). Violence and hostility among families of Vietnam veterans with combat-related posttraumatic stress disorder. *Violence and Victims, 17*(4), 473–489.

Gold, J. I., Taft, C. T., Keehn, M. G., King, D. W., King, L. A., & Samper, R. E. (2007). PTSD symptom severity and family adjustment among female Vietnam veterans. *Military Psychology, 19*(2), 71–81.

Grieger, T. A., Cozza, S. J., Ursano, R. J., Hoge, C., Martinez, P. E., Engel, C. C., et al. (2006). Posttraumatic stress disorder and depression in battle-injured soldiers. *American Journal of Psychiatry, 163*, 1777–1783.

Hoge, C. W., Auchterlonie, J. L., & Milliken, C. S. (2006). Mental health problems, use of mental health services and attrition from military service after returning from deployment to Iraq or Afghanistan. *Journal of the American Medical Association, 295*(9), 1023–1032.

Jakupcak, M., Conybeare, D., Phelps, L., Hunt, S., Holmes, H. A., Felker, B., et al. (2007). Anger, hostility, and aggression among Iraq and Afghanistan war veterans reporting PTSD and subthreshold PTSD. *Journal of Traumatic Stress, 20*(6), 945–954.

Kline, A., Falca-Dodson, M., Sussner, B., Ciccone, D. S., Chandler, H., Callahan, L., et al. (2010). Effects of repeated deployment to Iraq and Afghanistan on the health of New Jersey Army National Guard troops: Implications for military readiness. *American Journal of Public Health, 100*(2), 276–283.

Kim, J., & Cicchetti, D. (2004). A longitudinal study of child maltreatment, mother–child relationship quality and maladjustment: The role of self-esteem and social competence. *Journal of Abnormal Child Psychology, 32*(4), 341–354.

Kulka, R. A., Schlenger, W. E., Fairbank, J. A., Hough, R. L., Jordan, B. K., Marmar, C. R., et al. (1990). *Trauma and the Vietnam War generation.* New York: Brunner/Mazel.

Lieberman, A. F., & Van Horn, P. (2008). *Psychotherapy with infants and young children: Repairing the effects of stress and trauma on early attachment.* New York: Guilford Press.

Lieberman, A. F., Van Horn, P., & Ozer, E. J. (2005). Preschooler witnesses of marital violence: Predictors and mediators of child behavior problems. *Development and Psychopathology, 17*, 385–396.

Levine, K. (2002a). *Little listeners in an uncertain world: Coping strategies for you and your child after September 11* [Brochure]. Washington, DC: Zero to Three.

Levine, K. (2002b). *Little listeners in an uncertain world: Coping strategies for you and your child during deployment or when a crisis occurs* [Brochure]. Washington, DC: Zero to Three.

Matsakis, A. (1988). *Vietnam wives.* Bethesda, MD: Woodbine House.

Maughan, A., Cicchetti, D., Toth, S. L., & Rogosch, F. A. (2007). Early-occurring maternal depression and maternal negativity in predicting young children's emotion regulation and socioemotional difficulties. *Journal of Abnormal Child Psychology, 35*, 685–703.

May, J. C. (2005). Family attachment narrative therapy: Healing the experience of early childhood maltreatment. *Journal of Marital and Family Therapy, 31*(3), 221–237.

National Military Families Association (NMFA). (2006). *Report on the cycles of deployment: An analysis of survey responses from April through September, 2005.* Alexandria, VA: Author. Retrieved January 11, 2010, from *support.militaryfamily.org/site/docserver/nmfacyclesofdeployment9.pdf?docid=5401.*

Office of the Deputy Under Secretary of Defense, Military Community and Family Policy. (2007). 2007 Demographics: Profile of the military community. Retrieved January 11, 2010, from *www.militaryonesource.com/portals/0/content/service_provider_tools/2007_demographics/2007_demographics.pdf.*

Osofsky, J. D. (Ed.). (2004). *Young children and trauma: Intervention and treatment.* New York: Guilford Press.

Parlakian, R., & Seibel, N.L. (2001). *Being in charge: Reflective leadership in infant/family programs.* Washington, DC: Zero to Three.

Pincus, S. H., House, R., Christenson, J., & Adler, L. E. (2010). The emotional cycle of deployment: A military family perspective. Retrieved January 11, 2010, from *www.hooah4health.com/deployment/familymatters/emotionalcycle.htm.*

Ramirez, J. (2009, June). Children of Conflict: Since 9/11, more than a million kids have had a parent deployed: Their childhoods often go with them. *Newsweek, 153*(24), 54–57.

Rentz, E. D., Marshall, S. W., Loomis, D., Casteel, C., Martin, S. L., & Gibbs, D. (2007). Effect of deployment on the occurrence of child maltreatment in military and nonmilitary families. *American Journal of Epidemiology, 165*(10), 1199–1206.

Rosenheck, R., & Fontana, A. (1998). Transgenerational effects of abusive violence on the children of Vietnam combat veterans. *Journal of Traumatic Stress, 11*(4), 731–742.

Saltzman, W., Lester, P., Pynoos, R., Mogil, C., Green, S., Layne, C., et al. (2009). *FOCUS for military families: Individual family resiliency training manual* (2nd ed.). Los Angeles: FOCUS for Military Families.

Schell, T.L., & Marshall, G. N. (2008). Survey of individuals previously deployed for OEF/OIF. In T. Tanielian & L. H. Jaycox (Eds.), *Invisible wounds of war: Psychological and cognitive injuries, their consequences, and services to assist recovery* (pp. 87–115). Santa Monica, CA: RAND.

Shanker, T. (2008, April 6). Army is worried by rising stress of return tours to Iraq. *New York Times.* Retrieved January 11, 2010, from *www.nytimes.com/2008/04/06/washington/06military.html?_r=1.*

Siegel, D. J. (1999). *The developing mind: How relationships and the brain interact to shape who we are.* New York: Guilford Press.

Siegel, D. J., & Hartzell, M. (2003). *Parenting from the inside out: How a deeper self-understanding can help you raise children who thrive.* New York: Tarcher/Penguin.

Slade, A. (2006). Reflective parenting programs: Theory and development. *Psychoanalytic Inquiry, 26*(4), 640–657.

Tronick, E. Z. (1989). Emotions and emotional communication in infants. *American Psychologist, 44*(2), 112–119.

Vasterling, J. J., Proctor, S. P., Amoroso, P., Kane, R., Heeren, T., & White, R. F. (2006). Neuropsychological outcomes of Army personnel following deployment to the Iraq War. *Journal of the American Medical Association, 296*(5), 519–529.

PART IV

■ ■ ■ ■

WORKING IN JUVENILE COURT WITH ABUSED AND NEGLECTED YOUNG CHILDREN OF SUBSTANCE-ABUSING PARENTS

INTRODUCTION TO PART IV

We begin this section of the book with a focus on understanding and implementing best clinical practices with drug addicted mothers and their infants. Stacey R. Bromberg and Karen A. Frankel provide important information relevant to clinical practice in courts settings, especially since substance abuse problems in parents account for between 40 and 80% of the young maltreated children who enter the court system (Boris, 2009). These authors describe a creative residential program for substance-abusing parents that provides a multidisciplinary system of care for these struggling parents and their vulnerable children. Recognizing the increased risk for "recovering mother–infant dyads" and the importance of providing intensive parenting intervention as part of substance abuse treatment, the Haven Mother's House program was started. This program integrates infant mental health into the treatment setting to attend to the needs of both mothers and infants. The program serves as a promising example of the application of theory to practice for addicted women and their young children. Moving from the clinical treatment setting to the court, there are many creative models with innovative judges in different courts throughout the country. Notable are the Miami–Dade County juvenile court–clinical–early intervention–education model (Katz, Lederman, & Osofsky, in press; Osofsky & Lederman, 2004) and the Zero to Three Court Teams for Maltreated Infants and Toddlers

(Gersch, 2009), two of which (San Francisco and Omaha) are described in chapters in this section. These three chapters describe the evolution and implementation of juvenile and family court programs for young maltreated children. As will be evident to the reader, the key to the effectiveness of these programs is judicial leadership and collaborative partners. I have used the title "Working in Juvenile Court ... Substance-Abusing Parents" for two reasons. The first is that two of the chapters focus specifically on innovative drug court and treatment programs. The second is that although innovative model programs for maltreated young children may not focus specifically on the fact that substance abuse is a major contributing factor to the maltreatment, as mentioned earlier, the data indicate that a majority of these young children have substance-abusing parents. Gwynneth Smith, Mary O'Grady, Donna J. Hitchens, Patricia Van Horn, and Alicia F. Lieberman describe the San Francisco Court Team, with judicial leadership from Judge Donna Hitchens, in the ongoing story of the efforts of the San Francisco Unified Family Court, in collaboration with public and private partners, to shift the focus of intervention with traumatized children and their families from punishment to amelioration and prevention. In the development of this program, judicial decision making, the traditional province of courts, was blended with outreach to families to provide a close support system for children. San Francisco's Court Team built on the previous work and collaboration between the Child Trauma Research Program at University of California, San Francisco, and the San Francisco Unified Court. In 2008, they broadened their work and collaboration with Zero to Three as part of a national effort by the Zero to Three Court Team Programs for Maltreated Children to bring early childhood expertise to interventions by courts and child welfare systems in cases of early childhood maltreatment and trauma. The ultimate aim of the program has been prevention: "to prevent the acts of violence that would transform our present generation of infants and toddlers into our next generation of juvenile offenders and adult criminals" (p. 235). Judge Jeri B. Cohen, Gayle A. Dakof, and Eliette Duarte in the Miami–Dade County Dependency Drug Court and the Engaging Moms Program for drug court counselors present an innovative drug court program. These authors discuss the key role of the dependency drug court judge in not only making the final decisions related to the direction for the dependent child but also establishing the tone and direction of the court. In this court setting, drug court counselors and key drug court partners (attorneys, treatment and other service providers, and child welfare caseworkers) are held to high standards, differences are resolved among partners, and the judge acts as a role model for all in the court setting. They bring this collaboration to life for the reader by describing the impact on a parent and young child. In the fourth chapter in this section, Douglas F. Johnson describes the Zero to Three Family Drug Treatment Court (FDTC) that he developed in the

Separate Juvenile Court of Douglas County (Omaha), Nebraska. It provides an interesting approach, with a focus on improving outcomes for substance-abusing parents and their children from birth to age 3. With Judge Johnson's leadership and empathic approach, Omaha's Zero to Three FDTC gives equal attention to parents and babies. He emphasizes, as is the case with most programs for young, vulnerable children who "have no voice," that to establish, grow, and maintain a Zero to Three specialty court is not easy. Funding can come and go in such programs, with changes in agency administration impacting the ability to deliver services. To ensure sustainability, Judge Johnson emphasizes the need for ongoing training that he has worked with collaborators to implement in Nebraska. In his courtroom, he recognizes the rights of the parent and the baby to due process, fair hearings, and timely decisions, leading to reunification or other permanent outcomes, such as adoption. These court programs integrating "state-of-the-art" clinical interventions and treatments, such as those described in Part II of this volume, are fine examples of efforts to interrupt the intergenerational cycle of abuse and neglect for the most vulnerable infants, toddlers, and young children.

REFERENCES

Boris, N. W. (2009). Parental substance abuse. In C. H. Zeanah, Jr. (Ed.), *Handbook of infant mental health* (3rd ed., pp. 171–179). New York: Guilford Press.

Gersch, J. S. (2009). *Evaluation of the court teams for maltreated infants and toddlers: Final report.* Washington, DC: U.S. Department of Justice, Office of Juvenile Justice and Delinquency Prevention.

Katz, L. F., Lederman, C. S., & Osofsky, J. D. (in press). *Child-centered practices for the courtroom and community: A guide to working effectively with young children and their families in the child welfare system.* Baltimore: Brookes.

Osofsky, J. D., & Lederman, C. (2004). Healing the child in juvenile court. In J. D. Osofsky (Ed.). *Young children and trauma: Intervention and treatment* (pp. 221–241). New York: Guilford Press.

CHAPTER 11

■ ■ ■ ■

Treating Drug-Addicted Mothers and Their Infants: A Guide for Understanding and Clinical Practice

Stacey R. Bromberg
Karen A. Frankel

For those of us who treat individuals and families tortured by drug addiction and its many sequelae, trauma is an undeniable part of our clinical work. For the infants and children of addicted caregivers, it is a way of life that often becomes all too familiar before effective interventions can be put in place. It is a world of extreme unpredictability, horror, violence, loss, distress, and fear, and one that continues generation after generation, without regard for the new young lives at stake. It is a world where a mother and child suffer in emotional distress as they are separated, without the skills or support to cope with the helplessness and hopelessness that ensue. A child is left with a stranger, afraid to trust and unwilling to attach, for his experience has been one of only fleeting security combined with the intense heartache of separation and loss. His mother is left alone with her own grief and a profound sense of vulnerability, with yet another experience to confirm that life is harsh and the world is a punitive place. In desperation, she seeks the only comfort she knows—her drug. It is the very reason behind her suffering and yet her only means to cope.

There are numerous substance abuse treatments available today. However, for specialized programs, for example, gender-specific, dually diagnosed criminals, the options seem far more restricted. Furthermore, despite our knowledge that treatment of babies and young children is best delivered in the context of the caregiving relationship (Gaensbauer, 2004; Lieberman, 2004; Lieberman & Van Horn, 2004a, 2008), for many years the standard of care in addiction treatment has been to separate the mother and young child. This standard of care involving the separation of drug-addicted caregivers and their children has been implemented with the intention of helping the mother first heal from addiction, after which she is then expected to return to her parenting role. Rarely is attention given to the caregiving relationship as a central focus of intensive treatment. While the standards of care today are certainly shifting toward a model of family-focused treatment for addiction (Boris, 2009; Werner, Young, Dennis, & Amatetti, 2007), substance abuse programs or resources that incorporate and integrate the needs of pregnancy and/or parenting young children remain difficult to access. Pregnant and parenting women with addiction are marked as particularly high risk, and attributes or labels, such as "multiple failed placements," "extensive drug abuse history," and/or "significant mental health concerns," often evoke fear reactions and worries for a child's safety. Therefore, recommendations are frequently made to separate mother and child for the duration of her treatment stay, or at least until a mother is more stable or has had some treatment time to get addiction "under control." Sadly, it is often this very decision that perpetuates the cycle of failed treatment attempts and relapse as women rush through needed addiction treatment to get back to their children. Relapse becomes inevitable as they simultaneously face the many typical challenges of mothering, with the additional stressors of recovery from addiction; the consequences of ruptured relationships at home due to behavior in addiction; and time away from loved ones.

There are significant barriers to effective substance abuse treatment related to mothering. Mothers, more than the general female population, avoid needed services or minimize the severity of their addiction because of their mothering status. Lack of appropriate child care, stigma, guilt, and fear of separation from children as a consequence of honest reporting of symptoms lead to inaccurate reporting of substance use, inaccurate information to medical and other treating professionals, and therefore, an underrepresentation of mothers in substance abuse treatment (Bromberg, Krow, & Frankel, 2010). For those who do enter into treatment, mothering women tend to be proportionally overrepresented in poor completion rates and premature termination of service due to factors associated with mothering (Finnegan, 1988; Grella, Joshi, & Hser, 2000, Scott-Lennox, Rose, Bohlig, & Lennox, 2000). There is evidence that pregnancy and parenting children in residence is associated with retention in drug treatment, especially when the setting is geared to such populations and the majority of residents are also mothering (Grella et al., 2000), and that longer stays in treatment lead to sustained abstinence (Greenfield et al., 2004). For this reason (and others), longer-term residential substance abuse treatment focused on treating women with their babies is an extraordinarily viable option for addressing women's addiction treatment needs in the context of their mothering role.

For some women, drug addiction and jail/prison time become synonymous (see Johnson, Chapter 14, this volume, related to this issue). Each story is unique in its details, but the general experience is a common one. A woman is drug-addicted and may be on the streets, eventually engaged in criminal activity to support an addiction that is out of control. She is finally caught by police, and sentenced by a judge who begins to know her all too well from multiple appearances in the same courtroom. She is released early from prison back to the streets or to a drug-abusing partner at home, then quickly returns to drugs and alcohol, leading to her next criminal charge. The pattern continues for months or years; then, eventually, she becomes pregnant. She now faces the possibility of delivering her baby in prison, shackled to a hospital bed and separated from her child within hours of the delivery. Her fate lies with the decision of the judge who can offer the possibility of treatment in lieu of prison and a chance to fight for a new beginning *with her baby*.

THE ISSUE OF SUBSTANCE ABUSE AND TRAUMA

There is a range of perspectives on the impact of substance abuse on infant development. Some focus on the effects of prenatal substance exposure for the developing fetus *in utero*, noting consequences for difficulties with sensory regulation, attention, and potential for lifelong social and learning difficulties (Batshaw & Conlon, 1997; Frank, Augustyn, Knight, Pell, & Zuckerman, 2001; Niccols, 2007; Shankaran et al., 2007). Others argue that the environmental correlates of addiction are most damaging, and focus on impoverished, drug-infused, and unpredictable living conditions; poor self-care (e.g., malnutrition, lack of basic medical and/or prenatal care); and a host of consequences associated with a volatile and unstable lifestyle (Killeen & Brady, 2000; Kim & Krall, 2006). Some concerns about physical living conditions in substance-abusing homes can include exposure and inhalation of toxic fumes, accessible drugs and drug paraphernalia (e.g., pipes or needles), and weapons. The combination of such hazardous materials and the lack of supervision due to unavailable caregivers create an environment that is precarious for babies and young children. In addition to the material hazards, the presence of and exposure of children without parental protection to dangerous, drug-addicted individuals leave children especially vulnerable to physical and sexual abuse (Bates & Hutson, 2007). For women, substance abuse is correlated with the incidence of domestic violence; some statistics allege that up to 70% of women who flee to shelters from abusive partners report that their children have also been victims of abuse by the same perpetrator (Bates & Hutson, 2007). For children who have not been assaulted themselves, witnessing their mothers' abuse often leaves them victimized and traumatized (Lieberman & Van Horn, 2004b; Schechter & Willheim, 2009).

These few examples illustrate the ways infants and children with substance abusing caregivers are at significantly increased risk for abuse and neglect. Furthermore, these examples show the way maladaptive patterns of relating are transmitted from generation to generation as the children exposed to substance abuse and/or domestic violence grow up to become addicted themselves. Without resources or models of nurturance and safety, these children often grow into adults who are unable to protect and effectively parent their own children. Providers who work with substance-abusing parents and their children consider not only the risk for abuse and neglect but also the disrupted relationships to be a result of life with caregivers who are less capable, less available, inconsistent, and who may have distorted or harsh parenting attitudes and high levels of parenting stress (Camp & Finklestein, 1997; Killeen & Brady, 2000; Lester, Boukydis, & Twomey, 2000; Nair, Schuler, Black, Kettinger, & Harrington, 2003; Tronick et al., 2005). These infants and children are at great risk for disrupted attachment patterns and negative parent–child interaction, with caregivers showing a lack of basic parenting knowledge, limited sensitivity, intrusiveness, severe parenting stress, and significant conflict in the dyadic relationship (Eiden, 2001; Swanson, Beckwith, & Howard, 2000; Velez et al., 2004). Furthermore, for children of drug-addicted caregivers, the risk of neglect is very high. Illicit drug use renders parents unable to supervise their children appropriately (often in the presence of dangerous conditions), to attend to basic caregiving and medical or developmental needs, or to provide the emotional attention necessary for children to thrive (Bates & Hutson, 2007). Often compounded by poor signaling about needs on the part of the infant born drug-exposed, a negative cycle of interaction for the dyad is initiated from the very start of the postnatal relationship between mother and baby (Velez et al., 2004). The tragic course of addiction and parenting that so often leads to ongoing trauma and victimization is set in motion, and the maladaptive patterns of relating that have pervaded generations before are perpetuated.

In contrast to previous biologically based conceptualizations of addiction, we now know that addiction is also heavily tied to adverse childhood experiences, with unrecognized early negative experiences as a major determinant for substance abuse (Feletti, 2004). The drug-addicted mother who is unable to care appropriately for her child was likely a child victim of trauma herself, turning to substances as a means of coping in the absence of alternatives. Without models of nurturance and safety, a woman is destined to repeat that which she experienced. However, these families can and do benefit from appropriate interventions, and early intervention can interrupt what is otherwise a guaranteed course of heartache and trauma for the babies and young children of addicted caregivers. For those of us working to repair and better the lives of young children and families, working within the world of substance abuse offers an unparalleled opportunity to effect change and save lives. There is an escalating demand for treatment and service provision amid scarce resources, and very few people are trained both to hear and to be the voices of the infants and children who need intervention. Even fewer are trained to recognize that, in many instances, it is the addicted parent who has also lost her voice and needs to be heard in order to reach the child most effectively and change the trajectory of development.

The challenges of working with substance-abusing mothers highlight the importance of a relationship-based approach to care, in which a perspective of mother and infant as inextricable provides the most valuable opportunity for intervention and subsequent change. That is to say, the whole (relationship) is greater than the sum of its parts (mother alone or infant alone) and must be looked at accordingly. The application of this perspective requires training that targets a comprehensive understanding of the infant and his or her caregiver as partners in the relationship, with attention to characteristics of both caregiver and infant, as well as the interaction of the dyad and family system. One program that provides such training is the Harris Program in Child Development and Infant Mental Health at the University of Colorado School of Medicine. With a focus on training advanced mental health professionals in infant mental health, the Harris Program's philosophy asserts that "all infant mental health professionals need to know how to understand the emotional, developmental, biological, temperamental, and interactional capabilities of an infant and its partner" (Frankel & Harmon, 2000, p. 325). Training includes developmental assessment work focused on use of standardized parent–infant and infant assessment tools, didactics focused on core principles of infant mental health, and both individual and group supervision of clinical cases. There is a deliberate emphasis on observation and analysis of parent–infant interaction to drive case conceptualization. The relationship between caregiver and infant as a focus of intervention is integrated into practice, with the understanding that the dynamics of these early relationships provide valuable information about a caregiver's internal working models of relationships based on childhood experiences, and a precious opportunity to interrupt intergenerational cycles of dysfunction.

The knowledge that the course of relationship-based treatment is not designed to be linear or prescribed is most important for substance-abusing mothers and their infants, where there may be wide variability in presentation and level of need for intervention. There must be attention and respect for the principal components to be considered in the treatment of this population, with the understanding that there can be great flexibility in application and approach. In our training of new infant mental health practitioners at the Harris Program in Colorado, we often emphasize the many ports of entry into relationship, and the importance of meeting clients' or families' needs to begin clinical work. The integration of infant mental health service into residential addiction treatment provides an extraordinary holding environment in which to offer the highest quality of care to mothers and their infants, with integrated attention to recovery from addiction and parenting. It is a home for the very clients who seem, at times, the hardest to reach, and a place of remarkable learning and transformation for clients and providers alike. As is often true, it is from our most difficult cases that we learn effective strategies and approaches about what our patients really need to be well. In an attempt to highlight some of the most important principles and intervention strategies for working with families and babies afflicted by substance abuse, we focus this chapter on one of the most daunting populations we serve in the Harris Program: pregnant and parenting women who are criminally involved in the justice system and mandated to residential treatment for substance abuse, and their very new babies. The chapter describes an existing program that integrates infant mental health into addiction treatment as a frame for treatment considerations, highlights those strategies and components most critical for clinical intervention with this population, and concludes with implications for providers working with families afflicted by substance abuse.

THE EVOLUTION OF THE PROGRAM: A RESPONSE TO A NEED

The increased risk for "recovering mother–infant dyads" warrants recognition of the importance of providing intensive parenting intervention as part of substance abuse treatment (Bromberg et al., 2010; Heffron, Purcell, & Schalit, 2007). The Haven at the University of Colorado School of Medicine provides the Haven Mother's House Program, with its attention to the needs of mothers and infants in the integration of infant mental health service into the treatment setting, which serves as a promising example of the application of theory to practice for addicted women (see Bromberg et al., 2010, for a more comprehensive description). It also serves to provide a framework for highlighting some of the most important treatment considerations and intervention strategies when working with this population.

The original Haven modified therapeutic community (MTC) opened its doors to meet the need for residential addiction treatment for women in 1992, operating as part of the Addiction Research and Treatment Services (ARTS) in the Department of Psychiatry. Typical for therapeutic community (TC) populations (see De Leon, 2004, for a more comprehensive description of TC), Haven women are admitted from the county jail or Department of Corrections, were previously homeless, and/or are referred by the Department of Human Services. All of the clients treated at the Haven have a severe, chronic addiction to substances, most typically methamphetamines, cocaine, or heroin. Residential treatment typically lasts for 9–12 months.

The perinatal period is a time when women may be more amenable to treatment, and evidence suggests that treatment of addicts may be most successful when its focus is on the parent–child relationship. Parental sensitivity to infant cues is given priority very early on in the parenting relationship or even prenatally (Pajulo, Suchman, Kalland, & Mayes, 2006; Suchman, Pajulo, DeCoste, & Mayes, 2006). With estimates of up to 70% of women entering treatment having children at increased risk of abuse, neglect, developmental problems, and development of substance abuse themselves (Werner et al., 2007), the addition of treatment for pregnant and mothering women was a theoretically logical and empirically supported extension of the existing residential treatment model at the Haven. However, within months of incorporating the admission of pregnant and parenting women into the Haven's modified treatment milieu, it became clear that successful treatment for this population would require yet further modification tailored specifically to the demands of pregnancy and parenting. In addition to the need for a separate physical space to accommodate the infants living in the treatment facility, the need for infant mental health consultation surfaced in response to the seemingly conflicting demands of addiction treatment and family-centered care. For instance, the more typical "in your face" and confrontational intervention so central to TC is an inappropriate practice from an infant mental health perspective. Even with gender-specific, trauma-informed modifications in place (e.g., softer tone for confrontation, attention to relational patterns of women as primary treatment concern), use of confrontation of a mother with a baby in her arms is still troublesome, as the infant can unnecessarily experience stressors related to the intervention. Expert infant mental health consultation to the MTC was required for not only the mothering clients but also the staff, which was well trained in addiction but came to the treatment milieu with little or no training in parenting or infant care.

Robert Harmon, MD, an eminent infant psychiatrist, had also recently become board certified in Addiction Psychiatry. He forged a partnership with the Haven and began as the attending psychiatrist to provide medication consultation for the women in treatment. Dr. Harmon's extensive background in infant psychiatry and his newer passion for addiction psychiatry enabled him to be a visionary and spokesman for the needs of the babies and mothers in treatment. He began informal consultation to the Haven administrators and staff about weaving mental health, infant mental health, and addiction psychiatry into a comprehensive program. At the time, Dr. Harmon was also the director of the Harris Program in Child Development and Infant Mental Health at the University of Colorado School of Medicine. With both a personal and a professional passion for recovery from addiction and infant mental health, Dr. Harmon provided resources through Harris postdoctoral fellows to realize a vision for specialized services targeting pregnant women and their infants. His enthusiasm and tenacity soon translated into investment and commitment from the Haven's director, and a lasting partnership and ongoing collaboration between the Haven MTC and the Harris Program were launched. Together, they were challenged to strike a balance between adapting Haven MTC treatment programming and the specific needs of women and infants, without sacrificing the inherent, core elements of addiction treatment. Dr. Harmon headed the Infant Mental Health Program at Haven until 2006, when he passed away suddenly. Fortunately, being a person of great vision and planning, he had mentored several junior faculty members, who were able to continue this work in his footsteps.

A DESCRIPTION OF THE HAVEN MOTHER'S HOUSE

The Haven Mother's House provides residential substance abuse treatment to a diverse group of adult women who reside *with* their infant children. The women typically range in age from 21 to 40 years, with the majority of women identifying as European American (69%), and others as African American (10%), Hispanic, or Native American origin (J. Rea, personal communication, July 2010). Despite efforts made to admit women as early in pregnancy as feasible, women enter the program in various stages of pregnancy or with a newborn infant in their custody. Babies' ages typically range from newborn to 18 months, and the majority of infants in residence are 12 months old and younger.

Located just a few buildings away from the Haven Mother's House, the Baby Haven provides concurrent child care. In order to allow mothers to attend treatment, the child care is open from 8:00 A.M. to 4:00 P.M., with opportunities for mothers to be with and feed their infants during lunch as part of programming. During this time, mothers are able to meet individually with child care staff to address concerns and receive parenting support (e.g., nutritional guidance). The child care staff members assist each young-ster in meeting his or her developmental milestones and receive consulta-tion as needed from the Harris program's on-site infant mental health spe-cialists for interactions that seem problematic or require more specialized attention. A typical day at the Haven Mother's House differs from that at many other residential treatment communities in its modifications related to the presence of children. Rather than going off-site for parent training or parent–child services, feedback and services around parenting are ever-present. Clients begin by waking early and preparing both their babies and themselves for the day at 6:30 A.M. They eat breakfast with their children, then walk them to Baby Haven. Following drop-off at day care, clients then return to the Mother's House for intensive programming focused on major lifestyle change and abstinence from all substances they have been abusing, similar to the programming for nonparenting women. At approximately 4:00 P.M., the clients walk back to the Baby Haven, where they reunite with their infants and satisfy requirements and responsibilities related to child care (e.g., chores, completing logs related to baby needs). From 5:30 P.M. to 8:30 P.M. clients spend "bonding time" with their infants, a family-focused time with programming and structure developed by the infant mental health specialists.

Much in the same way that the purpose of the intentional "bonding time" described earlier is to implement and further practice parenting skills focused on developmentally appropriate dinnertime, bath time, and bedtime routines, cornerstones of the Harris–Haven collaboration include a compre-hensive model of nurturance and relationship-based care of the pregnant and parenting women. In addition to the day-to-day, often minute-to-minute, concrete examples of feedback and parent "retraining" that occur, specific services are delivered by the infant mental health team to ensure that moth-ers and their infants receive balanced treatment with regard to addiction treatment and infant mental health. Each woman admitted to the Moth-er's House Program is assessed by a member of the Harris infant mental health team, which consists of a licensed psychologist, several postdoctoral fellows, and a forensic psychiatrist. An individualized treatment plan for infant mental health services is determined during this intake based on client need. For women who are pregnant, an individualized infant mental health plan includes obtaining appropriate prenatal care; a birth plan centered on a supported and healthy delivery of the baby; breast-feeding support; and immediate postpartum services, including care focused on attachment and bonding with the newborn, and screening and treatment for postpartum mood disorders.

Services also include individual sessions, mandatory infant mental health groups, infant developmental assessment, and questionnaires mea-suring indicators of perinatal and parenting stress in the mother. Mothers participate in infant mental health groups as part of their regular weekly MTC schedule. Infant mental health groups include a process therapy group ("New Additions") focused on addiction, mental health, and parenting needs, and an evidence-based, manualized parenting curriculum known as Partners in Parenting Education (Butterfield, 1996).

Some mothers require additional infant mental health support beyond group treatment, with referrals for more intensive and individualized care. Circumstances that warrant individual services include co-occurring mental health disorders, severe mental health concerns (e.g., postpartum depression, bipolar disorder) impacting the parent–child relationship, substantial grief/loss issues related to other children, safety concerns, ambivalence about parenting (e.g., considerations for adoption, outside placement), and relationship disturbances around basic caregiving with the infant currently in residence. Individual infant mental health sessions are then provided, with a focus on parent–infant psychotherapy (see Van Horn, Gray, Pettinelli, & Estassi, Chapter 4; Smith, O'Grady, Hitchens, Van Horn, & Lieberman, Chapter 12; and Johnson, Chapter 14, this volume, for more discussion of implementation of child–parent psychotherapy for a child welfare population and in court settings; Lieberman & Van Horn, 2008) as adjunct to standard milieu services and part of a client's individualized treatment plan. The orientation of parent–infant work is grounded in attachment theory and principles of infant mental health, incorporating many of the well-established, relationship-based infant mental health approaches, including "Ghosts in the Nursery" (Fraiberg, Adelson, & Shapiro, 1975), "Wait, Watch, and Wonder" (Cohen, Muir, & Lojkasek, 2003), infant–parent psychotherapy (Lieberman & Van Horn, 2008; Lieberman, Silverman, & Pawl, 2000), and interaction guidance (McDonough, 1993).

TREATMENT COMPONENTS

The Therapeutic Relationship

When treating drug-addicted women with their young children, the concept of the therapeutic relationship warrants particular respect and deliberate attention. This is especially true for women for whom relationships are a central vehicle for functioning, learning, being, and, thus, changing. It is addressed here as a primary concept for effective treatment, as there is no identifiable strategy or intervention that will work without its presence. For those struggling with addiction, however, the notion of relationship in its therapeutic sense is foreign. There is often a long history of betrayal (whether perceived or reality-based), and there is little reason to believe that *you,* the next professional in the long line of those "here to help," will be any different.

With a substance-abusing mother in treatment, it is not enough to "strive" for a therapeutic relationship. What is required is absolute honesty and a direct personal approach that leaves little room for "interpretation." For some treatment providers, being straightforward may be associated with being harsh or uncompassionate and can feel uncomfortable or inconsistent with that which is therapeutic. However, in this instance, precisely that approach communicates respect and is analogous to working with clients in their "native language." For clients struggling with addiction, and especially those with criminal involvement, direct and honest communication resonates more readily and leaves less room for mistrust and misunderstanding that results from the client having to "read between the lines." There needs to be respect for the client's transference and an expectation that she comes with the history of maladaptive, disappointing relationships and has endured traumatic experiences, often at the very hands of those who promised to care for her needs. This directness can be especially challenging for trainees and providers newer to this population, as the direct and honest communication often requires putting into words horrific experiences that the client has worked hard to avoid and forget, and making conscious that which has been unconscious for so long.

Family-of-Origin and Partner Relationships

There are many facets to addiction and the recovery process, and there are gender differences in the biological, psychological, and behavioral correlates of addiction, as well as engagement in treatment, access and utilization of services, and retention and relapse (Agrawal & Lynskey, 2008; Best, Walker, Foster, Ellis-Gray, & Day, 2008; Green, 2006; Sarin & Selhore, 2008). Women, particularly those involved in the criminal justice system, have significantly higher rates of mental health concerns involving depression, anxiety, posttraumatic stress disorder, and histories of physical and sexual abuse that impact treatment (Lewis, 2006; Peters, Strozier, Murrin, & Kearns, 1997). By the same token, the role of abusive partners and maladaptive familial relationships is often at the forefront of both the initiation of substance use and (when not appropriately addressed and specifically targeted in treatment) relapse, as women return to their abusive partners and quickly fail in their attempts at sobriety (Martin, English, Clark, Cilenti, & Kupper, 1996; McKay, Rutherford, Cacciola, Kabasakalian-McKay, & Alterman, 1996; Rubin, Stout, & Longabaugh, 1996). In treatment, interventions must be tailored to the specific relationship needs of women, paying particular attention to partner and family relationships, and the woman in the context of her relationships to others.

Thus, interventions must view sobriety and relationships as inextricable concepts, for one cannot be achieved without the other. The manner in which a client relates to her peers and family, reacts to providers, and approaches her baby provides a vast amount of information about her internal working models of relationships and her capacity to make the healthy connections required to be a successful mother in recovery from addiction. While this may seem intuitive and logical, it is not uncommon in practice to find an isolated treatment goal of "build healthy relationships" amid a list of goals on a treatment plan or a single, specialized group in addiction treatment addressing relationship issues. These are, in fact, important interventions, and the fact that such attention is being paid to relationships as a critical component of substance abuse treatment speaks to the evolution of the field. However, attention to relationships, both therapeutic and familial, must be infused in *all* aspects of treatment with this population.

Process Groups

For the purposes of this chapter, a "process group" is defined as an open-ended, dynamically oriented therapy group, with at least one group facilitator. Process groups in substance abuse treatment settings are purposefully different and contrast the curriculum- or topic-based groups that also exist. Both types of groups are critical to quality treatment. For women who are in substance abuse treatment and also parenting, the importance of a process group that includes women at different points in their recovery process, with few limitations to content, should not be underestimated. Because the groups comprise women who share experiences of both addiction and mothering, there are unique parallels to the recovery model of Alcoholics Anonymous (AA) that should be noted. Consistent with the AA tenet of "one addict helping another," peer process groups provide a context in which peers, together as women, as addicts, and as mothers, have an opportunity to learn that their own experience is not unique.

In process groups for this population, the notion of one addict helping another becomes intimately tied to the experience of "one mother helping another." The common struggle for survival as addicts and mothers provides a foundation for trust and shared experience central to both recovery from addiction and healthy mothering. For many, the holding environment of the process group becomes the first safe place in which a woman can share her story with others who truly understand and can relate to her experience on an emotional level. It is a place where empathic understanding of extremely personal material is expressed. For many women, the process group becomes a primary vehicle for personal healing and a place to experience some of the very concepts that are communicated as being essential to healthy parenting (e.g., active listening, turn-taking, empathy and understanding, acceptance).

The presence of women who are at different points in their struggle to recover and successfully mother, free of drugs and alcohol, provides an incredible foundation for practicing AA's 12-step concept of "carrying the message" and giving back to others (Seppala, 2001). Considered essential to continued sobriety and personal growth, the idea of giving back to others by telling one's story provides a sense of purpose to the women who are sharing their experiences. For those in the midst of the initial struggle and unsure about their commitment or ability to endure the journey of recovery and mothering, their peers become living examples of that which is possible, providing hope and motivation.

Although the parallels to the AA model are important and lend credence to the utility of process groups in treatment, there is an important distinction to be made with regard to facilitation and the role of the clinician in the type of process group discussed here. Twelve-step groups themselves are not run by professionals. With an absolute respect for the necessity of the peer-to-peer model for recovery and support, process groups for recovering women in treatment should include at least one trained mental health facilitator. For the addicted mother who is first experiencing relationships in the context of group and may be sharing traumatic material for the first time, the presence of a knowledgeable facilitator as a guide to the process is warranted and advantageous. In fact, with a well-trained provider who can contain affect and navigate complex content and process, the process group can be an exceptional therapeutic tool for the expression and resolution of traumatic material for women who might otherwise not disclose their experiences. Similarly, the process group may serve as a forum for the expression of relationship dynamics that may otherwise not surface as readily in other contexts or one-to-one therapy. Such a process then invites reactions that are representative of past interactions, providing a window into the internal working models of relationships that drive clients' behavior and provide a framework for mothering. It is often in these groups that clients are vulnerable enough to let their defenses down and engage in a genuine way. A course of transformation proceeds as women empathize with peers, share their own stories, and develop a new understanding of relationships and mothering to begin to heal themselves and feel emotionally available enough to focus on caring for their children.

Focus on Mothering

For *mothering* women, additional treatment considerations need to be addressed, over and above those relevant to the general, gender-specific concerns. Attention must be paid to the woman in relationship to her baby, and the mothering role must be considered as primary. For women sentenced to the residential treatment community with their babies, failure to complete programming likely means prison time. A woman is inevitably challenged with the decree to "succeed" simultaneously in parenting her infant and learning to live a life free of drugs and alcohol. Because it is unlikely that she has experienced supportive relationships for any consistent period of time in her own life, the task of developing a healthy relationship with her baby can be overwhelming, especially when she has been stripped of the only coping mechanism she has known (i.e., drugs). Nonetheless, in the treatment of women with their babies, the notion of attention to the "mothering" relationship as a separate matter (or a separate treatment goal) is naive. Relationships are not static, and while there is certainly value in carving out time and space for specialized attention to relationship patterns, a newborn's need to connect to his or her caregiver does not exist in isolation or remain frozen in time until his mother is deemed "ready." Thus, for women in treatment with their babies, the mothering relationship must be targeted in *every* intervention and remain at the forefront of case conceptualization, intervention, and daily practice from the very start of treatment.

Attention to mothering must start from the moment the pregnant woman enters treatment. The typical notion of a mother falling in love with her baby is one that is usually presented as a natural and effortless affair. The world is flooded with beautiful messages and images of pregnant mothers daydreaming with a smile as they plan for the arrival of their newest love, and with mothers and their newborns snuggled up together without worries or cares, gazing lovingly into one another's eyes. However, for women with the illness of addiction, the images and experience of pregnancy, childbirth, and the perinatal period may be quite disparate from those just described. Instead, the experience may be riddled with feelings of insecurity, fear, grief, and negativity. In the absence of intervention, it is an experience that inevitably mimics past relationships and interactions, with disappointing outcomes and the perpetuation of maladaptive relational patterns that have persisted throughout generations. Women fighting to recover from addiction do not find healthy or "good enough" (Winnicott, 1960) mothering to be intuitive, and an astonishing number of obstacles may interfere with the connection between a mother and her child.

Of particular relevance here is the risk for "hidden trauma" to these infants that results from the poor psychobiological regulation within the primary caregiving relationship (Schuder & Lyons-Ruth, 2004). The substance-abusing mother who struggles to regulate her own physiological and psychological responses is often limited in her capacity to respond appropriately to her infant's cues, with inconsistent and intrusive behavior associated with caregiver impulsivity (Boris, 2009; Swain, Lorberbaum, Kose, & Strathearn, 2007). Subsequently, these infants, who may already be struggling with their own neurobiological difficulties in organization and sensory processing as a result of *in utero* drug exposure (Arizona Supreme Court,

2007), are particularly vulnerable to experiencing a heightened response to stressors that would otherwise be managed well by a more capable and attuned caregiver. The relationship between the drug-addicted mother and her infant can become a primary source of stress and trauma, in sharp contrast to one of comfort and protection.

While it can be overwhelming to think about the level of risk associated with substance abuse and young infants, fortunately for providers, the perinatal period is also a time when women may be psychologically more vulnerable, emotionally accessible, and particularly motivated to use intensive support (Crittenden, Manfredi, Lacey, Warnecke, & Parsons, 1994; Pajulo et al., 2006). It is a time that is ripe for intervention and positive change. Particularly useful for intervening with substance-abusing mothers and their young children is the notion of Selma Fraiberg's "ghosts in the nursery" as a metaphor for the intergenerational transmission of trauma and maltreatment (Fraiberg et al., 1975). For families afflicted with drug addiction, it seems that the "ghosts" are ever-present and dangerous in their obscurity. There is often an alarming amount of unresolved grief and loss, and "ghosts" of previous pregnancies and perinatal loss that have never been uttered out loud impact a mother's entire perspective and approach to relating. Providers treating this population must make therapeutic space for even the scariest ghosts to present themselves, be respectfully acknowledged and confronted, and incorporated into understanding of parenting behavior. It is only then that the intergenerational cycle of addiction and maltreatment can be interrupted and altered. One of the major determinants of addiction is the presence of adverse childhood experiences that are unrecognized and hidden from awareness by shame, secrecy, and social taboo (Feletti, 2004). These are the traumas that do not heal and are transmitted to the next generation, often reflected in disrupted attachment and relationship disturbance between caregivers and infants. The "ghosts" of childhood that remain with adult women as they enter into relationships with their own infants must be called forth from the unconscious and invited into the treatment context to facilitate healing and change.

For the provider entering into a treatment relationship with a substance-abusing mother, the tremendous presence of the metaphoric "ghosts" can feel oppressive. However, newer conceptualizations of addiction that include the notion of heritability (Kendler, Myers, & Prescott, 2007) and risk for substance dependence as highly experience-dependent (Boris, 2009; Feletti, 2004) provide us with the necessary hope and motivation right from the start to intervene and prevent harm to the very young infants born into addiction. With appropriate attention and intervention, there is exceptional opportunity to change the trajectory for a mother–infant dyad and present a significant interruption to maladaptive intergenerational patterns of relating. The development of satisfying relationships between mother and child can help to reorganize the addictive reward system from reliance on substances to the positive associations of the relationship with baby and sustained abstinence (Collins, Grella, & Hser, 2003; Pajulo et al., 2006). Thus, "angels in the nursery" (Lieberman, Padrón, Van Horn, & Harris, 2005) also becomes an important metaphor in treatment. As "ghosts" are uncovered, "angels" must also be identified to provide a window into the positive experiences that will serve to influence parenting attitudes and behavior. We readily acknowledge that the "angels" may be much more difficult to identify in a life story of horror and heartache. Nevertheless, it is the provider's challenge to seek them out and deliberately name them for the client. This can serve as the beginning of a reframe for the client about her own experience and the possibility of something better for her child.

Parenting "Education"

In addition to infusing a focus on mothering into every aspect of the residential treatment setting, there is good evidence for the utilization of specific parent training and/or parent education as a part of treatment for this population (e.g., Velez et al., 2004). For purposes of applicability across treatment settings and circumstances, this chapter does not provide a review of available curricula but serves to point out some of the most important common strategies in choosing an appropriate curriculum and providing parenting education services to caregivers.

First and foremost, one must challenge the traditional notion of education when thinking about this population, with emphasis on efforts to "train" or "educate." If we understand what is required for a child to be successful in a traditional learning environment, it is clear that attendance, interest, attention, adult support, and positive experiences with learning are all crucial. While it is not true for all, for many women with addiction, education in its formal sense has been yet another venue for failure and disappointment. As a simple example, something like attendance can become an extraordinary challenge for a child whose parents are addicted (an experience that is not uncommon for the adult women now in treatment), who have been up all night, and who may still be asleep when it is time to leave for school. Without a routine at home that includes a regular sleep schedule and attention to developmental needs, concentration and interest in learning quickly take a backseat to survival. Lack of parental support that lead to learning difficulties or disabilities that went unnoticed can result in a loss of critical building blocks and foundations for growth. It is often difficult to expect adult women and mothers to now be "taught" something like parenting in the context of a traditional educational forum. Instead, the paradigm for teaching and learning needs to be one in which different levels of ability and understanding can be acknowledged and incorporated. Information is best presented in a way that is both palatable to the learners and integrated into their current framework of understanding.

Therefore, given what we know about previous parenting experiences and pervious exposure to parenting education for this population, the following assumptions seem prudent:

1. All women in treatment for addiction, regardless of previous experience, should be exposed to basic information about infant development and parenting practice, as if this is their first baby and they have had no previous experience or exposure to parenting.
2. The information that is "taught" needs to be of *interest* to the mother, practical in its content, and applicable to her current situation.
3. The use of evidence-based practice is certainly important, but it is crucial to implement a curriculum that allows for flexibility so that the information presented is in a *manner* that feels relevant to the mother.

The first component to consider in "educating" addicted mothers is the development of a basic fund of knowledge around parenting and early child development. For many women who find themselves in a residential treatment facility, particularly those who are mandated to treatment, this is not the first experience of "parenting class" and often is not their first experience as a parent. So what basics are presented to a woman who has already parented several other children? How does the information differ from that for a woman encountering her first mothering role? And how does one best present the information given the fact that most of the mothers have already taken (and often completed) parenting classes in other areas (e.g., human services)? It is easy to get caught up in trying to figure out exactly what mothers may need, or to make assumptions about what a woman likely already knows given her past educational and parenting experiences. But, in fact, one can confidently assume that these women have not sought out previous parenting classes on their own for the sheer sake of learning. Completion and satisfaction of another's requirements have usually been the primary goal. Moreover, we have learned from the women who have openly shared about their previous parenting education experiences, that if they did attend the class, the likelihood that they were sober was poor.

From this, we know that substance-dependent mothers almost always lack even the most basic knowledge related to newborn care and developmental tasks such as feeding, sleep, and appropriate play (with overstimulation noted as a particular concern for this population) (Velez et al., 2004). Furthermore, because children who are exposed to substances *in utero* may also present special needs or sensitivities, education that includes ways in which parents can better understand those needs must be incorporated. In addition to information about ways in which drug-exposed infants may require particular strategies in caregiving to facilitate healthy development, information about appropriate developmental expectations and milestones is important to address. This all must be done with the understanding that there is often tremendous guilt about substance use during pregnancy and hypervigilance on the part of the mother who is now very worried that she may have caused harm or irreparable damage to her baby *in utero*. Thus, facts regarding developmental milestones should be presented with great sensitivity. Opportunities for mothers to grieve if drug exposure has impacted their children's development should be made available outside of the content education, and support for linkages to early intervention and navigation of the system from the time of referral through service provision should be readily available.

Second, although there is a great deal of information available on infant and child development, the information that is presented to a student of child development (and the way it is presented) will likely (and should) look very different than the information presented to a recovering mother learning in the context of substance abuse treatment with her infant. In practice, this means asking about what she is *interested* in learning (a question that has likely not been asked before), then listening to questions and concerns from the mother, with the intent of incorporating answers to such questions, even modifying curricula when necessary in order to do so. The assumption that previous experience and/or knowledge translates to good-enough practice for drug-addicted women and their babies is dangerous. For many, this is their very first encounter with parenting clean and sober, and there is a significant opportunity to effect change in both the way the woman thinks about her young child and how she translates her understanding into parenting practice and interaction with her little one.

Third, without attention to the *manner* in which content is presented, the integration of learned material can be lost. This is true for any population, but it is especially true for mothers in recovery from addiction who are learning to parent. Thus, a critical component to parent education for women struggling with substance abuse is experience and the opportunity to practice learned material. For many, it is not enough to have the didactics of parenting, and for this population, it is a critical mistake to believe that "teaching" parenting translates into practice. Any parenting program addressing the needs of recovering women and their infants should include a style of learning that values the mother's perspective as an expert on her baby, while incorporating discussion and enactment into didactics, including conversations about the mother's understanding of the material. There must be a component to learning that is experiential, for both mother and infant. This is where the important concept of relevance comes into play, as content must be relevant not only to mothers' questions and concerns about their babies but also to their own experiences. How does the mother understand the material in the context of her own experience? Given her own experiences, how will she apply what she is learning to interaction with her baby? In the absence of appropriate and accurate information, a mother is left to draw on what is familiar or known to her in order to make decisions. For the general parenting population, which tends to have a variety of good strategies from which to draw, this is not typically a problem. For the drug-addicted mother, there is a wide range and variability of experience, in which those with little to draw on may be left making unsafe decisions in an effort to cope with stressful parenting demands.

CASE EXAMPLE 1

Sitting around the table with her peers for parenting group, Jennifer is extremely quiet as the facilitator asks questions about efforts to soothe crying babies and reviews the risks associated with shaken baby syndrome as part of the typical protocol for this parenting unit. When asked about the questions they hope to have answered, one mother talks about her interest in learning to wrap the baby in a blanket, to swaddle. Another mother asks if it is true that babies respond favorably to the vibration of the washing machine when they are crying. Still another asks if it is really acceptable to leave the baby alone in the crib when she feels frustrated or overwhelmed, or if she will get in trouble for doing so. The discussion becomes quite animated, as peers seem to become activated and anxious in response to this question, offering suggestions and strategies to calm the crying baby instead of leaving him or her alone to cry. The facilitator wonders with the group why a question about leaving a baby alone in a crib when a parent is feeling overwhelmed is so difficult. A rich discussion about "neglect" follows. The women begin to examine their own feelings about triggers associated with crying babies and remember strategies they employed while still active in their addictions to get their other children to quiet down. They begin to acknowledge that the sound of the baby's cries were agitating and interfered with their primary focus on continuing to get high. They disclose that any strategy that would help the baby quiet more quickly was preferred to allowing the baby to continue to cry. As the women talk about things like bouncing the babies, playing music, giving the baby to a friend or neighbor, or using bottles or pacifiers to try to quiet their crying babies, Jennifer, who has remained quiet throughout the conversation, begins to cry. She is hesitant to speak but soon reveals that she often feels completely overwhelmed in the evenings with her 6-week-old infant, and has intrusive thoughts and memories of her older daughter as she attempts to soothe her newborn. As she is asked to talk about what strategies she is using to try to soothe her new baby, she speaks of rocking, feeding, and singing to her infant. She is then asked to remember what strategies were helpful to her in parenting her last child, the older daughter she is now remembering in the darkness as she holds her newborn. She begins to cry and is reluctant to speak. A peer turns and reminds Jennifer that she is in a safe place, and that each one of them is here to learn something new and different, to parent clean and sober, and to make a better life for their babies. She quickly answers in a quiet and hesitant way, "I didn't have any strategies. I gave her my drugs," as she sobs and hangs her head in shame. With the group's support, she bravely goes on to talk about her lack of knowledge, her desperation both to help her young daughter in distress, and her selfishness and impatience in wanting to find a "quick fix" to make the crying stop, as others had described. She speaks of one particular memory of blowing marijuana smoke into her baby daughter's face to help her calm and quiet, then tells the group she is not comfortable sharing any more details. Some of her peers are speechless with eyes wide, but a few nod knowingly. She is not alone in her experience.

This example serves to highlight the importance of allowing room for discussion and mothers' expressions of their own experiences in parenting "education," and it reminds us of the power of group dynamics and peer support in reaching this population. In contrast to a "class" that "teaches" about the dangers of shaken baby syndrome and strategies to soothe or calm a crying baby, the open and supportive environment allows for a richer understanding of the material through discussion, and makes the information relevant (and thus memorable) for the women in the group.

CASE EXAMPLE 2

In the weekly staff meeting at the addiction treatment center, the infant mental health specialist asked for updates on daily parenting activities and areas notable for their need of increased attention during parenting groups. Staff members listed a few typical concerns related to age-appropriate expectations around sleeping and developmentally appropriate play, and a newer staff member followed with a question about "appropriate feeding." The staff member went on to report that some of the women continued to "prop the bottle" and leave babies unattended during feeding, and that others were feeding their children and "only paying attention when the milk is coming out the sides or the baby is choking." She was distressed by her observations and asked the clinician, "Please teach the ladies how to feed the babies." The clinician, in hearing this, was surprised to learn about this behavior, having just completed a parent education group centered on feeding. The group session included information about risks of ear infections for babies left with bottles in their cribs, proper positioning for feeding related to optimal digestion, and what felt like a rich discussion about feeding as a perfect opportunity for nurturance as mothers and babies connect emotionally and interact socially.

In the next parenting group, the clinician followed up with the clients regarding staff concerns, and clients indicated that they had many tasks to complete to be compliant with treatment and felt the babies were doing just fine with feeding while they also took care of other responsibilities. When pressed, they identified propping the bottles as "lazy addict behavior." Some women took responsibility for their inappropriate behavior and agreed to change. One of the other women, who was not propping the bottle, acknowledged that she was feeding her baby while also trying to tend to other tasks, and that when her baby sometimes "leaked the milk all over her," she would become frustrated. She went on to say that she was working on being more patient and understanding that "babies are just messy." The women were asked to imagine what the experience might be like for a baby left alone with a bottle propped or held flat, or tilted toward the floor during feeding (while his or her mother was multitasking), while milk streams from the sides of his or her mouth. The women giggled in response and rolled their eyes; one commented, "It's not as big a deal as you are making. We are feeding our babies!"

At the start of the subsequent group session (with babies to "practice" learned skills), the facilitator requested that the women pair up for an exercise without their babies (this was in sharp contrast to the typical start of group). She then asked one woman in each dyad to lie flat on her back on the floor. The facilitator handed a cup of water to each partner in the pair and asked that they feed the cup of water to their partner as they remain flat on the floor. She then asked them to switch roles and attempt to balance the cup of water on their partner's chest in a way that the woman could remain lying down and use only her hands, with her elbows still at her side, to help herself to drink the water. They were asked to leave their partner and go to the other room as she struggled to drink the water.

At the next staff meeting, the clinician followed up with staff regarding any updates or concerns related to parenting. There were no feeding concerns reported.

In contrast to the first case example, which demonstrates the use of one's own experiences in shaping parenting behavior (i.e., the identification of drugs as the only available coping strategy), this second example highlights the importance of the experiential component of parenting education that is so critical for this population. The fact that these women were even feeding their babies consistently was something of which they were in fact proud, and a skill that might contrast previous parenting behavior while addicted. Being "taught" about appropriate feeding techniques was interpreted as excessive and irrelevant to their practical parenting needs. Thus, information from their initial parenting group on this topic was seemingly disregarded and not integrated into practice. It was only in the moment when the mothers could themselves feel (i.e., experience) what inappropriate feeding techniques might be like for their babies that the capacity for empathy and the ability to take on the baby's perspective emerged. It was this experience, in contrast to the didactic information presented, that eventually transformed their behavior.

The opportunity to practice learned parenting concepts in a safe and supportive environment is a critical component of learning that we are promoting. True transformation and change occurs only in the moments when mother and infant both sense the impact of good parenting behaviors, and there is an interaction and exchange that resonates emotionally with a mother and her baby. For substance-abusing mothers and their babies, the magic moments of parenting and the stance of being emotionally available enough to apply learned information in a healthy way can be difficult. Mental health concerns, grief and loss related to other pregnancies or children, traumatic experiences in their own lives, and the many correlates of their addictive existence can make interaction with an infant overwhelming and scary. Thus, a focus on the parent–infant relationship and purposeful attention to positive parenting practices *in the moment* are essential. One core principle of recovery from addiction is a focus on the present and the ability to stay in the moment. This can be especially challenging for women with histories of addiction. Intrusive thoughts or memories can be triggered by seemingly benign interactions, and without a trained treatment provider to help a woman focus on what is happening in the moment, important positive interactions or overtures from the infant to his mother may be misinterpreted or altogether missed. The clinician becomes crucial in helping the mother to identify moments of connection and to *experience* her interaction with her baby in those moments. The power of the intervention then lies in the accumulation of such moments with the real-time realization of successful parenting, the recognition that her baby can and will respond to her attempts to connect, and the emotional adventure of falling more deeply in love with each successful interaction.

Videotaped Interaction

The use of videotape provides the capability to capture and conserve moments of interaction that might otherwise be lost. It is almost always helpful clinically to be able to return to and review session material, and the use of videotape can be especially useful for this population, in which moments of positive interaction and emotional connection can often get lost due to a mother's distraction (whether internal or external) and/or an infant's need for basic caregiving (e.g., feeding, diapering). In even a 30-second video clip, countless examples of positive interaction between a mother and her baby may go unnoticed during the live interaction. The video becomes a powerful mirror through which women can see a reflection of themselves as mothers, and often see their infants as others seem them, adorable and innocent. The precious dialogue around the interaction as it unfolds on the screen provides an important opportunity for joint attention, and a shared understanding between clinician and client regarding the interaction as the mother experienced it. A genuine relationship between the client and her therapist is again essential, as the successful use of videotaped interaction requires access to the mother's affect and experience. With the mother's emotional experience and narrative as critical to transformation, her cooperation and commitment to the process allow her to reveal the actual meaning of that which is observable on the screen, to uncover significant moments of interaction that tell the real story of the dyad.

CASE EXAMPLE 3

Cynthia was referred to the infant mental health team for parent–infant therapy after it was noted that she was "spoiling" her 3-month-old son Michael by continually holding him and rocking him to sleep. In the milieu, Cynthia had been getting in trouble for sleeping with her baby in bed, a practice against residential treatment policy due to safety concerns. While she had been responsive to other interventions in the addiction treatment milieu, she was not responding to interventions addressing her parenting. The parenting group facilitator noted that Cynthia had a difficult time engaging with her baby during group. Cynthia often quickly attempted one or two activities, only to report that her son was "exhausted" and needing to nap. The facilitator described "excellent" interactions as Cynthia would put the baby to sleep, noting that mother and baby seemed very connected in those moments. The facilitator also noted that Cynthia seemed "at peace" and "in a zone and calm" when rocking with her baby. The baby was described by child care staff members to be an "easy baby," who would just "hang out and watch" the other children in child care and cry only when he needed to feed or sleep. They noted that he did not smile much and seemed most content when left alone to observe others and play with toys. They mentioned that he would often startle or grimace, as if to cry, when someone approached him face-to-face.

When invited to be videotaped to learn more about her baby (a strategy we have found very useful in engaging mothers to be videotaped with their infants), Cynthia was initially resistant but agreed hesitantly to a trial. As the taping began, Cynthia grabbed a toy from the floor and started to shake it over her son, who was lying on the floor. Michael looked at her with wide eyes and began to wave his arms and legs. Then he grimaced, as if to begin to cry, but did not. She quickly put the toy down and frantically reached for a book, looking at the clinician with wide eyes and an expression of terror. With a gentle nod from the clinician to keep going, she sat next to her son (who was still lying on the floor) and began to read. After a page, she looked down to find him beginning to roll to his side toward the toy she had put down just a moment earlier. She picked him up and said, "Are you tired baby?" and patted his back gently as she put him over her shoulder and began to rock. She closed her eyes, and he fussed for only a moment; soon he, too, began to close his eyes, his hands falling to his side, with his head resting comfortably on her shoulder. In review of the video-taped interaction, the therapist asked Cynthia about her experience of the different moments on the screen. The therapist praised Cynthia for her initial choice of an age-appropriate toy, but Cynthia reported that it was disappointing that her son was not interested in playing. The thera-pist probed Cynthia about how she knew her son was not interested, and Cynthia referred to "that face he makes" as the therapist paused the video to show her son's grimace. Also frozen on the screen was Cynthia's grimace in that moment, something about which the thera-pist then inquired. Cynthia began to cry and identified her own look as one of worry and fear. Further replay of the video revealed that it was Cynthia who first grimaced in response to her son waving his arms and legs excitedly as she offered the toy. Within a fraction of a second (slow-motion replay is a wonderful tool), he grimaced in response to her, mirroring her affect. It was only in the replay of the video that Cyn-thia was able to see her son tracking and following the toy, interested and motivated enough to roll toward it, all during the short time it took for her to find the book to read as an alternative activity. As Cynthia and her therapist then watched together as Cynthia rocked her son to sleep on video, Cynthia remarked that she could "barely remember that." The therapist asked what it felt like to rock him to sleep, and Cynthia was unable to answer, looking perplexed and anxious.

As Cynthia worked with her therapist reviewing moments of vid-eotaped interaction, she was able to identify her son's expression of excitement in waving his arms and legs as a trigger for her own physical abuse on a variety of levels (his "out-of-control" movements as pos-sibly harmful to her somehow, misinterpreting his excited movements as those of distress and helplessness). She reported feeling "crazy" that her little baby could be a trigger for her own experiences, and that there was incredible guilt and worry that she would not be able to be a good parent to her son because she herself was so damaged. She described face-to-face interaction with her son as intense and "scary because I don't know what he wants from me and he is just looking at me for all of the answers." It was not long before she and her therapist were able to identify periods of dissociation associated with rocking her baby to sleep. Attention to Cynthia's symptoms of posttraumatic stress disor-der (PTSD) could then become a primary point of intervention for this dyad. The clinician became more actively involved in the interaction by helping Cynthia notice her "worry face" and work to smile more (even if forced sometimes) when face-to-face with her son, with the idea that his ability to mirror her grimace meant that he could also mirror her smiles. Her misinterpretations of her son's overtures for interaction and signs of "exhaustion" were discussed and "normalized" within the context of her own traumatic history. Her desire to be a good parent to her son was used as motivation to present to Cynthia the challenge of sticking with a single activity for an appropriate amount of time (even when uncomfortable for her). She was encouraged to hold her baby during waking periods to disrupt the routine of rocking him to sleep as the only point of physical connection, and a vehicle for her own disengagement and dissociation. Those peers who roomed with her were enlisted to help Cynthia notice her "worry face" and were asked to help Cynthia stay present in the moment when rocking her baby to sleep.

In addition to its support of the use of videotape, Cynthia's case is one that serves to highlight an important warning to those of us working with drug-addicted mothers and their very young babies. With the knowledge that drug addiction and trauma go hand in hand, one must be mindful that even those interactions that look good to the outside observer may be incongruent with the mother's (and baby's) experience of the interaction. Even in situations where parenting appears to be going smoothly, for drug-addicted women, it is not uncommon to have a mother report feeling "like the babysitter," to describe her baby as wanting to "see everything (or everyone)" when asked why her baby is always facing outward and not interacting face-to-face, or to report feeling a complete disconnect from her baby despite appropriate (or even "excellent") demonstration of parenting skills. This case example reminds us of the importance of assessing for signs of hidden trauma in infancy as another vehicle for understanding the dyadic relationship by attending to and inquiring about the infant's behavior in a variety of contexts, and with a variety of caregivers. Also attending to the mother's mental health concerns is of paramount importance, as substance abuse is often intimately linked to mental illness, and the risks associated with the perinatal period often render women with comorbid substance abuse and mental health concerns even more vulnerable. Screening for perinatal mood disorders, assessment for mental health concerns, and recognition of the importance of treating mental health symptoms (even if they are subclinical in their presentation) in conjunction with addiction treatment is imperative.

IMPLICATIONS FOR PROVIDERS

There are several ramifications and implications for clinicians seeking to provide the types of support, education, and therapies described earlier. Among these are the need to work in a comprehensive program that addresses sub-stance abuse, parenting, and infant well-being within a relationship-based context; the intensity and complexity of the work; and the need for reflective supervision and self-reflection. As outlined in the preceding pages, recov-ery and parenting need to be considered together. Programs focusing sepa-rately on each aspect miss the intricate interplay of parenting and recovery, of recovery and loss, of parenting and loss, and so forth. Therefore, staff members and clinicians must work together to integrate the various pieces of programming and communicate "between" programs about each client. Similarly, this type of multiple focus means paying attention to the "whole person" of both the mother and the infant, and the space in between. As seen in the previous case examples, these mothers and their babies pres-ent multiple challenges. They have mental health, trauma, addiction, and relationship concerns. Attending to all of these issues increases the level of clinical demand enormously for the clinician. It also requires "prioritiz-ing" and intensive team treatment planning to determine how and when to address different problems. Finally, these cases make it abundantly clear that clinicians have strong feelings about these mothers and babies from time to time. There is great stigma attached to drug addiction in our culture, and clinicians are not exempt from negative and judgmental feelings about addicts. Reflective supervision (Heller & Gilkerson, 2009; Parlakian, 2001) and case consultation are crucial to helping clinicians work effectively and ethically. For those drawn to the adorable babies and who feel dedicated to prevention and early intervention efforts to change lives for babies and young children, we close with this perspective.

These addicted mothers are the very babies who were once struggling, now grown up. They are those whose families were out of reach, and who were not fortunate enough to grab anyone's attention or receive interven-tion. They had no voice as infants or children, and now, as adults and moth-ers themselves, they continue to search for a voice that can be heard. In an absence of healthy models for relationships and with low self-esteem, they sought out partners who validated their images of no self-worth and a view of the world as a threatening place. They are living examples of the trauma and devastation that ensues for those families who are not identified or reached by prevention and early intervention efforts. And they are now the models by which our smallest and most vulnerable clients will learn to live and experience the world. They are responsible for providing safe and loving environments for their children to thrive when they themselves did not experience such love. They are asked to cope with extraordinary stres-sors that would cripple most people, and they are faced with the challenge of doing so without the appropriate support or resources necessary. Like all mothers, they want to be successful in making a life for their children that is better than the life they have lived. Yet, for these mothers (without intervention), repetition of past patterns and traumatic experiences seems inescapable. However, because they are now in treatment and because they have come for help, there is opportunity to effect change. There is an opening to serve as a model of a different experience and reveal the possibility of a better life for the mother and her baby. There is the privilege of being intimately involved in a process of transformation by witnessing a mother begin to heal, creating emotional connections and a new openness to learning, shedding light on the strengths and capacities that are already there, and establishing the safe and supportive holding environment that allows a mother and her baby to fall in love.

REFERENCES

Agrawal, A., & Lynskey, M. T. (2008). Are there genetic influences on addiction?: Evidence from family, adoption and twin studies. *Addiction, 103,* 1069–1081.

Arizona Supreme Court. (2007). Arizona CASA/FCRB Training (*azcasa.org*): Neonatal substance exposure/substance exposed newborns (SEN). Retrieved March 12, 2010, from *www.supreme.state.az.us/casa/prepare/neonatal.pdf*.

Bates, S., & Hutson, R. (Eds.). (2007). *Child abuse and neglect: An introductory manual for professionals and paraprofessionals.* Denver: Colorado Department of Public Health and Environment.

Batshaw, M. L., & Conlon, C. J. (1997). Substance abuse: A preventable threat to development. In M. L. Batshaw (Ed.), *Children with disabilities* (4th ed., pp. 143–162). Baltimore: Brookes.

Best, D., Walker, D., Foster, A., Ellis-Gray, S., & Day, E. (2008). Gender differences in risk and treatment uptake in drug using offenders assessed in custody suite settings. *Policing and Society, 18,* 474–485.

Boris, N. W. (2009). Parental substance abuse. In C. H. Zeanah, Jr. (Ed.), *Handbook of infant mental health* (3rd ed., pp. 171–179). New York: Guilford Press.

Bromberg, S. R., Backman, T., Krow, J., & Frankel, K. A. (2010). The Haven Mother's House modified therapeutic community: Meeting the gap in infant mental health services for pregnant and parenting mothers with drug addiction. *Infant Mental Health Journal, 31*(3), 255–276.

Butterfield, P. M. (1996). The Partners in Parenting Education Program: A new option in parent education. *Zero To Three, 17*(1), 3–10.

Camp, J. M., & Finkelstein, N. (1997). Parenting training for women in residential substance abuse treatment: Results of a demonstration project. *Journal of Substance Abuse Treatment, 14,* 411–422.

Cohen, N. J., Muir, E., & Lojkasek, M. (2003). "Wait, watch and wonder": A child-centered psychotherapy program for the treatment of conflicted mother–child relationships. *Kinderanalyse, 11,* 58–79.

Collins, C. C., Grella, C. E., & Hser, Y. I. (2003). Effects of gender and level of parental involvement among parents in drug treatment. *American Journal of Drug and Alcohol Abuse, 29,* 237–261.

Crittenden, K. S., Manfredi, C., Lacey, L., Warnecke, R., & Parsons, J. (1994).

Measuring readiness and motivation to quit smoking among women in public health clinics. *Addictive Behaviors, 19,* 497–507.

De Leon, G. (2004). Therapeutic communities. In M. Galanter & H. D. Kleber (Eds.), *The American Psychiatric Publishing textbook of substance abuse treatment* (3rd ed., pp. 485–501). Washington, DC: American Psychiatric Publishing.

Eiden, R. D. (2001). Maternal substance use and mother–infant feeding interactions. *Infant Mental Health Journal, 22,* 497–511.

Feletti, V. J. (2004). The origins of addiction: Evidence from the adverse childhood experiences study [English version of the 2003 article published in Germany as Ursprunge des Suchtverhaltens-Evidenzen aus einer Studie zu belastenden Kindheitserfahrungen]. *Praxis der Kinderpsychologie und Kinderpsychiatrie, 52,* 547–559. Retrieved March 12, 2010, from *www.acestudy.org/files/origin-sofaddiction.pdf.*

Finnegan, L. (1988). Management of maternal and neonatal substance abuse problems. *NIDA Research Monograph, 90,* 177–182.

Fraiberg, S., Adelson, E., & Shapiro, V. (1975). Ghosts in the nursery: A psychoanalytic approach to the problems of impaired infant–mother relationships. *Journal of the American Academy of Child and Adolescent Psychiatry,14*(3), 387–421.

Frank, D. A., Augustyn, M., Knight, W. G., Pell, T., & Zuckerman, B. (2001). Growth, development, and behavior in early childhood following prenatal cocaine exposure. *Journal of the American Medical Association, 285,* 1613–1625.

Frankel, K. A., & Harmon, R. J. (2000). Advanced training in infant mental health: A multidisciplinary perspective. In J. D. Osofsky & H. E. Fitzgerald (Eds.), *Handbook of infant mental health: Vol. 2. Early intervention, evaluation, and assessment* (pp. 313–333). New York: Wiley.

Gaensbauer, T. J. (2004). Traumatized young children: Assessment and treatment processes. In J. D. Osofsky (Ed.), *Young children and trauma: Intervention and treatment* (pp. 194–216). New York: Guilford Press.

Green, C. A. (2006). Gender and use of substance abuse treatment services. *Alcohol Research and Health, 29,* 55–62.

Greenfield, L., Burgdorf, K., Chen, X., Porowshki, A., Roberts, T., & Herrell, J. (2004). Effectiveness of long-term residential substance abuse treatment for women: Findings from three national studies. *American Journal of Drug and Alcohol Abuse, 30*(3), 537–550.

Grella, C. E., Joshi, V., & Hser, Y. I. (2000). Program variation in treatment outcomes among women in residential drug treatment. *Evaluation Review, 24,* 364–383.

Heffron, M., Purcell, A., & Schalit, J. (2007). Building a collaborative one day at a time: Integrating infant mental health in a residential drug treatment program. *Journal of Zero to Three, 27*(4), 34–40.

Heller, S., & Gilkerson, L. (2009). *A practical guide to reflective supervision.* Washington, DC: Zero to Three Press.

Kendler, K. S., Myers, J., & Prescott, C. A. (2007). Specificity of genetic and environmental risk factors for symptoms of cannabis, cocaine, alcohol, caffeine, and nicotine dependence. *Archives of General Psychiatry, 64*(11), 1313–1320.

Killeen, T., & Brady, K. (2000). Parental stress and child behavioral outcomes following substance abuse residential treatment: Follow-up at 6 and 12 months. *Journal of Substance Abuse Treatment, 19*, 23–29.

Kim, J., & Krall, J. (2006). *Literature review: Effects of prenatal substance exposure on infant and early childhood outcomes.* Berkeley: National Abandoned Infants Assistance Resource Center, University of California at Berkeley.

Lester, B. M., Boukydis, C. F. Z., & Twomey, J. E. (2000). Maternal substance abuse and child outcome. In C. H. Zeanah, Jr. (Ed.), *Handbook of infant mental health* (2nd ed., pp. 161–175). New York: Guilford Press.

Lewis, C. (2006). Treating incarcerated women: Gender matters. *Psychiatric Clinics of North America, 29*, 773–789.

Lieberman, A. F. (2004). Child–parent psychotherapy: A relationship-based approach to the treatment of mental health disorders in infancy and early childhood. In A. J. Sameroff, S. C. McDonough, & K. L. Rosenblum (Eds.), *Treating parent–infant relationship problems* (pp. 97–122). New York: Guilford Press.

Lieberman, A. F., Padrón, E., Van Horn, P., & Harris, W. W. (2005). Angels in the nursery: The intergenerational transmission of benevolent parental influences. *Infant Mental Health Journal, 26*(6), 504–520.

Lieberman, A. F., Silverman, R., & Pawl, J. H. (2000). Infant–parent psychotherapy: Core concepts and current approaches. In C. H. Zeanah, Jr. (Ed.), *Handbook of infant mental health* (2nd ed., pp. 472–484). New York: Guilford Press.

Lieberman, A. F., & Van Horn, P. (2004a). Assessment and treatment of young children exposed to traumatic events. In J. D. Osofsky (Ed.) *Young children and trauma: Intervention and treatment* (pp. 111–138). New York: Guilford Press.

Lieberman, A. F., & Van Horn, P. (2004b). *"Don't hit my mommy!": A manual for child–parent psychotherapy for young witnesses of family violence.* Washington, DC: Zero to Three Press.

Lieberman, A. F., & Van Horn, P. (2008). *Psychotherapy with infants and young children: Repairing the effects of stress and trauma on early attachment.* New York: Guilford Press.

Martin, S. L., English, K. T., Clark, K. A., Cilenti, D., & Kupper, L. L. (1996). Violence and substance use among North Carolina pregnant women. *American Journal of Public Health, 86*, 991–998.

McDonough, S. C. (1993). Interaction guidance: Understanding and treating early infant–caregiver relationship disturbances. In C. H. Zeanah, Jr. (Ed.), *Handbook of infant mental health* (pp. 414–426). New York: Guilford Press.

McKay, J. R., Rutherford, M. J., Cacciola, J. S., Kabasakalia-McKay, R., & Alterman, A. I. (1996). Gender differences in the relapse experiences of cocaine patients. *Journal of Nervous and Mental Disease, 18*, 616–622.

Nair, P., Schuler, M. E., Black, M. M., Kettinger, L., & Harrington, D. (2003). Cumulative environmental risk in substance abusing women: Early intervention, parenting stress, child abuse potential and child development. *Child Abuse and Neglect, 27*, 997–1017.

Namyniuk, L., Brems, C., & Carson, S. (1997). Southcentral Foundation—Dena A Coy: A model program for the treatment of pregnant substance-abusing women. *Journal of Substance Abuse Treatment, 14*, 285–295.

Niccols, A. (2007). Fetal alcohol syndrome and the developing socio-emotional brain. *Brain and Cognition, 65*(1), 135–142.

Pajulo, M., Suchman, N., Kalland, M., & Mayes, L. (2006). Enhancing the effectiveness of residential treatment for substance abusing pregnant and parenting women: Focus on maternal reflective functioning and mother–child relationship. *Infant Mental Health Journal, 27,* 448–465.

Parlakian, R. (2001). *Look, listen, and learn: Reflective supervision and relationship based work.* Washington, DC: Zero to Three Press.

Peters, R. H., Strozier, A. L., Murrin, M. R., & Kearns, W. D. (1997). Treatment of substance-abusing jail inmates: Examination of gender differences. *Journal of Substance Abuse Treatment, 14,* 339–349.

Rubin, A., Stout, R. L., & Longabaugh, R. (1996). Gender differences in relapse situations. *Addiction, 91*(Suppl.), 111–120.

Sarin, E., & Selhore, E. (2008). Serving women who use drugs in Delhi, India: Challenges and achievements. *International Journal of Drug Policy, 19,* 176–178.

Schechter, D. S., & Willheim, E. (2009). The effects of violent experiences on infants and young children. In C. H. Zeanah, Jr. (Ed.), *Handbook of infant mental health* (3rd ed., pp. 197–213). New York: Guilford Press.

Scott-Lennox, J., Rose, R., Bohlig, A., & Lennox, R. (2000). The impact of women's family status on completion of substance abuse treatment. *Journal of Behavioral Health Services and Research, 27,* 366–379.

Schuder, M. R., & Lyons-Ruth, K. (2004). "Hidden trauma" in infancy: Attachment, fearful arousal, and early dysfunction of the stress response system. In J. D. Osofsky (Ed.) *Young children and trauma: Intervention and treatment* (pp. 69–104). New York: Guilford Press.

Seppala, M. D. (2001). *Clinician's guide to the twelve step principles.* New York: McGraw-Hill.

Shankaran, S., Lester, B. M., Abhik, D., Bauer, C. R., Bada, H. S., Lagasse, L., et al. (2007). Impact of maternal substance use during pregnancy on childhood outcome. *Seminars in Fetal and Neonatal Medicine, 12,* 143–150.

Suchman, N., Pajulo, M., DeCoste, C., & Mayes, L. (2006). Parenting interventions for drug-dependent mothers and their young children: The case for an attachment-based approach. *Family Relations, 55,* 211–226.

Swain, J. E., Lorberbaum, J. P., Kose, S., & Strathearn, L. (2007). Brain basis of early parent–infant interactions: Psychology, physiology, and *in vivo* neuroimaging studies. *Journal of Child Pyschology and Psychiatry, 48*(3–4), 262–287.

Swanson, K., Beckwith, L., & Howard, J. (2000). Intrusive caregiving and quality of attachment in prenatally drug-exposed toddlers and their primary caregivers. *Attachment and Human Development, 2*(2), 120–148.

Tronick, E. Z., Messinger, D. S., Weinberg, M. K., Lester, B. M., Lagasse, L., Seifer, R., et al. (2005). Cocaine exposure is associated with subtle compromises of infants' and mothers' social–emotional behavior and dyadic features of their interaction in face-to-face still-face paradigm. *Developmental Psychology, 41,* 711–722.

Velez, M. L., Jansson, L. M., Montoya, I. D., Schweitzer, W., Golden, A., & Svikis, D. (2004). Parenting knowledge among substance abusing women in treatment. *Journal of Substance Abuse Treatment, 27,* 215–222.

Werner, D., Young, N. K., Dennis, K., & Amatetti, S. (2007). *Family-centered treatment for women with substance use disorders: History, key elements, and challenges.* Rockville, MD: Department of Health and Human Services, Substance Abuse and Mental Health Services Administration.

Winnicott, D. (1960). The theory of the parent–child relationship. *International Journal of Psychoanalysis, 41,* 585–595.

CHAPTER 12

■ ■ ■ ■

Partnerships for Young Children in Court

How Judges Shape Collaborations Serving Traumatized Children

Gwynneth Smith
Mary O'Grady
Donna J. Hitchens
Patricia Van Horn
Alicia F. Lieberman

There is little question that in the United States, instead of focusing on the needs of children for quality education, economic opportunities, safe and good homes, and loving families, all of which go a long way toward preventing violence, we more quickly opt for punishment after the fact. There is overwhelming evidence that many of the adolescents and young adults who first become delinquent and later develop into criminals were exposed earlier in their lives to much violence, disorganized families, poor education, and limited opportunities. What is needed is a shift in thinking and behaving in our society ... to helping children develop the values and respect that comes from within families and community.

—OSOFSKY (1997, p. 5)

THE IMPORTANCE OF FOCUSING
ON YOUNG CHILDREN IN THE COURT SYSTEM

Scholars and clinicians have long recognized that early childhood experience, particularly early traumatic experiences such as interpersonal violence, can negatively impact a child's development. While the degree to which trauma impacts a child's well-being is mediated by his or her level of development and ability to marshal internal or external supports to help with coping, the negative consequences are nonetheless significant. Research shows that early childhood trauma may alter the shape and functioning of the central nervous system and stress hormone system (De Bellis et al., 1999a, 1999b); interact with developmentally relevant wishes, impulses, and fears to shape the developing personality (Marans & Adelman, 1997); and continue to impact later development in the form of traumatic reminders and secondary adversities that flow from the original trauma (Pynoos, Steinberg, & Piacentini, 1999). As traumatic life experiences interact with the child's unfolding developmental processes, risks for psychopathology and other maladaptive outcomes increase (Cicchetti & Cohen, 1995; Osofsky & Scheeringa, 1997). Interventions that help children understand and process the terrifying events they have witnessed or experienced, and that help their caregivers restore a sense of order and safety to their worlds, diminish these risks (Cicchetti, Rogosch, & Toth, 2006; Lieberman, Ghosh Ippen, & Van Horn, 2006; Lieberman, Van Horn, & Ghosh Ippen, 2005; Toth, Rogosch, Manly, & Cicchetti, 2006).

However, despite all we know about the perils of trauma, the words that begin this chapter remain highly relevant. Children in our society continue to be frequent victims of violence, at the hands of both their caregivers and others. In 2008, nearly 530,000 children under the age of 19 were injured in acts of violence, and 1 in 13 of these injuries were sufficiently severe to require hospitalization (Centers for Disease Control and Prevention [CDC], 2008b). Homicide is the second leading cause of death for children in this group, although it is the number one cause of death among African American youth (CDC, 2008a). Moreover, child maltreatment continues to be widespread in our society. State child protective services agencies estimate that nearly 800,000 children are the victims of substantiated maltreatment each year (CDC, 2009). Certain children are more likely to be victimized than others. Ethnic minorities, including African American, Native American/Alaska Native, and multiracial children experience higher rates of abuse (CDC, 2009). Tragically, the youngest children are at highest risk of victimization, with nearly 32% of maltreatment cases and 76% of maltreatment fatalities occurring among children under age 4 (CDC, 2009; U.S. Department of Health and Human Services, 2009).

These early childhood adversities have long-term negative consequences for both children and communities. Consistent with research findings that traumatic life experiences place the developing child at risk for psychopathology, researchers have identified exposure to violence in the home and community as major risk factors for youth violence later in life (Thorton, Craft, Dahlberg, Lynch, & Baer, 2002). Abused and neglected children have been reported to have higher rates of arrest for both juvenile and adult criminal behavior than nonabused children (Ryan & Testa, 2005; Windom & Maxfield, 1996). Violence among our youth continues to be a disturbing trend. Following a decline in the late 1990s, the number of young people involved in gangs has steadily increased to over 750,000 nationally in 2007 (National Youth Gang Center, 2009). Nearly 100,000 young people were arrested for violent offenses in 2007, a 5% increase since 2003. Over that same time period, the number of juvenile arrests for intentional homicides increased over 25% (Puzzanchera, 2007).

As a society, we continue to respond to the path from victim of violence to violent offender in punitive rather than ameliorative ways. The states spend, on average, nearly three times more per prisoner each year than they do per public school pupil (Children's Defense Fund, 2008b). In California, the authors' home state, a shocking 20 times more money is spent per youth in a state juvenile facility than is spent per public school pupil (Children's Defense Fund, 2008a). This egregious underinvestment in our youngest citizens continues despite compelling evidence from leading economists that investment in young human capital not only helps individuals but also improves state and national economies, with an estimated 7–8% overall return on investment (Rolnick & Grunewald, 2007).

Because of our tendency to focus on punishment later in life, the response to violent youth is centered in the criminal courts, where increasingly even very young children may be tried as adults. Over 50% of states permit children under age 12 to be tried as adults in criminal court, while 22 states plus the District of Columbia permit children as young as age 7 to be transferred to adult criminal court. Of note, over 50% of these children tried as adults are African American (Deitch, Barstow, Lukens, & Reyna, 2009). If our attention to punishment and our inattention to education, violence prevention, and support for families continue, we can expect that frightened young children will continue to grow into frightening youth and adults.

This chapter tells the ongoing story of one court's efforts, in collaboration with public and private partners, to shift the focus of intervention with traumatized children and their families from punishment to amelioration and prevention. We describe in depth the processes that the San Francisco Unified Family Court followed as it developed a model in which judicial decision making, the traditional province of courts, was blended with outreach to children's closest support systems: their families. Although the court's many initiatives have focused on intervention with youth and parents of all ages, the overarching philosophy has been that by supporting youth and families, the court could strengthen the nurturing environment for the youngest children. The ultimate aim throughout has been prevention: to prevent the acts of violence that would transform our present generation of infants and toddlers into our next generation of juvenile offenders and adult criminals.

Our focus is the process that San Francisco's Unified Family Court followed as it developed its philosophy of family-focused service and violence prevention, with special attention paid to the court's newest initiative, the Court Team for Maltreated Infants and Toddlers Project (hereinafter "the Court Team"). First we discuss the unique and crucial role juvenile courts can play in intervening with at-risk children and families. Next we briefly review several collaborative initiatives of the past 15 years, including the "unification" of San Francisco's Family Court, that exemplify the court's focus on children and families (for a more detailed discussion of these past initiatives, see Van Horn & Hitchens, 2004). Finally we discuss in detail the development and functioning of the Court Team, from its inception to its current docket of over 40 cases.

WHY INVOLVE COURTS IN COLLABORATIONS TO SERVE CHILDREN?

Although courts are sometimes viewed as coercive systems set apart from more traditional service organizations, family court can also be a natural collaborative partner with other agencies and community-based organizations to help children and families. First, courts are among the institutions in society where troubled children and families are most likely to be found. Children who are abused or neglected, who are delinquent, or who witness domestic violence are more likely than children who do not face similar stresses to need advocacy and mental health services. Their parents also need services to improve their parenting skills, to deal with their own mental health or substance abuse issues, to help them escape from dangerous environments, or to minimize the danger in their current environments.

Many of these children and their families come to court, and if their strengths are not affirmed and their problems not understood or adequately addressed, they will come back again and again. Abusive parents will not reunify successfully with their children; delinquent youth will repeat their harmful behaviors; parents in violent relationships will continue to be hurt and to expose their children to frightening conflict and violence. When troubled families come to a court that has formed good collaborative relationships with community service providers, the court is able to recommend interventions that can break destructive patterns before they become entrenched. This is particularly the case in families with infants, toddlers, and preschoolers. The needs of such young children may be overlooked in these highly stressed families. Parents may not have the skills required to read their young children's signals of distress; they may be so overwhelmed with their own problems that they assume their young children will be "resilient" and not remember the hardships they suffered at an early age. Together courts and their collaborative service providers can give voice to young children who might otherwise be overlooked.

In addition, courts are uniquely situated to move beyond merely recommending services. Under some circumstances, courts can use their power to compel participation in recommended programs. Traditionally, criminal courts and dependency courts have used this power to compel adults or children to take part in services. For example, criminal domestic violence courts now routinely require adult batterers to participate in intervention programs as a condition of their probation. Dependency courts routinely require parents who have abused or neglected their children to take part in substance abuse or mental health treatment as a condition of reunification. They may also compel assessments or treatment for dependent children (see Osofsky & Lederman, 2004, for an example of court-ordered intervention to benefit young children).

SAN FRANCISCO UNIFIED FAMILY COURT: TRACING THE DEVELOPMENT OF A CHILD- AND FAMILY-FOCUSED APPROACH

San Francisco Unified Family Court has a history of innovation with respect to the development of initiatives that focus on better serving young children and their families who come to court, whether because of child maltreatment, juvenile delinquency, domestic violence, or parental separation. In order to serve these children better, to maximize their chances of success, and to minimize the detriment posed by the circumstances that brought their families to court, judges and service providers have sought to collaborate and seek solutions together. Central to this philosophy of community collaboration and focus on the needs of children was the unification of the family court system in San Francisco, and this is where the story begins.

The Unification of the Family Court

In 1997, Judge Donna J. Hitchens (one of the authors of this chapter) began a process designed to move San Francisco toward the model of "one family–

one judge." Until that time, the departments of the court that served youth and families were physically and departmentally divided and communicated with each other poorly, if at all. Dependency judges and commissioners presided over cases in which the child protection system had petitioned the court to assume jurisdiction over children who were victims of abuse or neglect. Delinquency judges oversaw cases involving youth who were adjudged delinquent because of criminal behavior. Family law judges and commissioners presided over civil petitions for separation and dissolution of marriage, for domestic violence protective orders, and for orders regarding child custody and visitation. Still, additional commissioners presided over petitions for child support brought by the county in cases where the custodial parent had received public assistance, or where foster care reimbursement enforcement funds were sought. The adjunct systems that served families within the court were also divided. There were, for example, two groups of mediators: one that mediated disputes for families whose children were dependents of the court because of abuse or neglect, and another that carried out mediations required by law in cases where issues of child custody or visitation were disputed by parents. In fact, the mediators were in separate buildings and did not even know each other.

This departmental separation and lack of communication drastically affected the way that the court heard cases and how families were served. For example, a single family experiencing problems with both the child welfare system and domestic violence (an extremely common occurrence) would have each case heard in different courts by different judges, who did not necessarily know of the family's involvement with the other judge. The involvement of multiple departments meant that families were often burdened with multiple court appearances to resolve related issues. It also increased the risk that different departments would make conflicting orders.

The unification of all of the noncriminal Superior Court departments that serve families was designed to remedy these potential conflicts and to make appearing before the court less burdensome and confusing for families. Unification presented a major challenge for judges and commissioners. Before unification, each judge and commissioner had presided over a department that dealt with a limited range of legal issues. The judge or commissioner could become an expert in those issues that most commonly arose and the law he or she needed to understand in order to resolve them. Movement toward a model of "one family–one judge" meant that each bench officer would need to understand the whole range of issues that might affect the family. The bench officer would be the expert not in a particular area of the law, but in the particular family and its needs.

Moving in the direction of placing the necessity of understanding the needs of individual families on the same level of importance as the necessity of ruling on legal issues involving members of the family has opened the door for the possibility of creating a court that will act as a collaborative partner to support the individuals before it, even as it exercises the necessary restraints on their behavior.

Kids' Turn and the Rally Project

Even before the formation of the Unified Family Court, the family law department of the San Francisco Superior Court was pioneering collaborative new ways to serve families. In 1989, a family law judge, in cooperation with a few mental health professionals and attorneys, founded Kids' Turn, an agency that offers psychoeducational groups to children between the ages of 4 and 14 whose parents are divorcing, together with groups to help parents learn conflict resolution skills and focus on their children's needs following the breakup of the family. Kids' Turn has since expanded its curriculum to add a series of "Early Years" groups for divorcing parents whose children are 3 years of age or younger. The family law department was also instrumental in the foundation of the Rally Project, a center that offers supervised visitation exchange services in cases where there is high conflict or violence between separating or divorcing parents.

Increased Collaboration with the University of California, San Francisco, Child Trauma Research Program

In 1997, the Unified Family Court further solidified its focus on young children when it entered into a collaborative relationship with a university-based research and service program, the Child Trauma Research Program (CTRP) at the University of California, San Francisco. This collaborative relationship served as the foundation upon which several subsequent initiatives, including the Court Team model, have been based. CTRP provides clinical services to children younger than 6 who have witnessed domestic violence or experienced other interpersonal traumas, including child abuse and neglect. The process of the court and clinicians working together to serve at-risk children and families was not without challenges. Inevitable questions arose along the way concerning, among other things, the process of identifying and referring cases for treatment, whether and how service providers would give feedback to the court, the limits of therapeutic confidentiality, and how to obtain informed consent in a clinical research setting when working with families from the court.

Resolving these issues has been an ongoing process requiring flexibility, dedication, and openness on all sides. Court personnel have visited the CTRP clinic to learn more about the treatment process. Clinicians have attended court hearings and mediations to better understand the legal process. Engaging in the hard work to surmount these challenges has helped to construct the essential framework of collaboration: mutual understanding and respect for one another's needs, strengths, and limitations. This work also has made it clear to both CTRP and the court that together we are stronger and more effective than either of us would be alone.

Family Court Jamborees

The Unified Family Court established its willingness to collaborate with a broad range of partners in the community by holding two Family Court Jamborees. The court invited attorneys, mental health professionals, child welfare workers, mediators, bench officers, child custody evaluators, and parents to spend the day together working in small groups to solve problems related to making the Unified Family Court more accessible and effective. Topics ranged from the way the court handles domestic violence cases, to parent orientation, to improving the court process for self-represented litigants. These events were successful and important beyond the goal of devising recommendations to improve the Unified Family Court's service to the community. They firmly established the reputation of the Unified Family Court as a group of jurists willing to listen to and incorporate ideas from litigants, attorneys, and others with a stake in the court's operation. The court's willingness to change in response to the needs of those who appear before the court, rather than insisting that all involved accommodate themselves to the court's way of being, made it clear to the community that this court would be a genuine collaborative partner.

Youth Family Violence Court

In 2000, the Youth Family Violence Court was established to work with adolescents adjudicated to be delinquent because they had assaulted dating partners or members of their family. The vision was to bring together a group of professionals that could provide comprehensive services to the youth, their victims, and in cases in which the youth had children of their own, to those children. This was a much broader vision than one generally sees in treatment courts because it encompassed wraparound services for not only the youth but also those family members and dating partners whose lives have been touched by the youth's behavior. The supervising judge was particularly aware that a substantial number of the youth who would appear before the court were already the parents of babies and young children, or soon would be. She wanted to prevent violence from cycling through another generation by providing interventions that would help such youth understand the impact of their behavior on their young children. To accomplish this goal, she also included agencies that serve young children, Kids' Turn and the CTRP, on the planning team for the Youth Family Violence Court. Youth with children under age 6 who have witnessed domestic violence are also referred when necessary for treatment at CTRP.

Safe Start Initiative[1]

This broad initiative was established to bring sorely needed services and assistance to children under the age of 6 (and their families) whose lives have been affected by violence. Making this project a reality required extensive organizational and community collaboration, and the court worked closely with local government agencies, law enforcement, community-based child advocacy groups, and domestic violence service providers. Within this initiative, a family services provider employed by the court, and funded by Safe Start, works to help the court identify families with multiple legal needs and to facilitate their referral to Safe Start's network of advocates and mental health providers located in neighborhood-based family resource centers and mental health clinics.

THE COURT TEAM:
THE NEWEST CHILD- AND FAMILY-FOCUSED INITIATIVE[2]

The most significant and successful strategies for addressing early childhood trauma have resulted from collaborations among juvenile courts and infant/toddler mental health experts. Systemic changes have occurred for dependency families in the Unified Family Court due to the persistent efforts of creative and dedicated psychologists, primarily from the CTRP, to educate judicial officers, court mediators, and dependency attorneys on the importance of healthy attachment and the effects of trauma on the very youngest children who come into the child welfare system. These educational efforts have provided the catalyst for the court to expand its role in promoting the best possible outcomes for infants and toddlers.

This section describes the impetus and goals underlying the establishment of San Francisco's Court Team, the ingredients that are crucial to its success, and how the court operates on a daily basis. Even as the Court Team continues to evolve and improve, it has already yielded tangible results for babies and toddlers in foster care in San Francisco.

Zero to Three and the Focus on Babies and Toddlers

San Francisco's Court Team was developed as part of a national effort by the Zero to Three organization to bring early childhood expertise to bear on interventions by courts and child welfare systems in cases of early childhood maltreatment and trauma. This special focus on the youngest children is supported by research showing that this group is both highly vulnerable and highly resilient when successful interventions can be put in place.

Babies and toddlers are maltreated at higher rates than older children, more frequently enter the child welfare system, and have a higher chance of returning to foster care once removed. Nearly 32% of maltreatment cases involve children under age 4, with 76% of child maltreatment fatalities occurring in this age group (CDC, 2009; U.S. Department of Health and Human Services, 2009). Over one-third of all children entering into care in 2008 were age 3 years or younger (U.S. Department of Health and Human Services, 2008), and after one removal, infants in foster care stand a one in three chance of returning to the child welfare system later on (Wulczyn, Brunner Hislop, & Jones Harden, 2002). Half of babies who enter foster care before age 3 months spend an average of 31 months or longer in placement (Wulczyn & Hislop, 2002).

In addition to higher rates of maltreatment and removal, the effects of trauma on very young brains may be particularly devastating. From birth to age 3, children develop foundational capabilities in all domains of functioning, including cognitive, emotional, social, moral, and regulatory domains (National Research Council and Institute of Medicine, 2000). Maltreatment and instability at an early age act as "toxic stress," sometimes permanently impacting the neurophysiology and chemistry of the developing brain (Middlebrooks & Audage, 2008). And although babies and toddlers are tremendously resilient, the notion that they do not remember or are less affected than older children by maltreatment and instability is a fallacy. Research has shown that babies only months old can develop depression, are adversely affected by witnessing and experiencing trauma, and can easily sense the mood and emotions of caregivers (DYG, Inc., Civitas, Zero to Three, & the Brio Corporation, 2000).

Luckily the vulnerability experienced by babies and toddlers in the child welfare system can be tempered by their resilience when effective interventions are applied. At-risk children who are provided with effective, early interventions have dramatically improved outcomes on cognitive, scholastic, and social measures well into adulthood (Berrueta-Clement, Schweinhart, Barnett, Epstein, & Weikart, 1984; National Research Council and Institute of Medicine, 2000, pp. 342–343). Thus, for at-risk children, the early years of childhood are both a time of great vulnerability and a window of opportunity within which troubled trajectories can be altered.

It was with this in mind that Zero to Three, in partnership with San Francisco and other localities, sought to pilot the Court Team model to foster better outcomes for very young, traumatized children in the child welfare system. The Court Teams project has two related goals. The first goal is to increase awareness among all professionals working with babies and toddlers in the child welfare system about the consequences of maltreatment and trauma on these young children. The second is to use this knowledge to change local systems to improve outcomes and prevent future court involvement for these children (Zero to Three, 2008). In 2008, this model was brought to San Francisco.

Establishing the Court Team

A congressional allocation to National Zero to Three authorized the Court Team in San Francisco. The funding provided an experienced child welfare Community Coordinator to work directly with the court. The Community Coordinator initially assisted the court in bringing together a multidisciplinary team of over 20 professionals, from the nonprofit and government sectors, who provided services for infants and toddlers. The resulting team included psychologists, the Human Services Agency, pediatricians, Early Head Start, parent educators, the coordinators of the regional center serving children with developmental delays, public health department, San Francisco Court-Appointed Special Advocates (CASA), the Supervising Judge, and court staff and attorneys. For several months, the team met to identify existing gaps in services, how to ensure that a child's needs were properly assessed, how services could be quickly accessed, and how a dedicated Zero to Three Court might function. These initial collaborative meetings, as well as the breadth and depth of expertise embodied by the members, has set the tone for the Court Team going forward. Members of the Court Team continue to meet on a regular basis to advise the court, coordinate efforts among themselves, identify gaps in services, and collectively work to close the gaps.

The Functioning of the Zero to Three Court

After the initial planning process, the dedicated court was formed. The case of every child who is the subject of a child abuse/neglect petition between birth and age 3 years and placed in San Francisco is sent to this dedicated court. Early in the process, a dedicated Zero to Three court officer is named to work with the Community Coordinator to identify cases that fit the Zero to Three criteria before the detention hearing is even held. This enables the Zero to Three Community Coordinator to be notified of the case, to review the file, and to attend the first hearing, thereby bringing to bear the resources of Zero to Three to the child and family from the very start. The goal, as much as possible, is to join collaboratively with all parties at the start to focus on the needs of the child rather than the contentions of the legal process. To this end, the Community Coordinator seeks information from parents of children who have been removed to help the children feel as comfortable as possible during a difficult time. Questions like "Does your child have a favorite food?"; "How does he or she like to sleep?"; and "Does your baby have a nickname?" acknowledge the expertise of parents and helps them to feel invested in the process.

With the formation of this court, the Community Coordinator also assumed additional case management duties, ensuring that for each child there is a complete medical, developmental, and psychological assessment within 2 weeks of the child coming into the system. The Community Coordinator then works with the child's social worker to make sure the child has been connected to all appropriate services. As part of assessing each child's needs upon entering the system, the Community Coordinator conducts a home visit to meet each child and caregiver, discuss what services are necessary to foster healthy outcomes for the child, and to understand how visitations are going. If caregivers have concerns regarding a child's functioning or health, the Community Coordinator sets up consultations with Zero to Three medical professionals to address the child's needs. Finally, he or she works directly to assist the parents in connecting with services, provides encouragement, and facilitates visitation. Many of the parents also participate in Dependency Drug Court, and the Community Coordinator works closely with that program.

Cases in the court also have greater judicial oversight and intervention. A case can be on calendar as often as twice a month, depending on the individualized needs of the case. For example, in situations where a placement is not stabilized, concurrent planning has not occurred, services are not in place, or parental visitation is problematic, the case comes back to court more frequently. Prior to the calling of each court calendar, the Community Coordinator meets with the parents, all attorneys, the child welfare worker, and appropriate service providers to review services, parental participation in programs, the child's needs, and visitation. There is a collaborative approach to decision making and problem solving. Beyond the calendar meetings, the Community Coordinator works on an ongoing basis to monitor case progress with the child welfare worker, including a monthly check-in meeting for each case, and to work with all professionals to ensure the timely implementation of appropriate services.

The Children and Families in San Francisco's Court for Infants and Toddlers

As of January 2010, 41 children from 38 families were being served in San Francisco's Court for Maltreated Infants and Toddlers. As is typical of the child welfare system in general, both statewide and nationally, ethnic-minority children are significantly overrepresented. In San Francisco's court, 45% of the children are African American, 24% are European American, 15% are Latino, 14% are multiethnic, and 2% are Asian/Pacific Islander. The children the court serves are, in general, very young and have experienced significant adversities very early in life, including prenatally. The average age of the court children is 8 months, and for many, dependency is granted only days or weeks after birth. This is because many of these children are brought in to the system due to positive toxicology results at birth, alerting the agency to a parent's serious substance abuse problem. Eighty percent of the children have been removed for this reason. The other reasons the court in San Francisco has taken jurisdiction are equally grave, and include parental incarceration, severe parental mental health issues, domestic violence, abuse, and neglect. In addition, our parents themselves experienced significant adversity in their own childhoods, which has impacted their ability to parent successfully. Of 38 mothers, the parent the court most often has information about, 21 were once in foster care themselves. Two of the parents currently on the Court Team calendar are still minors and in the foster care system right now.

In order to better understand the court's families and the nature of the challenges they must overcome to reunify, if possible, with their children, we have included several case examples here. Not surprisingly, parents' inability to care adequately for young children so soon after they are born is indicative of extreme stress and challenges. But despite their gravity, the stories of our Court Team families also hold out hope, particularly in the way that additional case management, judicial oversight, and faster connections to appropriate services have had such an impact, allowing many families to make significant progress, and children to achieve stable permanency.

Case Example 1

Emma, a 30-year-old single mother, gave birth to her son Michael at a hospital in San Francisco. From the start, Michael's young life was challenging. He was born prematurely, with several very serious medical and genetic problems, including cerebral palsy, visual impairment, and motor difficulties. Because of his premature birth and the ensuing medical problems, Michael stayed in the hospital for over 2 months as the staff worked to address his medical issues and to help him get strong and healthy enough to go home with his mom.

Not surprisingly, this was a very challenging time for Emma. As Michael's hospital stay progressed, the staff became increasingly concerned about Emma's behavior. She sometimes missed visits and had a hard time following hospital rules, such as remembering to wear a hospital mask in the neonatal intensive care unit (NICU). Emma also had a hard time taking advice from hospital staff members as they taught her how to care for her medically fragile baby and often became impatient and angry. The staff members were concerned that Emma would not be able to meet Michael's needs upon discharge and ultimately made a referral to child protective services, unfortunately without telling Emma first. When she was unable to take her son home, Emma was furious and upset.

When the case was referred to the court, it was quickly apparent that one of the challenges of helping Emma to reunify with her son was her deep distrust of "the system." After several months of frequent communications and contacts between Emma, the Community Coordinator, the case manager, and the foster parent, the source of Emma's distrust became clear—she, too, had been a foster child. Her early childhood had been marked by unstable foster homes and reunifications with her birth mother. As an adolescent she had spent time in juvenile detention and had struggled with substance use and mental health issues. She had not trusted anyone enough to reveal this background for several months. Armed with this knowledge, the team set about trying to establish a collaborative relationship with Emma.

The team wanted to encourage visitations in the home of the foster parent, who initially was open to the idea but later became concerned as court hearings became contentious. When the team found out that visitations were occurring immediately after court, the visitation times were moved and the situation improved dramatically. The team also worked to keep Emma intimately involved with all of Michael's medical needs by having her sign all medical authorizations. Emma's relationship with professionals and the foster parent slowly began to improve. When Michael went in for surgery on his legs, his mother signed all of the paperwork and slept each night in the hospital with him, while the foster parent checked in daily. After 2 days in the hospital, Emma reached out to the Community Coordinator and asked her to come to the hospital and wait with her by Michael's bed. She cried and acknowledged what a difficult time this was for her. The team could see that after several months, the efforts to build trust were starting to work.

Case Example 2

Anna, age 25, was over 8 months pregnant when she began to experience severe respiratory problems. Anna's immune system was already weakened by a prior medical condition and she was diagnosed with pneumonia upon entry to the hospital. After several days it became tragically clear that Anna would not survive, and she was put into a drug-induced coma. Her baby boy, Patrick, was delivered successfully and survived. Anna died a few days later. Because the identity of Patrick's father was not known, he was placed with Anna's parents.

About 3 months later a young man named Thomas contacted the Human Services Agency and said that he had just learned of Anna's death and the birth of a baby boy. He believed that he was Patrick's father, which was later confirmed by paternity testing. Thomas had a long history of drug use, but he was currently in Narcotics Anonymous, had completed a substance abuse program, and was very involved with his sponsor, who had helped him find a job and housing. The Human Services Agency and the Community Coordinator met with him a number of times over the next 2 months. Patrick's grandparents were very anxious about the idea that he might be placed with his father because they had grown to love Patrick very much and were concerned about Thomas's stability. They filed for de facto parent status and wanted to fight to adopt him. However, even through this level of anxiety and uncertainty, they continued to work with the agency and Thomas on visitation. They allowed Thomas to have visits with Patrick at their home, occasionally had him over for dinner, and slowly began to forge a relationship with him.

Three months later, Thomas informed the court that he had relapsed and as a result had lost his housing and job. He continued to struggle significantly with his addiction. Even with these challenges, Patrick's grandparents continued to have a relationship with Thomas. He still visits their home to see his son. They have pledged to work with the Human Services Agency and the court to enable Thomas to remain in his son's life in an appropriate and safe way, even if he ultimately does not have physical custody of Patrick.

Case Example 3

Nicole, the young daughter of Jane and Bill, was born with a positive toxicology report. Jane and Bill both had a history of substance use and mental illness, but they wanted treatment and to work to retain custody of their baby. Soon after Nicole's birth, as part of their reunification requirements, the whole family entered a dual-diagnosis treatment facility where parents and children could be placed together during ongoing treatment. It soon became clear to the Human Services Agency and the court that these parents were having difficulty meeting their reunification targets, even with the close monitoring of the Community Coordinator and the court, and the extra support of the residential staff. Both parents were initially compliant with their treatment plan, but their relationship remained unstable. After approximately 3 months of treatment, Bill left the program and lost contact with the court and his daughter. Mother and daughter remained in the residential program, but the mother's behavior became increasingly erratic. One day, while the baby was being cared for by facility staff, Jane left the treatment program and disappeared. It was later learned that she had relapsed. Nicole was placed in a foster home. Despite extensive searches, neither parent could be located.

Because of the close contact between the Community Coordinator and the residential facility, it was discovered that, months earlier, Nicole's paternal aunt and uncle had sent her a gift of toys when they learned of her birth and her parents' efforts to recover. Armed with that knowledge, the agency went back and mined the files, ultimately finding and contacting Nicole's aunt and uncle. They had had no contact with their brother and were not aware that Nicole had been placed in foster care. The aunt and uncle quickly came to San Francisco to care for Nicole and have since filed to adopt her.

Early Successes

Although San Francisco's Court Team continues to evolve, dramatic results have been seen after just 6 months. In Court Team cases there are fewer placements, and concurrent planning occurs earlier. Comprehensive multidisciplinary assessments are more timely, narrowly tailored to the developmental needs of infants and young children, and results are communicated in a highly useable manner to caregivers. Parents and children alike are assessed and connected to appropriate services quickly, and their utilization of services is tracked via monthly check-ins and twice-monthly court calendars. The issue of consistent, frequent, and quality visitation between parents and children is especially crucial for the healthy development of babies and toddlers, and here, too, Court Team cases have shown improvement. Visitations are more frequent and increasingly occur in a collaborative manner between parents and caregivers. Pick-ups occur at the caregiver's home, parents regularly attend child medical and service appointments along with the caregiver, and visits sometimes take place in the caregiver's home. One hundred percent of parents in the court have visitations for 6 hours or more per week, including incarcerated parents, or those who have retained custody of their children through the dependency process. In one instance, when visitations to the jail became problematic, communication between the Community Coordinator and the Sheriff's Office resulted in an organized tour to orient attorneys and caregivers to the jail facility.

The ripple effects of the Court Team model are also being felt in the community at large as service providers work together to expand and target services to these vulnerable children. The Human Services Agency increased the number of caseworkers dedicated to work on Zero to Three cases and has worked to focus reports on the specific needs of babies and toddlers, including prenatal and birth history information that is crucial for caregivers. When gaps in services have been identified, particularly in services targeted toward parents, the Court Team model has fostered greater accountability for child development services in residential treatment programs. Similarly, some parents and attorneys have shared their appreciation for the Court Team model, giving feedback that the monthly meetings to discuss progress are helpful and steer cases in a positive direction. All in all, the benefits of Court Team far outweigh the cost of the Community

Coordinator staff position and have been felt across a range of services and professionals.

CONCLUSION

Not surprisingly, collaboration between the courts and community service providers is complex. Accurate and timely identification of families' needs and the effective connection to appropriate service providers is challenging, but it can be done. The task is made easier when the wide range of professionals who provide crucial interventions to young children and their parents in the child welfare system are in frequent contact and communication, and have a shared understanding of the special needs of young children.

When care is taken to identify gaps and to address issues that arise, involving courts in a collaboration of community agencies can be a powerful tool to serve families most in need of assistance. Courts can help service providers reach families that might otherwise not come to their attention. Providers can make it possible for courts to offer more than orders and punishment to families. In San Francisco we have seen many cases, like those described in this chapter, where the court, working with a cooperating agency, has intervened to protect our youngest children and to break the cycle of violence in families. The power of courts and clinicians together to improve outcomes for children is much greater than that of either group acting alone.

NOTES

1. The Safe Start Initiative was originally funded by the Office of Juvenile Justice and Delinquency Prevention of the U.S. Department of Justice, with continuation funding provided by the City and County of San Francisco, Department of Children, Youth, and Their Families, and the First Five Commission.
2. The Court Teams for Maltreated Infants and Toddlers Project is funded by the Office of Juvenile Justice and Delinquency Prevention of the U.S. Department of Justice. Considerable technical and advisory support is provided by Zero to Three: National Center for Infants, Toddlers, and Families.

REFERENCES

Berrueta-Clement, J. R., Schweinhart, L. J., Barnett, W. S., Epstein, A. S., & Weikart, D. P. (1984). Changed lives: The effects of the Perry Preschool Program on youths through age 19. Ypsilanti, MI: High Scope Educational Research Foundation. Retrieved February 11, 2010, from *www.eric.ed.gov/ericdocs/data/ericdocs2sql/content_storage_01/0000019b/80/1f/9e/e5.pdf.*

Centers for Disease Control and Prevention. (2008a). Web-Based Injury Statistics Query and Reporting System (WISQARS), Leading Causes of Death Reports, 1999–2006. Atlanta, GA: CDC, National Center for Injury Prevention and Control (Producer). Retrieved February 10, 2010, from *webappa.cdc.gov/sas-web/ncipc/leadcaus10.html.*

Centers for Disease Control and Prevention. (2008b). Web-Based Injury Statistics Query and Reporting System (WISQARS), Nonfatal Injuries: Nonfatal injury reports. Atlanta, GA: CDC, National Center for Injury Prevention and Control (Producer). Retrieved February 10, 2010, from *webappa.cdc.gov/sasweb/ncipc/nfirates2001.html.*

Centers for Disease Control and Prevention. (2009). Child maltreatment: Facts at a glance. Atlanta, GA: Author. Retrieved February 10, 2010, from *www.cdc.gov/violenceprevention/pdf/cm-datasheet-a.pdf.*

Children's Defense Fund. (2008a). Cradle to Prison Pipeline Campaign: California factsheet. Washington, DC: Author. Retrieved February 10, 2010, from *www.childrensdefense.org/child-research-data-publications/data/state-data-repository/cradle-to-prison-pipeline/cradle-prison-pipeline-california-2009-fact-sheet.pdf.*

Children's Defense Fund. (2008b). The state of America's children 2008. Washington, DC: Author. Retrieved February 10, 2010, from *www.childrensdefense.org/child-research-data-publications/data/state-of-americas-children-2008-report.pdf.*

Cicchetti, D., & Cohen, D. J. (1995). *Manual of developmental psychopathology.* New York: Wiley.

Cicchetti, D., Rogosch, F. A., & Toth, S. L. (2006). Fostering secure attachment in infants in maltreating families through preventive interventions. *Development and Psychopathology, 18,* 623–649.

De Bellis, M. D., Baum, A. S., Birmaher, B., Keshavan, M. S., Eccard, C. H., Boring, A. M., et al. (1999a). Developmental traumatology: Part I. Biological stress systems. *Biological Psychiatry, 45,* 1259–1270.

De Bellis, M. D., Baum, A. S., Birmaher, B., Keshavan, M. S., Eccard, C. H., Boring, A. M., et al. (1999b). Developmental traumatology: Part II. Brain development. *Biological Psychiatry, 45,* 1271–1284.

Deitch, M., Barstow, A., Lukens, L., & Reyna, R. (2009). From time out to hard time: Young children in the adult criminal justice system. Austin: The University of Texas at Austin, LBJ School of Public Affairs. Retrieved February 10, 2010, from *www.utexas.edu/lbj/news/images/file/from%20time%20out%20to%20hard%20time-revised%20final.pdf.*

DYG, Inc., Civitas, Zero to Three, & the Brio Corporation. (2000). What grownups understand about child development: A national benchmark survey. Retrieved December 20, 2010, from *www.buildinitiative.org/files/grown-ups.pdf.*

Lieberman, A. F., Van Horn, P., & Ghosh Ippen, C. (2005). Toward evidence-based treatment: Child–parent psychotherapy with preschoolers exposed to marital violence. *Journal of the American Academy of Child and Adolescent Psychiatry, 44*(12), 1241–1248.

Lieberman, A. F., Ghosh Ippen, C., & Van Horn, P. (2006). Child–parent psychotherapy: 6-month follow-up of a randomized controlled trial. *Journal of the American Academy of Child and Adolescent Psychiatry, 45*(8), 913–918.

Marans, S., & Adelman, A. (1997). Experiencing violence in a developmental context. In J. D. Osofsky (Ed.), *Children in a violent society* (pp. 202–222). New York: Guilford Press.

Middlebrooks, J. S., & Audage, N. C. (2008). *The effects of childhood stress on health across the lifespan*. Atlanta, GA: Centers for Disease Control and Prevention, National Center for Injury Prevention and Control. Retrieved February 10, 2010, from *www.cdc.gov/ncipc/pub-res/pdf/childhood_stress.pdf*.

National Research Council and Institute of Medicine. (2000). *From neurons to neighborhoods: The science of early childhood development* (Committee on Integrating the Science of Early Childhood Development, J. P. Shonkoff & D. A. Phillips, Eds., Board on Children, Youth, and Families, Commission on Behavioral and Social Sciences and Education). Washington, DC: National Academy Press.

National Youth Gang Center. (2009). National Youth Gang survey analysis. Tallahassee, FL: Author. Retrieved December 5, 2009, from *www.nationalgangcenter.gov/survey-analysis*.

Osofsky, J. D. (1997). Children and youth violence: An overview of the issue. In *Children in a violent society* (pp. 3–8). New York: Guilford Press.

Osofsky, J. D., & Lederman, C. (2004). Healing the child in juvenile court. In *Young children and trauma* (pp. 221–241). New York: Guilford Press.

Osofsky, J. D., & Scheeringa, M. S. (1997). Community and domestic violence exposure: Effects of development and psychopathology. In D. Cicchetti & S. Toth (Eds.), *Rochester Symposium on Developmental Psychopathology: Vol. 8. Developmental perspectives on trauma* (pp. 155–180). Rochester, NY: University of Rochester Press.

Puzzanchera, C. (2007). Juvenile arrests. Washington, DC: Office of Juvenile Justice and Delinquency Prevention. Retrieved February 10, 2010, from *ojjdp.ncjrs.org/ojstatbb/crime/qa05101.asp?qadate=2007&text=*.

Pynoos, R. S., Steinberg, A. M., & Piacentini, J. C. (1999). A developmental psychopathology model of childhood traumatic stress and intersection with anxiety disorders. *Biological Psychiatry, 46,* 1542–1554.

Rolnick, A. J., & Grunewald, R. (2007, Fall). The economics of early childhood development as seen by two fed economists. *Community Investments,* pp. 13–14.

Ryan, J. P., & Testa, M. F. (2005). Child maltreatment and juvenile delinquency: Investigating the role of placement and placement instability. *Children and Youth Services Review, 27,* 227–249.

Thorton, T. N., Craft, C. A., Dahlberg, L. L., Lynch, B. S., & Baer, K. (2002). *Best practices of youth violence prevention: A sourcebook for community action.* Atlanta, GA: Centers for Disease Control and Prevention, National Center for Injury Prevention and Control.

Toth, S. L., Rogosch, F. A., Manly, J. T., & Cicchetti, D. (2006). The efficacy of toddler–parent psychotherapy to reorganize attachment in the young offspring of mothers with major depressive disorder: A randomized preventive trial. *Journal of Consulting and Clinical Psychology, 74*(6), 1006–1016.

U.S. Department of Health and Human Services, Administration on Children, Youth and Families. (2009). *Child Maltreatment 2007*. Washington, DC: U.S. Government Printing Office.

U.S. Department of Health and Human Services, Administration on Children, Youth and Families, Children's Bureau. (2008). The Adoption and Foster Care Analysis and Reporting System (AFCARS). Washington, DC: U.S. Government Printing Office. Retrieved February 10, 2010, from *www.acf.hhs.gov/programs/cb/ stats_research/afcars/tar/report14.htm*.

Van Horn, P., & Hitchens, D. J. (2004). Partnerships for young children in court: How judges shape collaborations serving traumatized children. In J. D. Osofsky (Ed.), *Young children and trauma: Intervention and treatment* (pp. 242–259). New York: Guilford Press.

Windom, C. S., & Maxfield, M. G. (1996). A prospective examination of risk for violence among abused and neglected children. *Annals of the New York Academy of Science, 794*, 224–237.

Windom, C. S., & Maxfield, M. G. (2001). An update on the "cycle of violence." Washington, DC: U.S. Department of Justice, Office of Justice Programs, National Institute of Justice. Retrieved February 10, 2010, *from www.ncjrs. gov/pdffiles1/nij/184894.pdf*.

Wulczyn, F., & Hislop, K. (2002). Babies in foster care: The numbers call for attention. *Zero to Three Journal, 22*(4), 14–15.

Wulczyn, F., Brunner Hislop, K., & Jones Harden, B. (2002). The placement of infants in foster care. *Infant Mental Health Journal, 23*(5), 454–475.

Zero to Three. (2008). Changing the odds for babies: Court teams for maltreated infants and toddlers. Washington, DC: Author. Retrieved February 11, 2010, from *www.zerotothree.org/site/docserver/court_teams_final_fact_sheet. pdf?docid=3881*.

CHAPTER 13

■ ■ ■ ■

Dependency Drug Court

An Intensive Intervention for Traumatized Mothers and Young Children

Jeri B. Cohen
Gayle A. Dakof
Eliette Duarte

Trauma is no stranger to the women and children involved in dependency drug courts (DDCs). Young children of addicted mothers are at high risk of physical and emotional neglect (Erickson & Tonigan, 2008); often they witness or are victims of family violence (Magura & Laudet, 1996; Walsh, MacMillan, & Jamieson, 2003), and they are likely to receive neglectful and punitive parenting (Hein & Miele, 2003). The research is unequivocal: Infants and toddlers exposed to trauma display significant behavioral and emotional problems (e.g., Maughan & Cicchetti, 2002; Osofsky, 1995), and are at high risk for poor developmental outcomes throughout childhood and adolescence (Osofsky, 2004; Windom, 2000). Moreover, the mothers of these young children are themselves often trauma victims (Banyard, Williams, & Siegal, 2003). Many were neglected and abused as children, and as adults have suffered the exigencies of poverty, violence, and despair (Gara, Allen, Herzog, & Woolfolk, 2000).

The problems associated with child maltreatment and maternal substance abuse constitute a public health concern of the utmost importance (Magura & Laudet, 1996). It is estimated that as many as 80% of children involved in the child welfare system have a drug-dependent parent (Barth, Courtney, Duerr, Berrick, & Albert, 1994; Curtis & McCullough, 1993; Locke & Newcomb, 2004). Although there are interventions for adult substance use, interventions for infants and toddlers exposed to traumatic circumstances, and interventions designed to improve parenting practices of mothers involved in the child welfare system (e.g., Casanueva, Martin, Runyan, Barth, & Bradley, 2008; Suchman, Pajulo, DeCoste, & Mayes, 2006), these services are often not coordinated, integrative, or holistic. In many dependency courts, service providers for the parents and service providers for the children rarely, if ever, communicate or approach the case with a coordinated case plan that seeks a symbiosis between the services. By offering intensive and integrated multidisciplinary services aimed at addressing the dual problems of child maltreatment and maternal addiction, DDC offers a unique and distinct approach to handling child abuse and neglect cases involving addicted, frequently dual-diagnosis parents. DDCs, adapted from the adult drug court model, were established to serve "the best interests of the child" by helping parents "become emotionally, financially, and personally self-sufficient and to develop parenting and coping skills adequate for serving as an effective parent on a day-to-day basis" (Office of Justice Programs, 1998, p. 5). DDCs address parental addiction, mental health, and trauma, as well as child safety and permanency (Edwards & Ray, 2005; Green, Furrer, Worcel, Burrus, & Finigan, 2009), and, as such, offer a unique opportunity to change the lives of children—to break the intergenerational cycle of substance abuse, poor mental health, and violence—and to prevent future trauma exposure for mother and child.

Although research on DDC is limited, a small number of studies indicate that drug court has promise (Boles, Young, Moore, & DiPirro-Beard, 2007; Dakof, Cohen, & Duarte, 2009; Dakof et al., in press; Green, Furrer, Worcel, Burrus, & Finigan, 2007, 2009; Haack, Alemi, Nemes, & Cohen, 2004; Worcel, Furrer, Green, Burrus, & Finigan, 2008). Most DDCs share key elements, including a nonadversarial relationship among the participating partners, comprehensive assessment of service needs, frequent court hearings and drug testing, intensive judicial supervision, enrollment in substance abuse treatment programs designed to improve parenting practices and other necessary services, and the administration of judicial rewards and sanctions. In order to graduate from DDCs, participants must have successfully completed substance abuse treatment, remain compliant with mental health services, have a specified period of continuous abstinence, show evidence of a safe and stable living situation, spend a substantial period of time adequately performing the parental role, and have a life plan initiated and in place (e.g., employment, education, vocational training).

DDCs frequently include drug court counselors, who refer clients to substance abuse treatment and other court-ordered services, develop a recovery service plan, and monitor and report clients' ongoing progress to the court (Edwards & Ray, 2005). Although there are numerous components to DDCs, the contributions of the drug court judge and counselors to the effectiveness of drug court are undeniable (Dakof et al., 2009: Edwards & Ray, 2005; National Association of Drug Court Professionals [NADCP], 1997).

MIAMI–DADE DEPENDENCY DRUG COURT

The State of Florida 11th Circuit Judicial Juvenile Court in Miami, Florida, established a DDC in 1999. In order to be eligible for DDC, parents must be (1) 18 years or older, (2) with at least one child adjudicated dependent; (3) have a diagnosis of substance abuse or dependence, (4) have a potential for family reunification; and (5) after consultation with their attorney, voluntarily enroll in drug court.

The DDC is a 12- to 15-month program organized into four phases. Progression through the phases is related to the mother's level of substance abuse treatment and compliance with court orders. An assessment of the mother (using the Addiction Severity Index, as well as other structured instruments) is conducted immediately upon acceptance into drug court, and placement in appropriate substance abuse treatment is commenced, in many instances, even before the arraignment of the case. Whenever possible, children are kept with their parents in maternal or family addiction programs. When this is not possible, visitations occur frequently in order to maintain mother–child bonding. Thus, with very young children, visitation may occur three times per week. Parents are drug-tested (urine screens) at each court hearing and in their substance abuse treatment programs. These programs are required to report progress or lack thereof to the court. During the first month of drug court, mothers attend weekly drug court hearings. Thereafter, if reports to the court indicate that the mother is progressing well, court hearings are reduced to twice monthly. During Phase 2 of the program, which lasts approximately 3 months, clients continue to attend twice-monthly hearings. In Phase 3, which lasts another 3 months, the frequency of hearings is reduced to once per month. In the final Phase 4, which extends to graduation from drug court, clients attend hearings every 6–12 weeks.

This multiphase process includes a collaborative team approach that involves attorneys, drug court counselors, child welfare workers, treatment providers, parent educators, and other social and health care service providers, as needed. Drug court counselors have contact with their clients, either in-person or on the phone, on a weekly basis through Phase 2, reducing to biweekly in Phase 3, and monthly in Phase 4. Counselors are available more frequently on an as-needed basis. The caseload for drug court counselors is between 10 and 15 active cases. All cases have both dedicated child welfare workers and drug court counselors. Along with the attorneys, the drug court counselors, child welfare caseworkers, and treatment providers meet weekly to staff the case.

ENGAGING MOMS PROGRAM FOR DEPENDENCY DRUG COURT COUNSELORS

Counselors in the Miami–Dade DDC have been implementing the Engaging Moms Program (EMP) for over 5 years. This program is based on the theory and method of multidimensional family therapy (Liddle, Dakof, & Diamond, 1991). EMP was designed to help mothers succeed in drug court by complying with all court orders, such as attending and benefiting from substance abuse treatment, parenting intervention programs, and other services ordered by the court (e.g., domestic violence counseling, psychiatric care). EMP counselors do whatever it takes to facilitate recovery and stability, and enhance a mother's capacity to parent her children. EMP has shown considerable promise in the DDC context (Dakof et al., 2009, in press), specifically by increasing the likelihood of positive child welfare and parent outcomes when compared to standard drug court case management. EMP has been shown to reduce the number of parental rights terminations, placement in the foster care system, and overall risk for child abuse; and to improve the mother's mental and physical health status.

EMP counselors focus on six core areas of change: (1) mother's motivation and commitment to succeed in drug court and to change her life; (2) the emotional attachment between the mother and her children; (3) relationships between the mother and her family of origin; (4) parenting skills; (5) the mother's romantic relationships; and (6) coping and problem-solving skills. Mothers achieve change by participating in a series of integrated individual and family sessions with the drug court counselors (e.g., individual sessions with mother, individual sessions with family/partner, family and couple sessions).

EMP is organized in three stages: Stage 1, Alliance and Motivation; Stage 2, Behavioral Change; and Stage 3, Launch to an Independent Life.

In Stage 1, the counselor focuses on two goals: (1) building a strong therapeutic alliance with the mother and her family, and (2) enhancing mother and family motivation to participate in drug court and to change their behavior. EMP counselors provide support to both the mother and her family. They empower and validate; highlight strengths and competencies; build confidence in the program; and are very compassionate, loving, and nurturing. To enhance motivation, the EMP counselor highlights the pain, guilt, and shame that the mother and her family have experienced, and the high stakes involved (e.g., losing a child to the child welfare system), while simultaneously creating positive expectations and hope.

Stage 2 focuses on behavioral change in both the mother and her family/spouse focusing especially on drug use, parenting, and romantic relationships. EMP has several goals for this stage. First, counselors enhance the emotional attachment between the mother and her children by working individually with the mother to help her explore her maternal role. Mother and children sessions designed to enhance the mother's commitment to her children are also provided. Equally important is enhancement of the attachment between the mother and her family of origin and/or spouse. This is accomplished by helping the family restrain from negativity and offer instrumental and emotional support to the mother. Considerable attention is devoted to repairing the mother's relationship with her family, which frequently has been damaged by past hurts, betrayals, and resentments. Romantic relationships, typically with men, have often been a source of pain and distress for many of the mothers involved in the child welfare system. Hence, the EMP program addresses these relationships by helping the mother conduct a relationship life review, including examination of tensions between having a romantic relationship and being a mother. The counselors help the mother examine the choices she has made, and continues to make, in terms of romantic relationships, and teach her how to make better decisions for herself and her children. EMP counselors also help the mother address slips, mistakes, setbacks, and relapses in a nonpunitive and therapeutic manner (i.e., forward looking). Finally, in Stage 2, the EMP counselor facilitates the mother's relationship with court personnel (judge, child welfare workers, and attorneys) and treatment or other service providers. The EMP counselor conducts "shuttle diplomacy" between the mother and service providers to prevent and resolve problems, and helps the mother take full advantage of the services provided to her. With respect to the court, the drug court counselors facilitate therapeutic jurisprudence in the courtroom by preparing mothers for court appearances and advocating for the mother in front of the judge and at weekly drug court case reviews.

In the final launching phase (Stage 3), the EMP counselor helps the mother prepare for an independent life by developing a practical and workable routine for everyday life; addressing how the mother will balance self-care, children, and work; outlining a plan to address common emergencies with children and families; and addressing how the mother will deal with potential problems, mistakes, slips, and relapses.

THE WORK OF THE DEPENDENCY COURT JUDGE

Being an effective DDC judge requires considerable knowledge, skill, and experience. Obviously, the role of the DDC judge is key because he or she not only makes all the final decisions concerning graduation or discharge, child placement, and whether or not to terminate parental rights (TPR) but also establishes the tone and direction of the court, holds drug court counselors and key drug court partners (attorneys, treatment and other service providers, child welfare caseworkers) to high standards, resolves differences among partners, and functions as a role model. If the judge is well-organized and efficient, then the partners will be well-organized and efficient; and if the judge works to a high standard of excellence, then so will the partners. Finally, if the judge is highly involved in the daily functioning and workings of the drug court, clearly articulates the mission and values of the dependency drug court, and embraces a leadership style that is both collaborative and firm, then drug court counselors, partnering agencies and institutions, and even the DDC mothers will have an opportunity to function at an extremely high level of competence and cooperation.

Drug court is a collaborative effort among the various professionals and stakeholders involved in child welfare; this includes not only the judge but also the attorneys (defense and state); child advocates, such as the guardian *ad litem,* child welfare caseworkers, substance abuse treatment providers, parenting intervention providers, other service providers (e.g., child psychologists and psychiatrists), day care agencies, and schools; physicians; and, of course, the DDC counselors. Sometimes the sheer number of professionals involved can be overwhelming and counterproductive (i.e., "Too many cooks spoil the brew"), but the needs of the mothers and young children involved in DDC are vast, and it is frequently necessary to have a large number of professionals involved in the life of a single family. Without strong judicial leadership there would be chaos, inefficiency, and ineffectiveness.

The judge not only establishes the direction of the court, convenes the necessary stakeholders, monitors progress or the lack thereof, and demands respect for due process but also functions as an inspirational leader. Given the natural conflict between the long tradition of an adversarial legal system and the nonadversarial nature of drug court, a strong judicial leader is necessary to speak for the mission of drug court and to create an environment where mutual trust is nurtured. Each partner is essential to drug court, and the judge, of course, must rely on all the stakeholders. Thus, the DDC judge first needs to convene a highly competent and dedicated group of partners and stakeholders, then to respect each member's expertise and turf in the context of very strong judicial leadership.

Given the complex nature of DDC, the judge's training as an attorney is not sufficient. The judge in this setting needs to develop considerable competency in the fields of substance abuse and early child development, mental health and trauma, parenting practices, and family functioning (Lederman & Osofsky, 2008). This seems like a tall order, but it is our experience that the more the judge knows about these areas, the better he or she is able to determine which services and types of care are necessary. The judge will also be better able to monitor the delivery of services and use his or her position to demand higher quality services for mothers and young children, and to negotiate with the providers for enhanced services.

Dependency courts generally, and DDCs in particular, have a distinctly comprehensive perspective on young children involved in the child welfare system. The DDC focuses not only on the immediate family but also the extended family and anyone else who comes into contact with the child. The ultimate goal is to break the intergenerational cycle of substance abuse, untreated mental illness, domestic violence, and child neglect and abuse. The most effective DDC judges are widely read on child development, addiction, and trauma; they seek out educational opportunities and demand excellence in every aspect of their court, including the implementation of evidence-based practices (Lederman, Gomez-Kaifer, Katz, Thomlison, & Maze, 2009). With knowledge comes judicial leadership and innovation.

Cleary, DDC is a cooperative and collaborative effort, and it is the judge's responsibility to ensure that all the parties involved in the court work as a team. Achieving a truly cooperative and nonadversarial drug court is not an easy task, and it does not happen without strong and consistent teamwork. Many actions can be taken to inspire and maintain teamwork. First, all partners need to be aware of what other partners on the team are doing. Second, the judge cannot be biased and should show respect toward all partners. Third, all parties should be encouraged to attend monthly drug court meetings and weekly staffings designed to facilitate staff dedication to the court and its mission, and to solicit a discussion of problems and solutions.

Key ingredients of an effective DDC involve strong judicial leadership based on (1) knowledge about drug court, legal issues, child development and maternal addiction; (2) a clear and consistent mission; (3) competent partners who embrace evidence-based practices; (4) the creation of an atmosphere of respect and teamwork; (5) and a demand for excellence. It is the drug court judge who is responsible for integrating all the disparate parts of DDC into a comprehensive and integrated whole, ultimately leading it to its success or failure.

CASE ILLUSTRATION

What follows is an illustration of how DDC can produce positive developmental outcomes for young children involved in the child welfare system.

In this illustration we focus on how the judge and drug court counselors facilitate improvement in the young child through adequate assessment and placement in appropriate interventions, and improved parenting practices. It is important to recognize that since the mission of DDC is to sustain the mother's recovery from drug use and improve her overall functioning, as well as to improve parenting practices and child functioning, this illustration is necessarily partial. We do not delineate how the judge and drug court counselor help the mother (1) develop better coping, problem-solving, and communication skills; (2) sustain her sobriety; (3) improve her relationships with her family of origin and romantic partners; and (4) develop a life plan to balance her own individual needs with the demands of being a parent.

Our focus is on 2-year-old Reggie, exposed before birth to cocaine and benzodiazepines, and his 38-year-old mother Brianna. Prior to Reggie's birth, Brianna had her parental rights terminated on four children because she repeatedly failed to complete substance abuse treatment and demonstrate sufficient skills and capacity to parent her young children adequately. It was alleged in the dependency petition that Reggie frequently accompanied his mother while she was under the influence of drugs and engaged in prostitution. Child welfare records revealed that Brianna had five prior abuse reports concerning Reggie; the whereabouts of Reggie's father were unknown; and Brianna did not have family members who were willing to assist her. A level of care (LOC) assessment to determine psychosocial, medical, and developmental functioning revealed that Brianna had been using drugs for 29 years; dropped out of high school in the 10th grade; and was exposed to multiple traumas, including sexual abuse and domestic violence. She was diagnosed with major depression.

With respect to Reggie, the petition stated that he had severe developmental delays, specifically that he "is retarded and does not speak." Multiple sources reported that he did not respond to his name, speak or make sounds, follow directions, feed himself, or make eye contact. He banged his head repeatedly and generally failed to interact with others. Indeed, a teacher at the day care center described Reggie as "being in his own world." Psychological tests revealed that he had pervasive developmental delays, particularly in communication, fine motor skills, and problem-solving, personal, and social skills. The only domain in which he was not delayed was gross motor skills. While Reggie was medically stable, he did suffer from asthma requiring a nebulizer.

Child welfare workers who observed a visitation between mother and son reported that Brianna was overintrusive and smothering, and Reggie was detached and rejecting: "Reggie's mother swept him off his feet when he first arrived, hugging and kissing him. She did not let go of him for several minutes, and he had his head turned away from her the entire time. Reggie did not reciprocate the affection, and his body became stiff while his mother was hugging him. ... She was hyperverbal and remained in close proximity to Reggie's face. ... Reggie allowed his mother to hold him but did not return affection."

In dependency court, in contrast to DDC, this case would have gone to expedited termination of parental rights. Indeed, the mother had failed to complete prior substance abuse programs; was unemployed, with a low educational level; engaged in prostitution; and had little family support. She had lost four other children and appeared incapable of using good judgment and/or learning from past mistakes and experiences. Most significantly, it was thought that the severity of Reggie's developmental delays were, at least in part, attributable to extensive maternal neglect. Although a high percentage of children ages 0–3 come into the dependency court system with significant developmental delays in at least one domain, few come into the system with pervasive delays such as Reggie's. Given the facts of the case, the drug court judge was skeptical about the mother's ability to make significant progress within the Adoption and Safe Family Act time lines, and believed the prognosis for the mother's recovery to be extremely poor given any amount of time. However, instead of simply rejecting Brianna and Reggie from drug court, the judge decided to give Brianna and Reggie a chance. The judge made this decision on the basis of several factors: (1) the possibility that Reggie's assessment was not adequate, (2) the fact that Brianna was already enrolled in residential substance abuse treatment, and (3) Brianna's age. She was 38 years old, and in the court's experience, older women do better in treatment; they seem ready to change.

The judge immediately ordered a comprehensive neurological evaluation of the child, along with occupational, speech, and play therapy. The court was anxious to ascertain whether the delays were the result of severe neglect or an organic syndrome on the autism spectrum. Indeed, several assessors voiced the opinion that the child might be autistic. Nonetheless, the judge was willing to wait for the neurological examination before making a final decision regarding expedited TPR.

While waiting for the results of the neurological examination, mother and child were enrolled in drug court. The initial goal for the DDC counselor and judge was to retain the mother in treatment and ensure that she benefited from the program by enhancing her motivation to complete treatment; noticing and providing praise for all her accomplishments no matter how small; highlighting what she had to lose and gain from treatment; strengthening her self-examination, coping, problem-solving, emotion regulation, and communication skills; and addressing barriers to success, including her relationships with men. The judge requested weekly status reports from the drug court counselor, child welfare worker, and treatment provider. Frequent court hearings were held not only to praise the mother but also place high expectations on her (e.g., a sustained recovery, improvement in parenting skills, a stable living situation). The drug court counselor, as is prescribed in EMP Stage 1, focused on developing a strong therapeutic alliance with the mother ("I am behind you 150%"); preventing and solving problems that frequently arise in residential substance abuse programs, such as conflict among the residents and dissatisfaction with the facility and counselors; and advocating for the mother in court. The DDC counselor helped Brianna recognize that Reggie might be her last chance to be a mother, and that doing well with him offered her a chance to redeem herself and reduce the guilt she felt as a result of losing four previous children to the child welfare system.

Although Brianna was diagnosed with major depression, other symptoms were observed during the weekly court appearances and individual sessions with the drug court counselor, including disorganized thoughts, pressured speech, and odd mannerisms. It is important to recognize here that only through close contact by both the judge and the drug court counselor with the mother were these other behaviors observed. The drug court team began to question the accuracy of the original diagnosis, and the judge ordered a second evaluation.

Both mother and child were provided with a case plan. Unfortunately, but not unusual in the child welfare system in the United States, the psychiatric reevaluation for the mother and the neurological evaluation for her son were completed 4 months after the original court order. Given that Brianna's initial psychiatric evaluation did not appropriately diagnose her, the court lost valuable time in ordering appropriate services. Without the support of her drug court counselors, she would never have been able to remain in treatment and sober while waiting for professionals to diagnose her. As part of her case plan, Brianna was required to (1) remain in her substance abuse treatment program, (2) participate in frequent Narcotics Anonymous meetings with a sponsor, (3) obtain appropriate mental health care, (4) provide thrice-weekly drug tests, (5) participate in weekly EMP sessions with the DDC counselor and weekly court hearings in front of the DDC judge, and (6) complete a comprehensive, evidence-based parenting program.

Although Brianna was complying with her case plan, progress was slow, and she, like most people who are attempting a major life change, was ambivalent about her desire to change, and at times felt discouraged and hopeless that she would succeed in drug court. Normally, the EMP drug court counselor would reach out to any family members (mothers, fathers, sisters) living in the community and facilitate rapprochement with the mother and her family. In this case, because no family members in South Florida were willing to engage with Brianna at that time, the drug court counselor resurrected Brianna's relationship with her deceased mother. The counselor helped Brianna realize the importance of her relationship with her mother (hence, how important she was to Reggie), how proud Brianna's mother would be of her efforts to be a good parent to Reggie, and how it was possible to get off drugs and have a good life, since her mother, too, had been an addict but was able to reach and maintain sobriety. Moreover, the drug court counselor highlighted Brianna's strengths and accomplishments, such as remaining in treatment, participating in visits with her son, as well as what she had to gain by all this hard work: having a relationship with her son and being an important part of his life and development ("He needs you. You need him."). The counselor never forgot to emphasize how much she believed in Brianna, and that she had her full support and would do whatever it took to help Brianna get what she wanted (to be a full-time parent to Reggie). The counselor praised every small accomplishment and gradually Brianna improved her parenting practices. Visitations became more satisfying for both mother and child, Brianna felt extremely proud of herself, and Reggie was more responsive to her.

The case plan called for Reggie to receive a neurological exam, as well as a comprehensive array of services, including occupational, speech, and play therapy. The results of the neurological examination and review of medical records on both mother and child revealed no organic abnormality. The mother smoked and drank "mildly" during pregnancy, and tested positive for cocaine at Reggie's birth. The neurologist found Reggie to be "extremely overactive and distractible, with no specific language." Significantly, however, after nearly 5 months in foster care, he was able to respond to his name, repeat some words, and follow simple directions. He mimicked applause and could place objects in their proper receptacles. His fine motor skills appeared normal with small objects, and he attempted to dress himself and put on his socks. The neurologist reviewed all historical documents available on Reggie and determined that his social interaction had greatly improved. He was now interacting with his peers, smiling, and making good eye contact. In fact, he was found to be affectionate with people rather than object-oriented. Reggie was diagnosed with pervasive developmental disorder but not autism.

Despite the recommendations from the neurology report, it was difficult to get the appropriate wraparound services in place for Reggie. Even with the involvement of dedicated and committed drug court counselors and child welfare workers, the drug court judge was forced to intervene from the bench on numerous occasions in order to obtain the vital services. In addition, Reggie was moved twice before he was placed with an appropriate and loving foster mother, who was willing to work with the biological mother. Finally Reggie was placed in a suitable and high-quality program, where he has flourished. Additionally, he received other needed services, such as dental care, immunizations, well-child checkups, and an ear, nose, and throat (ENT) audiology examination. Genetic testing was also undertaken to rule out any genetic abnormality. When Reggie turned 36 months old, an Individual Educational Staffing was performed in order to plan for his educational future in the public school system.

After receiving the neurologist's report and hearing a verbal opinion from the neurologist that the child's delays were the result of neglect, the judge was inclined to move toward TPR. The mother was staying sober, but her mental health was deteriorating and her presentation in court was volatile, in that she presented with anxiety, pressured speech, and a somewhat fragmented thought process. The drug court counselor advocated strongly against TPR. In collaboration with the mother's defense attorney, the drug court counselor rallied support among the professionals involved in drug court, including treatment providers, the guardian *ad litem*, the child's day care provider, the foster mother, and the child welfare caseworker and attorney. Led by the drug court counselor, this group appealed to the judge to allow the family to remain in drug court at least until the mother received appropriate mental health care. After considering the testimony from all these interested parties, the judge decided to give the mother a three-month case plan.

As the judge and drug court counselor suspected, the mother's second psychiatric evaluation resulted in a diagnosis of bipolar II disorder. Brianna was placed on medication for this disorder, and a few months later her functioning had improved tremendously. It was evident during the court hearings that her thought process had become coherent and goal-oriented, and her speech had an even quality to it. Moreover, she had completed the first part of the parenting program, started dyadic therapy, successfully completed residential substance abuse treatment, and moved first to a halfway house, then to her own apartment, and was employed. She was actively attending outpatient treatment. After leaving her residential program, Brianna continued to attend outpatient substance abuse treatment; provide urine samples three times per week; and attend individual counseling, dyadic therapy, and daily meetings. Brianna found a sponsor and became actively involved in working the 12-step program. She continued to call and meet with her drug court counselor and to attend all court hearings on a bimonthly basis.

It is important to recognize that the court ordered Brianna to have not only regular supervised visits with Reggie but also to accompany him to most of his medical appointments and all therapy sessions, and to maintain regular and close contact with the foster parent, the day care program, and any other professionals working with Reggie. It is worth noting that many foster care systems isolate the parent from the child and his or her treatment and treatment providers while the child is in care, even when a reunification case plan exists. For obvious reasons, in a case such as this, reunification would have been impossible without the mother actively participating in the child's treatment and interacting with the professionals. Especially with young children, courts should encourage parents to attend all appointments for their children and interact frequently with the foster parents. This provides the court with a window into the parents' parenting skills, builds efficacy in the parent/child relationship and allows the parents to model the foster parents' parenting techniques.

Brianna completed an evidence-based parenting program, and reports to the court from the parenting program that compared pre- and posttreatment observational visits between Brianna and Reggie indicated tremendous growth of both mother and child in their relationship. Whereas at the pretreatment parenting observation Reggie was aggressive and sought distance from his mother, at the posttreatment observation he physically sought his mother out and wanted to be close to her. Brianna encouraged Reggie in a child-friendly tone, and laughed and interacted with him in a calm and relaxed manner, without being verbally or physically intrusive. While Reggie showed much affection toward his mother, at times he hit her and became aggressive. When she told him not to hit Mommy, he immediately relented and caressed her face. Play was reciprocal and Brianna was able to follow her child's lead. Reggie was permitted to explore at his own pace, and Brianna assisted him in transitioning from one activity to the other.

As is evident, Brianna was engaged in numerous services and her obligations were many. This can wear anybody down. The drug court counselor worked with Brianna to sustain her motivation, advocate for her in the courtroom, reduce or rearrange some of the service demands, and assist her in benefiting from the interventions she received. For example, the drug court counselor discussed the benefits of these services with Brianna, and how those services were designed to assist her in realizing her stated goals (being an involved and good parent to Reggie). The drug court counselor worked on diminishing Brianna's frustration toward required/recommended service and service providers.

Reggie's and Brianna's functioning continued to improve. Parenting program counselors, Reggie's occupational therapist, child welfare workers, and the foster mother all had nothing but praise for Brianna. It was reported she was better able to regulate emotions and behaviors, and this was contributing to Reggie's ability to regulate his behavior. Indeed, the occupational therapist described her as nurturing, appropriate, consistent, reliable, and loving. The parenting program dyadic therapist reported, "Brianna and Reggie's relationship continues to evolve from an insecure relationship to a healthy, secure attachment. The mother has been able to provide amazing consistency with her visitation with her son in child care and with the parent–child psychotherapy. ... Reggie has made drastic changes in his interactions with his mother, laughing with her and molding his body into hers when he plays with her. ... The transformation has been amazing." The foster mother, who became a preadoptive placement for Reggie, reported that she was "so proud" of Brianna and was willing and pleased to communicate with her and assist her. The drug court counselor advocated for increased independence for the mother, and the drug court team recommended daytime unsupervised visits and one overnight, which the judge granted. Ultimately, the mother and child were fully reunified. Today, Reggie lives with his mother Brianna, who provides a stable and loving family environment.

CONCLUDING REMARKS

Drug abuse and mental health comorbidity among women with children is a serious social and public health problem that not only impairs the mother but also places her children at risk of abuse, neglect, and numerous social, health, and behavioral problems (Brady, Back, & Greenfield, 2009). Moreover, mothers involved in the child welfare system who have substance abuse problems are more likely than non-drug-using child welfare–involved mothers to have their parental rights terminated (Marcenko, Kemp, & Larson, 2000). Thus, there is increasing urgency to develop new ways of working with substance-abusing parents involved in the child welfare system (Kerwin, 2005; Maluccio & Ainsworth, 2003; Marsh & Cao, 2005; Young, Gardner, & Dennis, 1998). Judicial and child welfare systems throughout the nation have turned to drug courts as a setting where parents can acquire the tools needed to turn their lives around and become productive, drug-free members of society (Tauber & Snavely, 1999). The Miami–Dade DDC embraces a model in which the drug court judge and counselors are the key change agents within the DDC content: The drug court counselor is the leader and coordinator of individual cases, and the drug court judge is the leader of the court as a whole. This collaboration is the foundation and scaffolding that facilitates building a successful DDC. The DDC judge and counselors collaborate to create an effective multidisciplinary intervention designed to ameliorate maternal addiction and child maltreatment with (1) a therapeutic jurisprudence vision of the mission of DDC; (2) clearly delineated and therapeutic roles; (3) strong leadership; and (4) implementation of evidence-based interventions both within and outside of drug court, thus achieving the promise of the judicial–mental health partnership proposed by Lederman and Osofsky (2008) "to establish more effective interventions when a child comes into care and is adjudicated dependent ... it is crucial that we begin to develop and implement interventions that will make a difference for these families especially those that will interrupt the intergenerational cycles of abuse and neglect" (pp. 44–45).

DDC generally, and perhaps the Miami–Dade DDC model in particular, appears to be a promising intervention not only to ameliorate the trauma associated with maternal addiction and child maltreatment but also to produce better child welfare outcomes (Dakof et al., 2009, in press). This, we hope, will help to reduce the risk of young children of addicted mothers for ongoing exposure to chronic trauma, especially physical and emotional neglect. We believe that DDC offers a unique opportunity to integrate and coordinate high-quality service delivery to young children and addicted mothers involved in the child welfare system and, hence, finally to provide the kind of services necessary to change the lives of families who come in contact with the child welfare system. Judicial leadership, with its demand for accountability and excellence coupled with the implementation of evidence-based drug court counseling (e.g., EMP), evidence-based parenting interventions, and substance abuse and trauma treatment seem to be the best hope to prevent poor developmental outcomes for young children of addicted mothers and to begin to change the life trajectory for both mother and child (Lederman et al., 2009).

ACKNOWLEDGMENTS

Completion of this chapter was supported by a grant from the National Institute on Drug Abuse (Grant No. RO1 DA016733).

REFERENCES

Banyard, V. I., Williams, L. M., & Siegal, J. A. (2003). The impact of complex trauma and depression on parenting: An exploration of mediating risk and protective factors. *Child Maltreatment, 8,* 333–349.

Barth, R. P., Courtney, M., Duerr Berrick, J., & Albert, V. (1994). *From child abuse to permanency planning: Child welfare services pathways and placements.* Hawthorne, NY: Aldine de Gruyter.

Boles, S. M., Young, N. K., Moore, T., & DiPirro-Beard, S. (2007). The Sacramento Dependency Drug Court, development and outcomes. *Child Maltreatment, 12,* 161–171.

Brady, K. T., Back, S. E., & Greenfield, S. F. (Eds.). (2009). *Women and addiction: A comprehensive handbook.* New York: Guilford Press.

Casanueva, C., Martin, S. L., Runyan, D. K., Barth, R. P., & Bradley, R. H. (2008). Parenting services for mothers involved with child protective services: Do they change maternal parenting and spanking behaviors with young children? *Children and Youth Services Review, 30*(8), 861–878.

Curtis, P. A., & McCullough, C. (1993). The impact of alcohol and other drugs on the child welfare system. *Child Welfare, 72*(6), 533–542.

Dakof, G. A., Cohen, J. B., & Duarte, E. (2009). Increasing family reunification for substance abusing mothers and their children: Comparing two drug court interventions. *Juvenile and Family Court Journal, 60,* 11–23.

Dakof, G. A., Cohen, J. B., Henderson, C., Duarte, E., Boustani, M., Blackburn, A., et al. (2010). A randomized pilot study of the engaging moms program for family drug court. *Journal of Substance Abuse Treatment, 38,* 263–274.

Edwards, L. P., & Ray, J. A. (2005). Judicial perspectives on family drug treatment courts. *Juvenile and Family Court Journal, 56*(3), 1–27.

Erickson, S. J., & Tonigan, J. S. (2008). Trauma and intraveneous drug use among pregnant alcohol/other drug abusing women: Factors in predicting child abuse potential. *Alcoholism and Treatment Quarterly, 26,* 313–332.

Gara, M. A., Allen, L. A., Herzog, E. P., & Woolfolk, R. L. (2000). The abused child as parent: The structure and content of physically abused mothers' perceptions of their babies. *Child Abuse and Neglect, 24,* 627–639.

Green, B. L., Furrer, C., Worcel, S., Burrus, S., & Finigan, M. (2007). How effective are family drug courts?: Outcomes from a four-site national study. *Child Maltreatment, 12,* 43–59.

Green, B. L., Furrer, C., Worcel, S., Burrus, S., & Finigan, M. (2009). Building the evidence base for family drug treatment courts: Results from recent outcome studies. *Drug Court Review, 6,* 53–82.

Haack, M., Alemi, F., Nemes, S., & Cohen, J. B. (2004). Experience with family drug courts in three cities. *Substance Abuse, 25,* 17–25.

Hein, D. A., & Miele, G. M. (2003). Emotion-focused coping as a mediator of maternal cocaine abuse and antisocial behavior. *Psychology of Addictive Behaviors, 17,* 49–55.

Kerwin, M. E. (2005). Collaboration between child welfare and substance-abuse fields: Combined treatment programs for mothers. *Journal of Pediatric Psychology, 30*(7), 581–597.

Lederman, C., Gomez-Kaifer, M., Katz, L. E., Thomlison, B., & Maze, C. L. (2009, Fall). An imperative: Evidence-based practice within the child welfare system of care. *Juvenile and Family Justice Today,* pp. 22–25.

Lederman, C., & Osofsky, J. D. (2008). A judicial–mental health partnership to heal young children in juvenile court. *Infant Mental Health Journal, 29,* 3–47.

Liddle, H. A., Dakof, G. A., & Diamond, G. S. (1991). Adolescents and substance abuse: Multidimensional family therapy in action. In E. Kaufman & P. Kaufman (Eds.), *Family therapy approaches with drug and alcohol problems* (2nd ed., pp. 120–171). New York: Gardner.

Locke, T. F., & Newcomb, M. D. (2003). Childhood maltreatment, parental alcohol/drug-related problems and global parental dysfunction. *Professional Psychology, Research, and Practice, 34,* 73–79.

Magura, S., & Laudet, A. B. (1996). Parental substance abuse and child maltreatment: Review and implications for interventions. *Children and Youth Services Review, 18,* 193–220.

Maluccio, A. N., & Ainsworth, F. (2003). Drug use by parents: A challenge for family reunification practice. *Children and Youth Services Review, 25,* 511–533.

Marcenko, M. O., Kemp, S. P., & Larson, N. C. (2000). Childhood experiences of abuse, later substance use, and parenting outcomes among low-income mothers. *American Journal of Orthopsychiatry, 70,* 316–326.

Marsh, J. C., & Cao, D. (2005). Parents in substance abuse treatment: Implications for child welfare practice. *Children and Youth Services Review, 27,* 1259–1278.

Maughan, A., & Cicchetti, A. (2002). Impact of child maltreatment and interadult violence on children's emotion regulation and socioemotional adjustment. *Child Development, 73*(5), 1525–1542.

National Association of Drug Court Professionals (NADCP). (1997). Defining drug courts: The key components. Washington DC: Department of Justice, Drug Courts Program Office. Retrieved from *www.ndci.org/sites/default/files/ndci/keycomponents.pdf.*

Office of Justice Programs. (1998). Juvenile and family drug courts: Profile on program characteristics and implementation issues. Washington, DC: American University. Retrieved from *www.ojp.usdoj.gov/dcpo/familydrug/.*

Osofsky, J. D. (Ed.). (2004). *Young children and trauma: Intervention and treatment.* New York: Guilford Press.

Osofsky, J. D. (1995). The effects of exposure to violence on young children. *American Psychologist, 50*(9), 782–788.

Suchman, N. E., Pajulo, M., DeCoste, C., & Mayes, L. C. (2006). Parenting interventions for drug dependent mothers and their young children: The case for an attachment-based approach. *Family Relations, 55,* 211–226,

Tauber J. J., & Snavely, K. R. (1999). *Drug courts: A research agenda.* Alexandria, VA: National Drug Court Institute.

Walsh, C., MacMillan, H. L., & Jamieson, E. (2003). The relationship between parental substance abuse and child maltreatment: Findings from the Ontario Health Supplement. *Child Abuse and Neglect, 27,* 1409–1425.

Windom, C. S. (2000). Childhood victimization: Early adversity, later psychopathology. *National Institute of Justice Journal, 242,* 2–9.

Young, N., Gardner, S., & Dennis, K. (1998). *Responding to alcohol and other drug problems in child welfare: Weaving together practice and policy.* Washington, DC: CWLA Press.

CHAPTER 14

■ ■ ■ ■

Zero to Three Family Drug Treatment Court

Douglas F. Johnson

On May 3, 2005, the Zero to Three Family Drug Treatment Court (0–3 FDTC) opened in the Separate Juvenile Court of Douglas County (Omaha), Nebraska, with a focus on improving outcomes for substance-abusing parents and their children from birth to age 3. This chapter traces the origins of the 0–3 FDTC, the philosophy supporting the program, the framework, and how and why the FDTC operates as it does. Because goals of FDTC are to help parents become sober and fit caretakers for their children, some people think FDTC is all about the parents. Some FDTCs focus primarily on the parents (Edwards & Ray, 2005). However, Omaha's 0–3 FDTC gives equal attention to both parents and babies, and recognizes the rights of the parent and the baby to due process, fair hearings, and timely outcomes leading to reunification or other permanency, such as adoption. While research has not yet examined the efficacy of 0–3 FDTC, plans are under way to develop an evaluation for the program. To date, the qualitative data from the program indicate much success for babies and parents going through Omaha's 0–3 FDTC program.

THE DEVELOPMENT OF THE ZERO TO THREE FAMILY DRUG TREATMENT COURT

Prior to May 2005, the docket for cases involving abused and neglected children was extremely busy. The juvenile court in Douglas County, consisting of five judges in the most populous county in Nebraska, hears one-third of all child welfare cases in the state. As the court began to convene meetings with governmental and private agencies about the possibility of an FDTC focusing on infants, toddlers, and their parents, many court stakeholders were concerned about whether the addition of another court improvement program would be possible, especially one of this magnitude. After much discussion leading to consensus about moving forward, a presentation was made in 2002 to Nebraska Supreme Court Chief Justice John Hendry on the merits of piloting a 0–3 FDTC, and the presentation was received positively. Since the Supreme Court administers to all lower courts, it was crucial to have his approval in order to request implementation of the pilot project because it would require a reallocation of limited court resources and voluntary collaboration of court systems stakeholders. Encouraged by administrative permission to proceed, and the excitement and willingness of court stakeholders to participate, plans were made to create a new type of problem-solving court.

It is important to elaborate on how the decision was made to change court practice and focus specifically on cases involving children under age 3. Research shows that infants fare poorly even when the court and child welfare agency try to provide for their safety through removal from neglectful or abusive parents and placement into foster care. In fact, 1 in 5 foster care placements is an infant; once infants are in care, they remain twice as long as older children (Wulczyn & Hislop, 2002). In 2008, there were an estimated 1,740 child fatalities due to child abuse or neglect and more than three-fourths (78.1%) of these children were younger than age 4 (U.S. Department of Health and Human Services Administration of Children and Families, 2008). Unfortunately, children in the age group from birth to 1 year old suffer the highest rate of victimization at 21.7 per 1,000 children (U.S. Department of Health and Human Services Administration of Children and Families, 2008). There is scientific evidence that the first 3 years of a child's life are *the* most formative period for cognitive and emotional development (Shonkoff & Phillips, 2000). During this time, the infant's brain "hardwires" for learning, language, self-esteem, motor skills, and social relationships. Babies develop best with a consistent, nurturing, caring, and loving parent or caregiver (Dicker & Gordon, 2004).

Prior to starting the 0–3 FDTC in Omaha, the most vulnerable children suffered foster care "drift," being moved by the child welfare agency from foster home to foster home up to 8–10 times in a single year (Wulcyzn & Hislop, 2000). Also, each additional placement a child experiences reduces the odds of obtaining permanency within the year by 32% (National Clearinghouse on Child Abuse and Neglect Information, 2005). The Nebraska Department of Health and Human Services (DHHS) provided supervised visitation between parent and child once or twice a week for 1 or 2 hours. No one knew what a "Part C" (early intervention) evaluation[1] was, and none were ordered by the court. Parents did not receive any rehabilitative services until after adjudication (90 days from the filing of the petition),[2] and not until disposition (60 days from the adjudication under favorable conditions).[3] A "petition" is a pleading, with allegations of parental abuse or neglect; an "adjudication" is the trial of the allegations; and the "disposition" is the hearing in which evidence is offered as to services to correct the abuse or neglect and to meet the best interests and well-being of the child. The court process regularly required between 4 and 6 months before the young child and parent(s) received any intervention or treatment services. These families were being treated like "files" instead of persons. The court process and the reasonable efforts services of DHHS[4] were failing both the baby and the parent.

As one judge in collaboration with legal professionals, DHHS, and service providers, we were determined to create an alternative to "business as usual" for families in situations where substance abuse played a major role in the allegations of maltreatment. The science of early childhood development showed the court that these children may already have suffered developmental damage or delays when they come into foster care (Leslie, Hurlburt, Landsverk, Barth, & Slyman, 2004). The existing court process and lack of knowledge of the science of early childhood development meant that these children's developmental needs were not being properly addressed, and indeed, the court might be causing further trauma for the children (see *ohiocandokids.org*; *nctsn.org*). The rehabilitative needs of the parents were also not being met in a timely way. Nationally, parental substance abuse and mental health issues account for 70–80% of all children in foster care (Foster, 2001), and the parents of the babies in our court were no different. Our goal was to help the youngest children and to provide them with a better opportunity for well-being, safety, healthy development, and timely permanence, and to give their parents a better opportunity for timely rehabilitation services and possible reunification.

GETTING STARTED

In spring 2002, the court and agency stakeholders convened service providers and legal professionals to create an FDTC planning team that included the following:

- A DHHS Child Protective Services worker to serve as the case manager
- The Douglas County Juvenile County Attorney

- The Douglas County Public Defender
- A guardian *ad litem* (child's best interest attorney)
- Court-Appointed Special Advocate (CASA) for Douglas County
- Family Connections, Inc., a nonprofit corporation to facilitate the collaborative and comprehensive provision of child welfare and behavioral health services

Fortuitously, in December 2002, the Separate Juvenile Court of Douglas County was selected to become a National Council of Juvenile and Family Court Judges (NCJFCJ) Child Victims Act Model Court, and I became the Lead Judge.[5] The Court had worked with the NCJFCJ since 1994, and had already implemented many recommended court systems reforms from its two landmark publications, *Resource Guidelines: Improving Court Practice in Abuse and Neglect Cases,* and *Adoption and Permanency Planning Guidelines: Improving Court Practice in Abuse and Neglect Cases,* which included the following:

- Avoiding unnecessary separation of children and families.
- Permanency planning for timely reunification or other permanency plans when reunification is not feasible.
- Meaningful and timely hearings in child abuse and neglect cases.
- Making timely decisions in child abuse and neglect cases.
- Oversight role of the juvenile and family court judge—judicial leadership on and off the bench.
- One family–one judge—for continuity of judicial decision making.
- Direct calendaring by the judge, credible court dates, time management, and notice to the parties on the record.
- A no-continuance policy to prevent delays in decision making.
- Court collaboration with systems stakeholders—judicially led collaborative meetings and educational trainings for court systems reform and improvement.

Through participation of one court in the Model Courts project, additional federally funded NCJFCJ technical assistance, training, crossover court site visits, and participation in the Annual NCJFCJ All Sites Conferences was available for the program. In fact, the 0–3 FDTC pilot project was identified as an Omaha model court goal at the 2004 NCJFCJ All-Sites Conference. A great deal of new information was available from other model court sites that had existing dependency drug treatment courts showing positive outcomes, and assimilated some of their protocols that fit our local community. In this way, the Douglas County Juvenile Court could benefit from and build on knowledge gained in other jurisdictions, which allowed the court to build on precious experience.

In addition, several model court judges were focusing special attention on infants and toddlers in foster care, albeit not with an emphasis through FDTC. We worked closely with Judge Cindy Lederman from Miami–Dade County Juvenile Court in collaboration with Joy Osofsky in developing the model in Douglas County Juvenile Court.

To gain additional knowledge from the promising preliminary results from Miami–Dade Juvenile Court, utilizing our model court training funds, the court invited Judge Cindy Lederman, Dr. Joy Osofsky, and Dr. Vicky Youcha to present in Omaha a daylong training session in August 2002, entitled "Infant and Toddler Well-Being in the Child Welfare System." In addition to learning about the Miami Juvenile Court model, the court was introduced to child–parent psychotherapy and relationship-based assessments in order to begin implementing these evaluation and treatment models. All court systems stakeholders were invited to attend this training at no cost, and more than 200 people participated. The collaborative team from Miami, with Dr. Youcha from Zero to Three, presented information on the science of early childhood development, the Florida Infant Mental Health Pilot Program, and the intervention and treatment model being implemented in Miami Juvenile Court,[6] which provided relationship-based assessments and child–parent psychotherapy.

After this training, the court decided to combine this model of evaluation and treatment with an FDTC focusing on babies. This holistic approach could provide help for infants and their mothers. If fathers were involved with the child, then they, too, were encouraged to be involved and learn how to care for and nurture their babies.

FACILITATED PREHEARING CONFERENCES

Another vital element in the 0–3 FDTC process was instituting facilitated prehearing conferences in 2004. The facilitated prehearing conference, which modified the existing protective custody hearing,[7] was another goal of the Omaha Model Court.

The protective custody hearing is the first hearing where parents, the legal professionals, and DHHS come to court for a hearing to discuss whether a child can safely be returned to the parents and upon what conditions, or whether the child must remain in temporary foster care. Typically, protective custody hearings in Omaha were held between 3 and 12 days after children were removed from their homes. For 15 minutes, the court heard from attorneys about what the outcome of the hearing should be in a highly contentious proceeding. Because they were seen as the cause of child maltreatment, parents were not viewed as potential partners in finding or building on family strengths to meet the best interest of their children. The brief hearing did not come close to the *Resource Guidelines'* recommendation of 1 hour for a problem-solving atmosphere and meaningful hearing.

It was apparent that the protective custody hearing was not meeting the needs of parents, their children, or the court. Therefore, after partnering and training with the Pima County Model Court in Tucson, Arizona, the court assimilated their model of a facilitated prehearing conference, which occurs prior to the protective custody hearing and focuses on providing a meaningful opportunity to build on family strengths and talk about issues that meet the best interests of the child. Facilitated by a neutral mediator, conference participants include the parents, other family members or friends, legal professionals, child welfare workers, and other interested parties. Although the judge addresses the participants and sets an encouraging, problem-solving tone, the process is completely off the record, and the judge and court reporter are not present. By state statute, the parental participation and discussion cannot be used against the parent to prove the child maltreatment case. The only exception is mandatory child maltreatment reporting. Whenever a child is placed into foster care, DHHS has the legal duty to assess the family and maltreatment with regard to what rehabilitative services might correct those issues.

Through this problem-solving process, greater respect is shown to the family and all involved, and parents are more likely to deal voluntarily with issues. During the 1-hour facilitated prehearing conference, the participants establish early on the needs of the children and the rehabilitative needs of the parents. Within days after this hearing, parents can receive services and have safe family time (visitation) with their children. Parents are now active participants at the beginning of proceedings. Some even admit to the child maltreatment allegations at this first hearing in order to improve parental inadequacies and get their children home sooner. The prehearing conference is not only a problem-solving tool to help all children and their parents but also an excellent opportunity to introduce appropriate families to 0–3 FDTC.[8]

The court's plan to combine these programs as a way of better meeting the needs of infants, toddlers, and their parents continued to progress as funding was received for both skills-based training related to starting an FDTC and to hire an FDTC coordinator.[9] After several years of patient planning, training, and collaboration, the court was prepared to start seeing babies and their parents in 0–3 FDTC in May 2005.

ESSENTIALS OF THE ZERO TO THREE
FAMILY DRUG TREATMENT COURT

Mission Statement

Like most FDTCs, the Omaha 0–3 FDTC has a mission statement to help it stay focused and to support a consensus that fits the community:

Douglas County 0–3 Family Drug Treatment Court seeks to achieve healthy, safe, permanent homes for infants and toddlers in state custody due to parental substance abuse. It provides for the timely resolution of child maltreatment for the benefit of children, families, and society through intense supervision and special collaboration of the court, child welfare, community, and treatment providers.

The mission statement reminds all the participants that the 0–3 FDTC serves both baby and parent. A parent not only has to overcome substance abuse within a reasonable time frame according to the Adoption and Safe Families Act, but also she must be able to properly care for her baby. Providing care and nurturance for her baby may include resolving issues of housing, legal source of income, domestic violence, and all other issues necessary to parent her infant independently. Each baby deserves a nurturing, caring, loving, stable, and consistent parent. If the parents cannot fill that role, the prosecutor will file a termination of parental rights pleading. In that case, we refer the family for mediation of the permanency issue. Mediation has proved successful, with the majority of parents voluntarily relinquishing their parental rights, which frees the baby for adoption.

The Role of the Judge

The role of the judge is critical in any juvenile or family court. Juvenile and family court judges, compared to judges in other courts, have an especially challenging jurisdiction given the complexities of not only the law but also family life. The court works with experts in mental health, substance abuse, medicine, child abuse, sociology, education, domestic violence, housing, legal income, and other areas. The judges do not sit as disinterested magistrates. Rather, they work on and off the bench in the community to ensure that children and family needs are met. All of the stakeholders are held accountable pursuant to our state and federal laws. Child welfare recommendations are not "rubber-stamped" child welfare recommendations. Rather, the court follows through with necessary findings to determine whether a child can safely be returned to his or her parents, whether reasonable efforts have been offered to prevent removal of a child or to return the child to the parents, and ultimately whether a parent's rights to a child should remain intact or be terminated. In my view as a judge, such work is more important than civil litigation of any other kind. The court is dedicated to improving the lives of children and their parents.

At 0–3 FDTC, as in all my other cases, as a judge, I strive to set a problem-solving tone by acting and speaking with respect, dignity, and civility to all involved, and I expect the same of them. Judges are ethically responsible to ensure that this occurs. Parental improvement is encouraged by using affirmation with accountability. The smallest correct step that a parent has made is recognized. Even if a parent missteps (e.g., sees old friends and smokes marijuana), the parent is encouraged with compliments for calling the caseworker, therapist, and sponsor, and owning up to what occurred. The parent is supported for coming to court and not avoiding responsibility. A fundamental principle of the 0–3 FDTC is to focus on strengths, while dealing with weaknesses. The court believes that it is in a child's best interest to have a permanent caring parent, and parents are reminded of that every time they are in court. While some FDTCs measure success by the number of parents who graduate (or "commence," as the 0–3 FDTC terms it), the Douglas County FDTC court does not do so. The goal is reunification; however, the measure of success is related to whether the infant or toddler gained a permanent caring caregiver in a timely manner, and without multiple foster placements. The court works diligently to make the first placement the last. Timely adoption is a successful outcome when reunification is not possible.

Finally, it is the role of the judge to collaborate with organizations and stakeholders such as NCJFCJ, Zero to Three: National Center for Infants Toddlers and Families, Early Interventionists, the child welfare agency, service providers, all court systems stakeholders, and a host of others to promote ongoing improved practice and outcomes. Collaborative work is time consuming. However, for professionals with the desire to be of service to infants, toddlers, and their parents, that duty is recognized and willingly fulfilled.

Goals for Infants and Toddlers

Each infant or toddler must achieve a safe, secure, permanent home in a timely fashion according to the Adoption and Safe Families Act (ASFA),[10] defined as no later than the 12th month after having entered foster care. This aspect of ASFA notes the paramount concern for a child's well-being and safety, and for a permanent caregiver. Children are not meant to languish in foster care, which is why ASFA set deadlines for permanency. If a child is still in foster care at the 12-month Permanency Planning Hearing, a compelling reason must be documented by the child welfare agency in order to grant more parental rehabilitative time. If additional time is granted, a similar hearing must occur within 30 days after the 15th month in foster care. Evidence must be presented as to why more time is needed (i.e., either the parent has not had time to avail herself of services, the child has been placed with a relative, or a compelling reason exists not to terminate the parental rights).

When a baby must be placed out of the parental home, we seek a secure, nurturing, caring, and loving caregiver who is willing to adopt the baby. In many instances we place the baby with a relative because of information gained at the prehearing conference. We strive for the first placement to be the last one. We know it is in the baby's best interest to have as few placement disruptions as possible.

Whenever possible, we enable infants and toddlers to live safely with their parents, with the help of safe and supportive relatives or providers. Ideally, a mother lives with her baby, if it can be done safely. However, a parent who is an active substance user presents an obvious danger to her baby. If that safety concern can be met, through others who can ensure the baby's safety, we can encourage bonding and attachment. If a relative is interested, foster care training and licensing is offered. This option has been successful in most instances.

Another resource in Omaha is the "Family Works" program through Heartland Family Services, an original partner in starting 0–3 FDTC. Through a federal grant and private donations, this provider offers apartment-style living for pregnant mothers or mothers with a child 1 year old or younger. As long as this requirement is met, older siblings are welcome, too. All of the mother's treatment needs are met in this setting. This provider also offers relationship-based assessments and child–parent psychotherapy for mother and baby. With time, the mother learns to fulfill all of her parental duties in a supportive environment.

Compared to how the court operated before 0–3 FDTC, infant and toddler developmental needs are now identified and met through medical, hearing, vision, and dental, evaluations; Early Development Network and Part C evaluation and services to the child and parents; Early Head Start; Head Start; relationship-based child assessments; child–parent psychotherapy; and parent training. We encourage training of local clinicians in relationship-based evaluations and child–parent psychotherapy in order to provide the same type of therapeutic help to infants and parents in 0–3 FDTC.

As mentioned earlier, 0–3 FDTC is not just about the parent. For that reason, concurrent permanency planning is implemented (i.e., reunification and adoption) from day one, which is allowed under ASFA. While this approach sometimes "unnerves" parents' defense attorneys, it reminds the parent that the ASFA permanency clock is ticking, and that the infant has the right to a fit parent in a timely way. The court emphasizes to the parents that there is no "perfect" parent, and perfection is not required. The court also emphasizes that the parent must be able to fulfill parental duties within a reasonable amount of time. If not, a contingency plan is in place so that the child will not suffer from foster care drift (i.e., moving the child from home to home, without a clear plan for permanency).

Goals for Parents

Parents who agree to participate in 0–3 FDTC must actively participate in the program and be responsible for their life choices. Trainings have indicated that there is a difference between a parent's *inability* to comply with court-ordered rehabilitative services and a parent's *unwillingness* to do so. Trained clinicians working with the parent on substance abuse recovery need to know the difference. We also have learned that many, if not most, of these mothers are very young—late teens to early 20s—and were already in the court system due to their parent's abuse or neglect of them. These young mothers come to the court with a history of trauma. The earlier traumatic experiences include growing up in foster care, or being the victim of child sexual abuse or domestic violence. Many of the young mothers suffer from untreated anxiety or depression. The court works with gender-specific mental health and substance providers who are sensitive and effective with this population. Treatment must be sensitive to the parent's needs and cannot be the same for women and men. If the interveners or therapists are not trained to work with trauma and the services are not delivered sensitively and well, the result can lead to potential failure of services and a finding by the judge that the child welfare agency did not offer reasonable efforts.

To be successful, parents must achieve adequate parenting skills and demonstrate the ability to provide a safe, healthy family environment for their children. Especially for parents coming from abusive and limited environments, such skills development takes time. These parents must learn about components of adequate parenting skills, including putting the baby's best interest and needs first; responding to developmental needs; providing for the young child's medical, dental, vision, and educational needs; and learning how to cook, budget, and provide a safe and decent home.

In order to help the parent achieve a sober lifestyle and mental well-being, early substance abuse and mental health evaluations, participation in gender-specific treatment, sober supports, and work with a sponsor with at least 5 years of sobriety are provided by the program. The parent must complete treatment and aftercare, and maintain ongoing support and counseling as needed. Mothers who are compliant with the program are learning to live life again. For these parents, the journey is a process much more like a "marathon than a sprint."

Additional Concerns for Parents

The 0–3 FDTC provides due process and fair hearings. Before the implementation of this program in the court, we studied several FDTCs around the country to learn more about their process of conducting hearings and disputed matters. The situations were not handled as expected. At time, parents would disagree with what the FDTC team stated was noncompliance, or had what seemed to be a good reason to deviate from what they were supposed to do. For example, one mother was ordered to enter inpatient substance abuse treatment. But due to the length of time it took for the availability of an open bed, rather than enter inpatient treatment, the mother enrolled herself and was participating in intensive outpatient treatment. When this became apparent to the FDTC team, the sanction of jail was recommended. The mother told the judge that she enrolled in intensive outpatient treatment because no inpatient bed was available, had negative drug screens for drugs or alcohol, was maintaining a job, and was paying the mortgage on her home. Nevertheless, the judge stated the mother was not in compliance, and she was sent to jail for several days.

As a judge, I was troubled by the use of jail as a sanction. Much criminal drug court training, as well as some FDTC training, calls for immediate sanctions for noncompliance. This can include jail time, if a parent is noncompliant with program requirements and, therefore, in contempt of court. Some FDTCs view the jail time as a "retreat," a "wake-up call," or a way to show the parent that the court "means business." While respecting this different view, the 0–3 FDTC is in fundamental disagreement with the propriety or appropriateness of such a sanction, especially since parental maltreatment of a child is a civil action. Research suggests that imprisonment should not be used as a sanction for a number of reasons, including the lack of evidence that jail sentences produce better results and the negative impact that jail sentences can have on the child's life, leading to possible temporary placements and loss of visitation with their parents (Edwards, 2010). Treatment considerations should guide decisions concerning parental failure; since imprisonment is not treatment oriented, the court believes it is an inappropriate sanction (Edwards, 2010).

Recently, the California Supreme Court held that contempt of court and incarceration are not permissible sanctions in child protection cases (*In re Nolan W.*, 2009). It is possible that other state Supreme Courts may follow suit, if an appeal is heard. The California Supreme Court reasoned that the law in child welfare cases focuses on the child's well-being, best interest, and permanency, and the ultimate sanction is termination of parental rights. The court noted that a parent does not have to participate in services if she or he does not want to.

In training provided by NCJFCJ, substance abuse and mental health issues have been described as diseases. If a substance-abusing parent suffers from anxiety or depression, has a relapse, or otherwise makes a mistake and is held in contempt and jailed, would it not follow logically that a non-substance-abusing parent who has neglected or abused a child would be more culpable and also deserve such a sanction? Yet common practice is that they do not suffer the same consequences. Our court does not think this response is fair or helpful.

Affirmation motivates parents to improve. Drug court professionals generally agree that rewards and other positive incentives enhance the effectiveness of collaborative courts (Meyer, 2007). Some literature notes that awarding small tokens worth only a dollar for some parental progress is often successful in helping parents overcome methamphetamine abuse (Join Together, 2005). Omaha's FDTC has never used jail as a sanction and will not in the future. The 0–3 FDTC is collaborative, encouraging, and affirming with accountability. In cases where reunification is not likely, mediation related to the issue of permanency is offered, and the court has found that the mother usually chooses to relinquish parental rights voluntarily because she was treated with respect, dignity, and affirmation. The result is few terminations of parental rights hearings in 0–3 FDTC.

Eligibility Criteria

There are a few requirements to participate in 0–3 FDTC. Since the primary focus is children from birth to age 3, at least one child of the parent must be in that age range. We also accept siblings. Our court follows NCJFCJ's protocol of one family–one judge for continuity of judicial decision making and familiarity with the family. It does not make sense to separate older siblings to another docket or to have another judge hear that part of the case. In training provided by NCJFJ, we learned that other FDTCs have some families on the FDTC docket who also remain on the docket of origination, resulting in two judges reviewing the case. The FDTC judge reviews the case under that program's protocols, which are normally intensive, with frequent appearances in court. The judge in whose court the case started retains the case for 6-month review hearings.[11] Our court did not follow that practice because often it is inefficient and not helpful to families.

Participation in 0–3 FDTC is not mandatory; families are accepted into our program if they have entered into voluntary adjudication (an admission to the allegations in the petition without trial). This shows a willingness on the part of parents to accept responsibility for their substance abuse issues that resulted in the removal of their children and placement into foster care. Most parents' love for their child is unquestioned. That love is a strong motivating factor for a parent to want to get better, which is why focus is placed on parental strengths, even small ones, which are recognized publically in court. Our court affirms that the parent is worthwhile.

CASE EXAMPLE 1: AN ALTERNATIVE WAY
TO PARTICIPATE IN THE PROGRAM

There are some exceptions to voluntary participation in the program. On occasion, a parent's defense attorney has asked the 0–3 FDTC team to order the parent into the program. This occurs for a variety of reasons, not all of which are made known to the team or judge. For example, a mother delivered a baby, and both tested positive for methamphetamine. Child Protective Services gathered historical information about the mother from another state and discovered that the mother previously had had other children placed in foster care due to her substance abuse. The mother did not achieve reunification because she never gained sobriety or adequate parenting skills, and her parental rights had been terminated. Under ASFA, a prosecutor need only obtain a certified copy of the judgment of parental rights termination from any jurisdiction, register it, then file an immediate termination of parental rights action based solely on the prior termination. That is exactly what the prosecutor did in this case.

At the prehearing conference, as the judge, I did not shy away from the allegations that included termination of parental rights. There was not a foregone conclusion that the termination allegation would be granted because showing that there was a prior termination of parental rights is only one part of the prosecutor's burden. The prosecutor must also prove that it is in the best interest of the child to have her parent's rights severed. Such an action was not being heard at that time, but it might have in the future. I encouraged everyone to consider what services would help the mother deal with her methamphetamine problem and learn to properly care for her newborn.

Just as in other, similar cases, an array of rehabilitative services was identified and would be provided to the mother if she wanted to participate before the adjudication. The mother told me, against advice of counsel, that she just wanted to relinquish her parental rights. She had never been able to "beat meth" and at this point in her life did not want to try. Generally, I am patient and determined, so I encouraged her to consider 0–3 FDTC. Other mothers with similar drug and child protective histories had completed our program and were sober and successful parents. She told me she could not believe it, so I invited her to visit the next session of 0–3 FDTC. She came each Tuesday over the next 3 weeks, but in the end, she still wanted to relinquish her parental rights. Needless to say, she continued using methamphetamine. Finally, at the mother's fourth visit to 0–3 FDTC, her defense attorney stood up and asked me to order her client into 0–3 FDTC. The mother was shocked and upset. A situation like this had never occurred before. The defense attorney made a heartfelt plea for me to order her client into the program because it was the mother's only real chance to learn how to parent her baby, live substance-free, and be reunified with her infant. I agreed and ordered the mother to participate in 0–3 FDTC.

In this case, the mother succeeded in treatment, commenced from 0–3 FDTC, and was reunified with her baby. Her progress was the result of being in an intensive, affirming therapeutic court process that helped her learn to value herself over time. She had been self-medicating for years in order to stave off her depression. Her drug lifestyle and irresponsibility to prior children cut her off from family ties. Through 0–3 FDTC, those relationships were healed. Seeing this woman's desire to get better, along with participation in our program, helped her mother, the baby's grandmother, forgive her daughter and offer support, concern, and love. She also became a group leader at "Moms Off Meth," a sober support program for women. I remind parents every time they are in court that they can get better and must never give up on themselves or their baby.

CASE EXAMPLE 2: PROTOCOLS MUST BE FLEXIBLE

Generally, parents who have violent felony charges or convictions with lengthy incarceration are not allowed into 0–3 FDTC. This protocol was added because of the unlikelihood that there would be successful bonding and attachment between the child and parent. Moreover, reunification is an unlikely permanency objective in such a case, and often a termination of parental rights allegation is filed in the Petition, with a request that no reasonable efforts rehabilitative services be offered to the parent. When such cases occur, the family is referred for mediation of the permanency issue and usually results in voluntary relinquishment of parental rights to a relative.

There was one exception. A father was convicted of felony domestic violence assault on the mother of their baby. The parents' use of methamphetamine and domestic violence resulted in placement of their infant and toddler into foster care in my court. In this case, we allowed them into 0–3 FDTC because they were willing to participate, and because the criminal court judge would suspend the sentence of incarceration if the father graduated from the program. Both parents successfully completed 0–3 FDTC despite complex and multiple rehabilitative issues. Reunification of their infant and toddler occurred in a timely fashion.

Parents who suffer such severe, prolonged mental illness that improvement is unlikely are not accepted. Unfortunately, these parents usually are not able to develop a bond or form an attachment with their babies, and reunification is unlikely.

KEY ELEMENTS

As noted earlier, the prehearing conference and protective custody hearing provide the critical opportunity on day one to invite parents into a collaborative, problem-solving specialty court such as 0–3 FDTC. However, the prehearing conference and protective custody hearing are helpful no matter what brings the family to court. The first hearing is the most important and sets the foundation for all following hearings.[12] If done well, the protective custody hearing results in an informed judicial decision concerning whether or not a child can be safely returned home pending adjudication. Parental participation is strongly encouraged from the very beginning. Generally, the adage "nothing about us without us" applies to parents. By including the parents, we treat them respectfully, talking with them, not at them. This hearing is helpful in identifying parental strengths, relative support, and timely reasonable efforts and services at the earliest stage of the case.

This hearing focuses on discussing and resolving the following key protective custody questions:

- Should the child be returned home or kept in foster care prior to adjudication?
- What services will allow the child to remain at home safely? Is there a safety plan?
- Will parents voluntarily participate in services?
- Has DHHS made reasonable efforts to avoid out-of-home placement or to reunify?
- Are responsible relatives available?
- Is placement proposed by DHHS the least disruptive and in the most family-like setting?
- Does the Indian Child Welfare Act (ICWA)[13] apply? Who will send notice and when?
- Will implementation of the service plan be monitored? Are restraining orders needed?
- What infant, toddler, and parental examinations, evaluations, or other services are needed? When should they be done? What is the source of payment? What are the terms/conditions for parenting time and sibling time?
- Is a child support referral/hearing needed?
- Are there absent parties and a need for future hearings?
- Whether to set the next hearing in court.

The court believes that infants, toddlers, and their parents should receive a coordinated "emergency room–type" response. Families need a prompt and effective response from the court and system stakeholders to address the maltreatment issues that brought them to the court. Therefore, the court and team strives to offer these services:

- Access to immediate substance abuse and mental health evaluations, dual-diagnosis treatment and therapy, bonding and attachment-building opportunities, domestic violence programs, income, housing, and family support.
- A focus on a holistic child–parent relationship, well-being, and permanency—making sure the first placement is the last.
- Daily or near-daily parenting time (visitation) with safety plan.
- Parents and baby reside together as soon as safely possible.
- Fewest foster placement changes.
- Parent–child relationship assessments, evidence-based parenting services, and evidence-based child–parent psychotherapy treatment.
- Intensive judicial monitoring through frequent court appearances.
- Collaborative, nonadversarial court stakeholders supported by ongoing cross-training.
- Service plan based on incremental goals, expectations, and requirements.
- Use of graduated incentives and corrective actions to effect behavior change.
- Enhanced case management to monitor progress/facilitate.
- Free age-appropriate books and encouragement for parents to read to their babies/toddlers.
- Diet and exercise, and smoking cessation.
- Education, job skills, time management.
- Planned activities for the parent and child to include social interaction and healthy self-care.
- Help with safety planning regarding domestic violence, housing, relationships, friends, and family.
- Random, frequent, and observed drug testing—more in the beginning and less with phase progress.

PHASE STRUCTURE: 12–18 MONTHS

The court borrowed from other model court FDTCs a progression structure that sets achievable goals and rewards the parent for accomplishing them. The court learned, similar to other maltreatment cases, that overloading parents with too many tasks could cause them to give up. This is the structure of our program:

- Phase 1: Choice (45 days)
- Phase 2: Challenge (60 days)
- Phase 3: Commitment (90 days)
- Phase 4: Commencement/Graduation (90 days)
- Phase 5: Change (90 days)

These phases are not based simply on parental sobriety. The whole picture of the parent in relationship to the baby's well-being is always considered. The following question is addressed: Is this parent not only establishing sobriety but also becoming a skilled and caring parent for her baby?

INCENTIVES AND CORRECTIVE ACTIONS

FDTC training taught the court that incentives and sanctions are key elements of any program. As noted earlier, I disagreed about using sanctions of incarceration for contempt of court. However, when the program began, several stakeholders thought that this sanction should be included as part of the program. Although I reluctantly agreed, this sanction was never used in my court, as it did not seem helpful or appropriate, and it has not been part of 0–3 FDTC protocol since the first year. There is no statutory language in the Nebraska Juvenile Code using the term "sanction" with regard to child maltreatment cases. It seemed appropriate to use a different term when parents were not following the program protocols. In order to help parents be responsible for becoming the type of parent a baby needs and deserves, the court uses a more positive term—"corrective action." The following incentives and corrective actions are used in our 0–3 FDTC.

Incentives

- Praise in the courtroom by the judge and others—words of encouragement, applause.
- Forgiveness/accountability for mistakes: Encourage the next right step.
- "Treasure Chest"— parents can choose a child's book or developmental toy, diapers, a personal hygiene item, or toothbrush/toothpaste (depending on what has been donated).
- Gift certificates, sober support inspirational medallions, certificates for phase advancement.
- Fewer court appearances.
- Solo parenting time—no oversight by child welfare agency or others.
- Living safely with one's child.

Corrective actions

- Pay $10 fee or community service hours for missed, diluted, or positive drug tests.
- Setback in phase structure or zero days in phase level—depends on issue and can be set for evidentiary hearing.
- Increased level of treatment or therapy sessions, if recommended by the clinician.
- Write essay regarding child's life in foster care, child's view of missed family time because parent did not come; what kind of parent the child deserves and how to become that parent.
- Other community service—parent serves meals at a shelter to bring awareness and gratitude for the opportunity to turn her life around and become the parent her child needs.
- Observe a termination of parental rights hearing or Adult Drug Court sentencing—in the hope that these experiences help a parent make choices to avoid these outcomes.
- More frequent court appearances/drug tests—stepped-up court oversight, as in the beginning phase in order to encourage the parent to stay on point.
- Denial of parenting time (visitation) is never used as a corrective action. However, if a parent is under the influence of a nonprescribed, mood-altering substance, parenting time is delayed until it is safe for the child to be with this parent.

CHILD–PARENT RELATIONSHIP QUESTIONS FOR THE JUDGE

A critical part of 0–3 FDTC is asking parents questions about their relationship with their infant or toddler. It is important for parents to recognize their feelings, which they may have intentionally or unintentionally ignored while under the grip of substance abuse. By focusing on the parents' feelings toward the child, as the judge, I can draw attention to why we are in court: "This is about your baby waiting to see if you will become a fit parent." I ask different questions depending on what is appropriate for each mother. A judge has to be flexible, use common sense, and know what to ask (and what not to ask) at different times. Parents are encouraged to tell me something specific about their relationship with their babies. Here are some examples:

- "Describe one highlight/challenge of being a mother/father this past week. How did that feel?"
- "What is your child's favorite color? Food? Toy? Blanket?"

- "What frightens your child? What do you do to comfort/calm her? How does that feel?"
- "How does your child react when he sees you? How does that feel?"
- "Describe your child in one, two, or three words."
- "What books do you read to your baby? How does she react? What words does she say?"
- "Do you sing to your baby?" (Once a mother sang a made-up lullaby that all the other mothers then wanted to learn and sing to their babies.)
- "Describe the kind of father/mother your toddler needs. Are you that man/woman? Do you want to be? Are you getting there? What gets in the way?"
- "How does it feel to hold your child?"
- "What is your baby's bedtime routine?"

Parents light up when asked these sorts of questions about something as intimate and special as their baby. While parents are proud of staying sober, their progress as parents is what clearly is most important to them.

PROGRESS SO FAR

Our 15th Commencement was held March 23, 2010. As of April 2010, the Omaha 0–3 FDTC has had:

- 56 participants—48 mothers and 8 fathers.
- 25 parents who successfully reunified with their children.
- 35 children successfully reunified with their parents.
- Four mothers delivered drug-free babies while participating in FDTC. These four babies never entered foster care.
- Participants with independent housing at time of Commencement: 25.
- Participants gainfully employed or receiving a legal source of income at time of Commencement: 24.
- Number unsuccessfully discharged: 11, with five voluntary relinquishments and one termination of parental rights.
- 92 total children have received a timely permanency outcome, either reunification or adoption.
- Currently: 14 active cases with 14 mothers, 3 fathers, 36 children.

EXPANDING EFFORTS TO HELP INFANTS,
TODDLERS, AND THEIR PARENTS STATEWIDE

While the Omaha 0–3 FDTC has made great strides, more is needed for babies and their parents in Nebraska. Infant and toddler training need to be offered to juvenile courts and system stakeholders who do not have a specialty problem-solving court like the FDTC court. Greater awareness is needed about better court practice and the science of early childhood development, and what is possible using a community's existing resources. Moreover, many rural judges cover a great number of cases over vast geographic areas and do not have time for additional responsibilities such as 0–3 FDTC. After receiving approval from Nebraska's current Chief Justice Michael Heavican, I partnered with our state's Through the Eyes of the Child Initiative, NCJFCJ's Permanency Planning for Children Department, Zero to Three, DHHS, the Early Development Network (Nebraska's Part C/ Early Intervention System) and clinicians to plan a series of statewide training sessions called "Helping Babies from the Bench."[14]

In May 2008, the state began providing daylong, intensive, interactive training, free of charge, through court improvement funds and partners offering material and personal resources. System stakeholders who work in juvenile courts, child welfare, and early intervention are invited to learn about the science of early childhood development, including infant/toddler attachment and social–emotional development; the parent–infant relationship; meaningful parenting time (visitation); parental skills development; meaningful reasonable efforts services; NCJFCJ resources, such as *Resource Guidelines: Improving Court Practice in Child and Abuse and Neglect Cases,* with special emphasis on the facilitated prehearing conference and protective custody hearing; and Early Development Network Part C evaluations and resources. This information is integrated into the systems by forming small groups of multidisciplinary participants to discuss, analyze, and apply it to pragmatic case scenarios, with guided assistance by the trainers.

Evaluation responses have been overwhelmingly positive and appreciative, with many requests for more training on the subject. "Helping Babies from the Bench" has been presented in 13 communities throughout the state so far. Further trainings are being planned in 2010.[15]

CONCLUSION

To establish, grow, and maintain a specialty court such as 0–3 FDTC is not easy. Obtaining and maintaining funding for these programs is challenging and can "ebb and flow." Omaha's 0–3 FDTC recently received federal and local funding to be a Zero to Three court team, part of a broader national initiative, with Douglas County Court as the project sponsor. In all systems, child agency administrations change and new ones may not support a 0–3 FDTC. Because turnover is constant, training must be ongoing. Team volunteers are pressed for time and have other cases. Still, the science of early childhood development informs us that business as usual is unacceptable and can even be harmful to infants and toddlers. Judicial leaders can convene court system stakeholders, provide training, and improve court practice and services for these babies and their parents. What would practice look like if we treated all babies and their families like our own? Would we accept less than an urgent and excellent response for our own children?

The reader is invited to observe the 0–3 FDTC and facilitated prehearing conferences. Our court would love to host you and all others who are interested in attending.[16] Finally, this is not about the judge, the legal professionals, the child welfare agency, the CASA, or the service providers. It is always and only about those we serve: the infants, toddlers, and their parents.

ACKNOWLEDGMENTS

Many thanks to Joy Osofsky, PhD, Professor of Pediatrics and Psychiatry, Louisiana State University Health Sciences Center; to Sarah Zoellner, my extern from Creighton University School of Law; and to Jackie Ruffin, NCJFCJ Manager of Communications, for their generous assistance in editing this chapter.

NOTES

1. The Early Intervention Program for children under the age of 3 years, also known as Part C of the Individuals with Disabilities Education Act [IDEA; 20 U.S.C. Section 1431 (2000)] (Osofsky, Maze, Lederman, Grace, & Dicker, 2002).
2. Adjudication Hearing—In child welfare proceedings, the trial stage at which the court determines whether allegations of dependency, abuse, or neglect concerning a child are sustained by the evidence and, if so, are legally sufficient to support state intervention on behalf of the child. It provides the basis for state intervention into a family, as opposed to the disposition hearing, which concerns the nature of such intervention. In some states, adjudication hearings are referred to as "jurisdictional" or "fact-finding" hearings (National Council of Juvenile and Family Court Judges [NCJFCJ], 1995, p. 121).
3. Disposition Hearing—The stage of the juvenile court process in which, after finding that a child is within jurisdiction of the court, the court determines who shall have custody and control of a child; elicits judicial decision as to whether to continue out-of-home placement or to remove a child from the home (NCJFCJ, 1995, p. 121).
4. Reasonable Efforts—Public Law 96-272, the Adoption and Child Welfare Act of

1980 requires that reasonable efforts be made to prevent or eliminate the need for removal of a dependent, neglected, or abused child from the child's home and to reunify the family if the child is removed. The reasonable efforts requirement of the federal law is designed to ensure that families are provided with services to prevent their disruption and to respond to the problems of unnecessary disruption of families and foster care drift. To enforce this provision, the juvenile court must determine in each case where federal reimbursement is sought, whether the agency has made the required reasonable efforts [42 U.S.C. 671(a) (15), 672(a)(1)]. ASFA added a new requirement for reasonable efforts to find permanent homes for children who cannot safely be reunited with their parent or guardian (NCJFCJ, 2000, p. 86).

5. The Victims Act Model Courts are a group of more than 30 juvenile and family courts around the nation working with the National Council of Juvenile and Family Court Judges' Permanency Planning for Children Department (PPCD) and using the best practices bench book *Resource Guidelines: Improving Court Practice in Child Abuse and Neglect Cases* as a guide to systems reform. The model courts identify impediments to the timeliness of court events and delivery of services for children and families in care, then design and implement court and agency-based changes to address these barriers, with technical assistance and training from the PPCD (NCJFCJ, 2006).

6. Nebraska's Safe Start program provides early childhood mental health services specifically designed to meet the needs of children age 5 and younger, and their families, for a safe, secure, and developmentally appropriate home and family environment.

7. Protective Custody Hearing or Preliminary Protective Hearing—The first court hearing in a juvenile abuse or neglect case (referred to in some jurisdictions as a "shelter care hearing," "detention hearing," "emergency removal hearing," or "temporary custody hearing"), occurs either immediately before or immediately after a child is removed from the home on an emergency basis. It may be preceded by an *ex parte* order directing placement of the child; in extreme emergency cases it may constitute the first judicial review of a child placed without prior court approval (NCJFCJ, 1995, p. 123).

8. For a full discussion of the facilitated prehearing conference, please see Johnson (2009).

9. *Douglas County Zero To Three Participant Handbook* and other materials are available from the author.

10. ASFA—Adoption and Safe Families Act of 1997, Public Law 105-89, which amended Titles IV-B and IV-E of the Social Security Act to clarify certain provisions of Public Law 96-272 and to speed the process of finding permanent homes for children (NCJFCJ, 2000, p. 83).

11. Review Hearing—Court proceedings that take place after disposition, after the permanency hearing, or after termination of parental rights in which the court comprehensively reviews the status of a case, examines progress made by the parties since the conclusion of the prior hearing, provides for correction and revision of the case plan, and makes sure that cases progress and children spend as short a time as possible in temporary placement (NCJFCJ, 2000, p. 86).

12. NCJFCJ's *Resource Guidelines* (1995) provides a detailed description and a bench card checklist as a ready reference for any child abuse and neglect hearing.
13. ICWA—Indian Child Welfare Act, passed in 1978, addresses the removal of Indian children from their home and their placement with non-Indian families (NCJFCJ, 2000, p. 85).
14. The title was borrowed from Zero to Three's 2007 DVD of the same name. This free resource is available at *www.zerotothree.org.*
15. A sample agenda is available by contacting the author.
16. Contact the author at *douglas.johnson@douglascounty-ne.gov* regarding visiting the 0–3 FDTC or obtaining any related materials about the court.

REFERENCES

Dicker, S., & Gordon, E. (2004). Building bridges for babies in foster care: The Babies Can't Wait Initiative. *Juvenile and Family Court Journal, 55*(2), 29–41.

Edwards, L. P. (2010). Sanctions in family drug treatment courts. *Juvenile and Family Court Journal, 65*(1), 55–62.

Edwards, L. P., & Ray, J. A. (2005). Judicial perspectives on family drug treatment courts. *Juvenile and Family Court Journal, 56*(3), 1–18.

Foster, S. (2001, January 29). *Shoveling up: The impact of substance abuse on state budgets.* Presentation by the National Center on Addiction and Substance Abuse at Columbia University, New York.

In re Nolan W., 45 Cal. 4th 1217, 203 P.3d 454, 91 Cal.Rptr.3d 140 (2009).

Johnson, D. F. (2009). The role of the judge: Convene stakeholders for facilitated prehearing conferences in abuse, neglect, and dependency cases. *Juvenile and Family Justice Today, 18*(3), 20–23. Available at *www.ncjfcj.org/vdir/source.prehearing.*

Join Together. (2005, October 13). Rewards help keep patients in treatment, study says. Boston: Author. Available at *www.jointogether.org/y/0,2521,578419,00.html.*

Leslie, L. K., Hurlburt, M.S., Landsverk, J., Barth, R. P., & Slyman, D. J. (2004). Outpatient mental health services for children in foster care: A national perspective. *Child Abuse and Neglect, 28,* 697–712.

Meyer, W. (2007, April). Developing and delivering incentives and sanctions. Available at *www.georgiacourts.org/courts/accountability/2008conference.html.*

National Clearinghouse on Child Abuse and Neglect Information. (2005). Concurrent planning: What the evidence shows (U.S. Department of Health and Human Services). Available at *nccanch.acf.hhs.gov/pubs/issue_briefs/concurrent_evidence/index.cfm.*

National Council of Juvenile and Family Court Judges (1995). *Resource guidelines: Improving court practice in child abuse and neglect cases.* Reno, NV: Author.

National Council of Juvenile and Family Court Judges. (2000). *Adoption and permanency guidelines: Improving court practice in child abuse and neglect cases.* Reno, NV: Author.

National Council of Juvenile and Family Court Judges. (2006, January). *Model* courts: *Improving outcomes for abused and neglected children and their families*. Reno, NV: Author.

Osofsky, J., Maze, C., Lederman, C., Grace, M., & Dicker, S. (2002, December). *Questions every judge and lawyer should ask about infants and toddlers in the child welfare system*. National Council of Juvenile and Family Court Judges Technical Assistance Brief. Reno, NV: National Council of Juvenile and Family Court Judges.

Shonkoff, J., & Phillips, D. A. (2000). *From neurons to neighborhoods: The science of early childhood development*. Washington, DC: National Academy Press.

U.S. Department of Health and Human Services, Administration of Children and Families. (2008). Child maltreatment 2008. Washington, DC: Author. Available at *http://www.acf.hhs.gov/programs/cb/pubs/cm08/cm08.pdf*.

Wulczyn, F., & Hislop, K. B. (2000). *The placement of infants in foster care*. Chicago: University of Chicago, Chapin Hall Center for Children.

Wulczyn, F., & Hislop, K. B. (2002). Babies in foster care: The numbers call for attention. *Zero to Three Journal, 4*, 14–15.

PART V

■ ■ ■ ■

SPECIAL ISSUES

INTRODUCTION TO PART V

The final section of the book focuses on special issues that impact high-risk infants, young children, and families. Given my work with young children exposed to different types of traumas, I have contributed two of these chapters. These three chapters focus on best practices in special situations. In the first chapter in this section, I have stressed the impact on young children and their families traumatized by exposure to disasters. We have learned from our own work, and that of others, that children of all ages are traumatized when disasters strike; however, young children are particularly vulnerable because they are totally dependent on their caregivers, who may also be traumatized through displacement, loss, and lack of control. Unfortunately, with major disasters, separation of young children from caregivers and even loss of primary caregivers is not uncommon. Best practices in the area are described with illustrative examples of interventions with young children experiencing trauma in the aftermath of Hurricane Katrina. For the interested reader, the journal *Child Development* recently published a Special Section on Disasters and the Impact on Child Development (Masten & Osofsky, 2010). Betsy McAlister Groves and Marilyn Augustyn raise the reader's awareness of the common presentation of early childhood trauma. These authors, who work in pediatric settings, recognize that for many parents the pediatrician is the first and often the most trusted professional they seek out if their child has experienced an adverse event, or if there are worries about a child's behavior. Identification of childhood trauma can be a powerful form of prevention. Pediatric health practitioners, including doctors, physician's assistants, nurses, nurse practitioners, and others who work in pediatric settings, have an opportunity to identify and respond to early childhood trauma, if they are well informed. They must recognize the impact of exposure to trauma on young children and have both knowledge and effective interventions as part of their responsibility. Groves and Augustyn emphasize the importance of mental health–pediatric collaboration in enabling these settings to better serve families with young children affected by traumatic stress, a message that is consistent throughout all the systems discussed in this book.

In the final chapter in the book, I discuss the issue of vicarious traumatization, compassion fatigue, and/or burnout that occurs far too often among professionals from all disciplines who have to deal with traumatized young children. Whether it is the mental health professional trying to support children and families of a service member injured in combat, the judge who hears cases after case of young children experiencing abuse and neglect, or the child welfare worker or mental health professional with an overwhelming caseload, taking on the traumatic experiences of those we try to help is common. Experiencing vicarious traumatization can lead to impatience at work, difficulty sleeping and nightmares, crankiness, or in some cases, leaving a job. Self-care is crucial for all who work with traumatized young children. My chapter elaborates on steps that professionals who work with trauma can take to help support themselves.

REFERENCE

Masten, A. S., & Osofsky, J. D. (2010). Introduction: Disasters and their impact on child development: Introduction to the special section. *Child Development, 81,* 1029–1039.

CHAPTER 15

■ ■ ■ ■

Young Children and Disasters

Lessons Learned from Hurricane Katrina about the Impact of Disasters and Postdisaster Recovery

Joy D. Osofsky

> If I only had my old room back, I'd be good.
> —5-year-old after Hurricane Katrina

Disasters affect the lives of millions of children each year, causing immense hardship and suffering. The traumatic experiences for children and their families include displacement, loss of homes and personal property, economic hardship, loss of community and social supports, and, at times, injury and death of loved ones. Although frequently less emphasized, young children are particularly vulnerable to being traumatized by disasters, with the impact mediated by the responses of parents, caregivers, and other adults in their environment. With protection and support, most children are resilient following a disaster. However, because the environment during and after a disaster may be very confusing for young children, it is common for them to appear numb, unresponsive, and anxious. The behaviors and emotions that follow reflect their anxiety, with behavior and emotion dysregulation that is frequently interpreted by adults as misbehavior, leading to impatience and even harsh punishment. Planning effectively in responding to children's

295

needs and making preparations before disasters is very important to support resilience and recovery.

Hurricane Katrina struck the Gulf Coast on August 29, 2005, followed by the breach of the levees causing much physical destruction, loss of homes, property, toys, pets, and for many, a loss of community. The impact was both physical and psychological for children and families. Hurricane Katrina has been described as one of the worst natural disasters in U.S. history (Knabb, Rhome, & Brown, 2005), and, 5 years later, it continues to impact residents and communities in Louisiana. As this chapter is being written, the same families and communities impacted by Hurricanes Katrina, Rita, and Gustav are coping with the devastation caused by the Deepwater Horizon oil rig that exploded on April 29, 2010, killing 11 oil workers and injuring many others. With oil in the Gulf of Mexico, and uncertain impact on the fishing industry, the oil industry in the Gulf, and another hurricane season beginning, there is much anxiety and concern for children, families, and communities in this region.

Disasters with a slow recovery, such as Hurricane Katrina, can result in acute and chronic psychological effects (Kessler, Galea, Jones, & Parker, 2006; Osofsky, Osofsky, Kronenberg, Brennan, & Hansel, 2009; Weems et al., 2007) that negatively impact the child's normal developmental trajectory (Pynoos, Steinberg, & Piacentini, 1999; Shaw, 2000). Younger children are particularly vulnerable, especially if trauma and stress are making parents less emotionally available to their children. Large-scale disasters, such as Hurricane Katrina and the Deepwater Horizon Oil Spill are of particular importance related to children's development because they affect not only the individual but also multiple systems, including microsystems and exosystems, in which children develop (Bronfenbrenner, 1986; Masten & Obradovic, 2008). For many children affected by Katrina, their once thriving neighborhoods, grocery stores, and playgrounds were no longer functional; many children experienced multiple moves and changes in schools, as well as parental unemployment (Osofsky et al., 2009; Osofsky, Osofsky, & Harris, 2007). The families impacted by the Deepwater Horizon Oil Spill are being threatened with severe economic impact, as well as loss of their identities because they live and thrive by the water. For example, in St. Bernard Parish, an adjacent parish (county) to New Orleans that was devastated by Hurricane Katrina, at present, the oil spill is threatening the tranquil coastal fishing and wildlife areas of the parish. Lessons from the Exxon Valdez oil spill (*www.onearth.org/article/lessons-from-the-exxon-valdez*; Picou & Gill, 1996) showed the significant vulnerability of children over time, with significant impact on individual, family, and community identity. Outcomes for young children are still in question, and such uncertainties are common for all children exposed to a disaster with slow recovery.

WHAT WE KNOW ABOUT THE IMPACT
OF DISASTERS ON CHILDREN

Research on disasters has shown that the impact on children depends on the nature of the disaster, the age and vulnerability of the child, the types of resources available to the child, and family and community supports (Masten & Osofsky, 2010). Studies of older children can provide background for understanding the potential impact on younger children for whom less research is available. Traditionally, child-focused disaster research examines postdisaster symptomatology. For example, the majority of the literature on hurricanes indicates that children are at a high risk for symptoms of depression, anxiety, and posttraumatic stress disorder (PTSD) (Goenjian et al., 2001; Kessler et al., 2006; Osofsky et al., 2007, 2009). A number of disaster studies with older children have documented symptoms of PTSD in children who have experienced natural disasters, including earthquakes, tsunamis, and hurricanes (Goenjian et al., 2005; John, Russell, & Russell, 2007; Kolaitis et al., 2003; La Greca, Silverman, Vernberg, & Prinstein, 1996; Lonigan, Shannon, Taylor, Finch, & Sallee, 1994; Piyasil et al., 2007; Pynoos et al., 1993). Many of these studies have reported comorbid symptoms of depression in children following natural disasters. Although there is overlap in symptomatology of both PTSD and depression, including anhedonia, sleep difficulties, problems with concentration, irritability, and a restricted range of affect, the research has been clear in demonstrating the distinct presence of each disorder following disasters (Goenjian et al., 2001; Kolaitis et al., 2003; Roussos et al., 2005). For example, a study exploring PTSD and depression in children between the ages of 7 and 17, who experienced a supercyclone in India, found that although PTSD and depression were significantly correlated, most children with PTSD did not meet criteria for depression, and 55.7% of children with a diagnosis of depression did not meet criteria for PTSD (Kar et al., 2007).

The relation between PTSD symptoms and disaster-specific aspects of trauma has been well documented in the literature. For example, a study of 16- and 17-year-old children following a 1999 earthquake in Greece (Roussos et al., 2005), as well as studies of 13-year-olds following Hurricane Mitch in Nicaragua (Goenjian et al., 2001, 2005), showed that exposure to a natural disaster was consistently related to increases in the severity of PTSD symptoms. In a study of over 5,000 children, ages 9 to 19, who experienced displacement and damage to their homes as a result of Hurricane Hugo, PTSD was associated with traumatic experiences (Lonigan et al., 1994). Similarly, Russoniello and colleagues (2002) found that 9- to 12-year-old children whose homes were flooded as a result of Hurricane Floyd were three times more likely to have symptoms of PTSD compared to those whose homes did not flood. Hamada, Kameoka, Yanagida, and

Chemtob (2003) reported that 6- to 12-year-old children who experienced Hurricane Iniki were more likely to report posttraumatic symptoms if they felt that their lives or the lives of others were threatened at the time of the hurricane.

Experiencing previous trauma plays an important role in severity of symptoms. Neuner, Schauer, Catani, Ruf, and Elbert (2006) assessed 64 tsunami survivors, ages 8 to 14, in Sri Lanka, and found that previous traumas, including exposure to war, domestic violence, community violence, medical treatment, physical abuse, and natural disaster, were associated with increased posttraumatic stress symptoms. Similarly, Garrison, Weinrich, Hardin, Weinrich, and Wang (1993) assessed 1,264 children, ages 11 to 17, following Hurricane Hugo and found that experiencing previous violent, traumatic events was associated with increased likelihood of PTSD. Unlike symptoms of PTSD, depression has not been found to be consistently related to level of disaster exposure or proximity. Depression has been associated with several different factors, including reported difficulties at home following the disaster (Roussos et al., 2005), death of a family member (Goenjian et al., 2001), and feeling that one's own life or the lives of family members were in danger (Thienkrua et al., 2006).

Research regarding how children express traumatic responses has been well established. Commonly observed traumatic reactions in school-age children include specific fears, separation difficulties, sleep problems, reenactment of the trauma in play, regression, somatic complaints, irritability, decline in academic performance, fear of recurrence of the trauma, and trauma-related guilt (Steinberg, Brymer, Decker, & Pynoos, 2004; Vogel & Vernberg, 1993). Adolescents, on the other hand, often express difficulties through individuation and identity development processes. Pynoos (1993) stated that "a trauma-induced sense of discontinuity can give a disrupting influence on the adolescent task of integrating past, present, and future expectations into a lasting sense of identity" (p. 222). Pynoos reaffirmed the Blos (1967) description of adolescence as a period of individuation, and elaborated that any threat to this process, through trauma, can potentially disrupt the developmental focus of this important period.

The Impact of Gender on Children's Psychological Responses to Natural Disasters

Research on children and adolescents has generally also shown a relationship between gender and reports of posttraumatic stress symptoms following exposure to natural disasters. The majority of studies have reported that females are more likely than males to develop PTSD symptoms (Bal, 2008; Giannopoulou et al., 2006; John et al., 2007; Pfefferbaum, 1997; Shannon, Lonigan, Finch, & Taylor, 1994). For example, following Hurricane Floyd,

9- to 12-year-old females were twice as likely as males to report symptoms of PTSD (Russoniello et al., 2002). Although much of the literature has described gender differences in psychological response to trauma, not all research is consistent on this finding. For example, Kar and Bastia (2006) reported no significant differences in depression and PTSD diagnoses for males and females in high school students following a supercyclone; however, they did report differences in the expression of symptomatology, with girls being more likely to report guilt and boys more likely to have increased worry, anhedonia, concentration problems, and academic problems. Shannon and colleagues (1994) also described gender differences in expression of symptomatology in 9- to 19-year-old children and adolescents, with females being more likely to report symptoms associated with emotional processing/emotional reactions, and males more often showing symptoms associated with cognitive and behavioral factors. While the disaster and trauma literature often reveals that females report more symptoms (Tolin & Foa, 2006), the interpretation of gender differences is complex, in that female adolescents and adults generally discuss feelings more openly and disclose symptoms of distress more easily, after they have experienced trauma (Crick & Zahn-Waxler, 2003).

The Impact of Hurricane Katrina on Children

Research data that are becoming available on the effects of Hurricane Katrina on children and adolescents reflect the unprecedented scale of the storm and complexity of the recovery. In a sample of 166 students in the 9th through 12th grades, Marsee (2008) found that 63% of students had symptoms of PTSD 15–18 months following the hurricane, and that the PTSD symptoms, together with high levels of aggression, were associated with emotional dysregulation. Weems and colleagues (2009) expanded the understanding of post-Katrina symptomatology, and found that, among 52 children with a mean age of 11 years in the 6–7 months following Katrina, level of posttraumatic stress symptomatology was related to hurricane exposure, female gender, and level of predisaster anxiety. Osofsky and colleagues (2009) found that variables including separation from a caregiver and evacuation to a shelter were associated with posttraumatic stress symptoms in 7- to 19-year-old students 2 years after Hurricane Katrina. In a study of 8- to 16-year-old students, Spell and colleagues (2008) found similar results, reflecting the importance of caregiver symptomatology in predicting a child's psychological status. Terranova, Boxer, and Morris (2009) provided further support for the importance of relationships in their study of sixth-grade students who were evacuated prior to Hurricane Katrina but did not experience significant flooding. In this group of children, negative peer interactions were associated with symptoms of PTSD 8 months following the storm. Kronenberg and colleagues (2010) found that younger children, ages 9–11, compared to adolescents, ages 15–18, and females compared to males were more likely to show continued symptoms. Furthermore, children and adolescents who reported school and family problems were three times as likely to show continued symptoms of depression and anxiety. Similarly, Shannon and colleagues (1994) reported that in a sample of 5th through 11th graders impacted by Hurricane Hugo, symptoms of posttraumatic stress were more common in younger than in older children. Scheeringa and Zeanah (2008) studied 3- to 6-year-old children impacted by Hurricane Katrina and found that hurricane-related PTSD was associated with caregivers' level of symptomatology. Based on the newly emerging literature, mental health symptoms following Hurricane Katrina, as in other disasters, appear common, and children's responses are associated with hurricane exposure, previous trauma, as well as environmental and relational factors.

FACTORS THAT AFFECT RESILIENCE AND RECOVERY AFTER DISASTERS

Recent theoretical research has focused on examining patterns of resilience and recovery related to developmental theories and trajectories for children. Important factors that support resilience in preparation for and following disasters include promotive and protective influences (Bonanno, 2004; Bonanno & Mancini, 2008; Layne et al., 2009; Masten & Obradovic, 2008). Masten (in press) considered promotive factors to predict better outcomes at all levels of risk or adversity, and protective factors to be more important when risk or adversity was high. These two perspectives are extremely important in understanding the effect of disasters on children. The impact of disasters and developmental issues that follow are influenced by the nature and severity of the exposure, the importance of pre- and post-disaster context for understanding disaster response and recovery, protective factors for positive recovery, and the possible role of age and gender (Masten & Osofsky, 2010). Pynoos (1993) discussed factors that influence poor long-term outcomes following disasters, including extended periods of high cumulative adversity related to breakdown of infrastructure, ongoing economic consequences, family stress, loss of life and property, and other aspects of slow recovery.

While parents play a key protective role for children of all ages related to preparedness, safety, communication, and role modeling adaptive behaviors, parents are particularly important for younger children, who are more vulnerable and dependent on adults. To ensure the protection of children during and following disasters, parents need education and information to carry out their caring roles most effectively. While relatively few available studies relate to factors that support resilience in younger children, a recent study by Kithakye, Morris, Terranova, and Myers (2010), which also includes predisaster adjustment, shows that self-regulation skills in preschoolers were associated with prosocial behavior in general and had an moderating effect on the impact of exposure severity on prosocial outcomes. Masten (2007) also has found that self-regulation skills can support a protective role for children.

An important part of disaster preparedness for children must involve parents' and caregivers' effectively planning and carrying out the roles of protection, communication, and safeguarding children under very difficult circumstances. As mentioned earlier, an additional risk factor for children is prior traumatic experiences and losses, which play a key role in how young children (or children and adults of any age) react to and cope with disasters. Children with prior difficulties and those who have experienced previous trauma or loss, and continue to experience postdisaster trauma and adversities, are at higher risk for mental health problems than those without these compounding difficulties (Bowlby, 1973; Laor et al., 1997; Osofsky, 2004; Pynoos, 1993; Pynoos, Steinberg, & Goenjian, 1996; Vogel & Vernberg, 1993).

ISSUES FOR YOUNG CHILDREN

For infants, toddlers, and young children affected by disasters, relatively little information and a paucity of both research and effective interventions are available, probably for two main reasons. First, as mentioned earlier, many people continue to believe that very young children are "too young" to be impacted. Second, it is often difficult to gain access to young children to provide evaluations, interventions, and services after a disaster. Young children are dependent on their parents or caregivers, and, in our experience, parents often tend to underreport symptoms and to seek out help for them well after the problematic behaviors occur. Older children are in school settings with teachers and counselors, who generally are more familiar with the classroom setting, and individual and student behaviors. They generally are easier to access, have more supports outside the family, including friends, and can communicate how they are feeling. Yet, as noted, infants and toddlers are exquisitely sensitive to the reactions, behaviors, and emotions shown by their parents or caregivers, particularly their stress level, and how they cope is very dependent on the reactions of others (Masten & Obradovic, 2008; Masten & Osofsky, 2010; Osofsky, 2004: Osofsky et al., 2007; Pine, Costello, & Masten, 2005).

Furthermore, the disaster and the postdisaster environment play an important role for children, families, and communities related to the issue of multiple adversities (Felitti, 2009; Klasen et al., 2010; Kronenberg et al., 2010; Pynoos, 1993). The co-occurrence of trauma and poverty can lead to increased vulnerability for children of all ages, and particularly for young children. These issues are significant following disasters and were illustrated poignantly in the aftermath of Hurricane Katrina by children and families in the Gulf South, for whom symptom severity was very high and has decreased only slightly in the years following the disaster (Kronenberg et al., 2010; Osofsky, Osofsky, & Harris, 2007). Fernando, Miller, and Berger (2010), in a study of tsunami survivors in Sri Lanka, discussed the role of daily stressors related to outcomes and coping, in addition to the actual exposure to a disaster. Although much of this work has involved older children, there are important implications for younger children, since more stress in families has a significant impact. Becker-Blease, Turner, and Finkelhor (2010) provided data on prevalence and incidence of exposure to disasters in a nationally representative sample in the United States for children ranging in age from 2 to 17 years. The data indicated that about 14% of children and adolescents reported experiencing some type of traumatic event in their lifetimes, with about 4% experiencing such an event in the previous year. A recent study by Chemtob and colleagues (2010) that highlighted the importance of parents' emotional state and availability to their children after a disaster showed that preschool children of parents with more PTSD symptoms and other mental health problems following the September 11, 2001, terrorist attack had more difficulties. Consistent with developmental theory, children who are not protected at the time of the disaster by supportive caregivers may be more vulnerable to the effects of the disaster.

As a result of the evacuation and displacement following Hurricane Katrina, some children who were separated from their parents experienced other disruptions in their primary relationships, family, child care, and other support systems. While few circumstances other than disasters cause such a massive disruption in the lives of young children, history has shown (Bowlby, 1973; Burlingham & Freud, 1942) that in times of stress, attachment behaviors are activated, with young children turning to their caregivers for comfort and security. During World War II, during the London Blitz, Burlingham and Freud (1942) observed young children being cared for at a residential nursery. Children who were separated from their caregivers showed regressive behaviors, aggression, and withdrawn and depressed behaviors. In 2003, Foster, Davies, and Steele studied the long-term effects of children's separation from caregivers during the London Blitz. They found that 60 years later, adults who were separated from their parents as children, compared to those who lived in London with their parents during the war and did not evacuate, were at increased risk for an insecure attachment style and were more likely to report low levels of psychological well-being. These results are consistent with the recent Adverse Childhood Experiences Study (Felitti, 2009). During Hurricane Katrina, children were confronted by multiple stressors, including the primary stressors of the storm, such as witnessing the devastation and destruction and sustaining injuries, and inability for some to access their primary attachment figures or other supports (e.g., their pets, familiar toys, and schools) in order to cope. When young children lack secure caregiving relationships, they are at risk for less optimal social and cognitive outcomes (O'Connor & McCartney, 2007; Rydell, Bohlin, & Thorell, 2005).

EFFECTIVE INTERVENTIONS FOR YOUNG TRAUMATIZED CHILDREN AFFECTED BY DISASTERS

Consistent with important intervention components discussed in different chapters (e.g., Cozza & Feerick, Chapter 8), young children impacted by disasters benefit from (1) support for the parents and caregivers, which includes reducing individual and family stress; (2) support for child, parent, and family functioning; and (3) helping parents and caregivers communicate with their young children related to the changes in their lives. For young children, it is important to recognize the importance of the family environment, supports for the family in the community, and attachment relationships that provide safety, routine, and a sense of normality in the young child's life. Suggested interventions for young children are presented with illustrative examples.

Psychological First Aid

Psychological first aid (PFA) is an evidence-informed intervention for disaster response and recovery (Brymer et al., 2006). Five key principles of PFA intervention emphasize (1) establishing a sense of safety, (2) promoting calming through distress reduction, (3) building a sense of self and community efficacy, (4) fostering connectedness, and (5) promoting a sense of hope. With young children exposed to disasters, these PFA principles can be implemented in disaster settings (e.g., shelters), and in family settings, community-based programs, family and parenting support programs, child care centers, and so forth. Those intervening with PFA can also provide support to others who relate to the young children.

PFA principles must be applied in a developmentally appropriate manner. For example, maintaining daily routines and physical proximity to a trusted adult are essential in establishing feelings of safety in infants, toddlers, and preschoolers. In addition to attending to safety, preschool children (3–5 years old) may have unique requirements for managing distress. Their lack of cognitive capacity to understand the situation fully or to describe their feelings necessitates nonverbal outlets. Young children gain mastery through play, practice, and repetition. Playing with developmentally appropriate toys can help children become more comfortable with the experiences of their parents. One resource related to disasters developed specifically for children at this age is the Sesame Workshop's Let's Get Ready *www.sesame-workshop.org/initiatives/emotion/*) and You Can Ask (*www.sesamework-shop.org/newsandevents/pressreleases/you_can_ask_online*).

Illustrative Example

Shortly after Hurricane Katrina, my husband and I were living with first responders in temporary housing on boats in New Orleans. The boats were provided to allow family reunification, since most first responders had lost their homes and many had displaced family members. I noticed an officer, his wife, and 4-year-old child in the cafeteria looking upset and frustrated. I walked over to them and introduced myself, said I was local, from the Louisiana State University Health Sciences Center, and asked if I could be of help to them. The father responded, "There is nothing you can do to help." I asked if I could sit down with them and handed the little girl a toy from my pocket. I said that I knew it was very hard for so many of the officers and their families who had lost their homes and possessions, and I wondered how things were going with their daughter. Then they started to talk about how hard it was on the boat with close quarters, how difficult it was to access the insurance money they needed to rebuild their home, and the lack of family support since their extended family could not return to New Orleans at this time. I asked what they did with their child during the day. On the verge of tears, the father replied that there were no child care centers, no work for his wife, and they did not know what they could do. After listening to them express their frustration, worries, and uncertainties, I acknowledged how hard it was and wondered about possible steps that we could take together. The father then started sharing more about their lives. He said that not only had they lost their home, but also his wife had lost her job. She described fears that all of their years of effort to create a safe, comfortable home for themselves and their daughter would be lost. They felt angry and hopeless. We were then able to sort out together what they could do for themselves and for their daughter. I was able to tell them that our team, together with volunteers, would be opening a child care program on the boat, and that the Red Cross and other groups would continue to bring clothes on the boat for families since they had all lost everything. We talked about their daughter being taken care of for part of the day, which would give them some time off to help organize their lives; there might also be possibilities of a job for the wife. I also said that our team would be bringing more donated toys on the boat, so that their daughter would have some toys to play with in the evening. Since it was early after the crisis, they were not ready to think about where they might live and whether they might rebuild their house. However, after talking together for 45 minutes and trying to problem-solve, they were able to see a "dim light" at the end of the empty tunnel. I told them I would be on the boat and they requested follow-up, feeling that it would be helpful. They now seemed more relaxed and smiled more with their daughter.

Child–Parent Psychotherapy

Child–parent psychotherapy (CPP), which engages the child and parent together, is an evidence- and relationship-based treatment (Lieberman & Van Horn, 2004, 2008) designed to support the child–parent relationship through interventions for children ages birth to age 5. It is used for young children who are showing emotional or behavior problems, including symptoms of posttraumatic stress, and those who have been maltreated and exposed to trauma (Van Horn, Gray, Pettinelli, & Estassi, Chapter 4, this volume, discuss principles of CPP in depth). CPP can be very helpful for young children exposed to disasters that include displacement, separation from parents or caretakers, and trauma that has disrupted usual routines and support. Together with the caregiver, the therapist works to help the child create a new narrative through words, pictures, and play, including an understanding that the caregiver will keep him or her safe. The therapist helps both child and parent understand the maladaptive behaviors that result from the traumatic experience, and supports the child's positive development, building on the strengths of the parent.

CPP is based on the premise that the child's relationship with the mother, father, or primary attachment figure represents the most important "port of entry" or opportunity for intervention to help support the child's development in all areas, with particular focus on social and emotional development. Furthermore, CPP works with parent and child to facilitate increased emotional and behavioral regulation. These issues are particularly important for children who have been traumatized and, as a result, are unable to show emotions and behaviors in appropriate ways, and instead display, for example, increased aggression or withdrawn behavior.

Illustrative Example

Three weeks after Hurricane Katrina, a 4-year-old child of a first responder was staying with his grandparents in temporary housing because he had lost his home in the hurricane and his father had to work. His father was his primary parent. The grandparents were concerned about his withdrawn behavior. They stated that he used to be happy and relaxed and now did not smile, play, or talk much. The mental health consultant sat down with the little boy and his grandfather, talked to him about Hurricane Katrina, and conveyed to him a wish to know more about his experience. The little boy started to talk, and his grandfather listened. He said he was in the Superdome on his birthday and waited and waited for his father to come with a cake—and he never came. He was very disappointed. He knew that his father would never forget his birthday, and he worried about his father. The therapist commented that he was sure his father also missed bringing him a cake for his birthday and the grandfather described that he had wanted to be there but could not get there because of the storm—but they would soon be together. As he talked, the boy began to brighten once he was able to share what was bothering him. He became engaged in the play and interactions with his grandfather. (The mental health professional knew that his father had been stranded at the Superdome during the flooding and could not communicate with his family, and that there were initial, but now resolved, concerns about his safety.)

Parental Guidance Related to Trauma and Developmental Expectations for Young Children

Often parents or caregivers may misunderstand that many difficult behaviors in young children can result from exposure to a traumatic event, such as a disaster. The child may be scared and anxious following the traumatic experience, showing it through behaviors and emotions that are difficult for parents and caregivers to understand and may lead to impatience and unresponsiveness. Parental guidance following trauma is designed to help the adult understand that a young child's behavior has "meaning," and to learn more about the relationship between emotions and behaviors.

Illustrative Examples

EXAMPLE 1

As noted, in November 2005, the Louisiana State University Mental Heath Trauma Team, together with Substance Abuse and Mental Health Administration (SAMHA) volunteers, established a child care center on the cruise ship that housed first responders and their families, 80% of whom had lost their homes during Hurricane Katrina and were living on the boat while they continued to do their work in New Orleans. The child care center was needed for these first responders, some of whom had to go to work and others who needed some respite from being with the children all day. The first game that the children wanted to play and repeat day after day was "Hurricane." It was very difficult for the parents to observe and join in their children's play involving repeated experiences during the hurricane. Education and support was needed to help the parents accept child behavior that was a normal part of working through the traumatic experiences. Furthermore, the therapists had to be mindful of the nature of repetitive traumatic play and, over time, together with the parents, help the young children understand their new life experiences after the hurricane, which included much displacement and loss, many new adjustments, and hopes for the future. This example illustrates how children play out traumatic experiences, and how difficult it can be for parents to see and experience this play.

EXAMPLE 2

A 2½-year-old lost his home in Hurricane Katrina and was evacuated with his two parents. Although the boy was safe and protected, his parents had to rebuild their home in an area that was totally flooded. He had a teddy bear that he took everywhere with him since Hurricane Katrina. When he was 4 years old at preschool, the teacher wanted him to take a nap without his teddy bear, and said that the teddy bear would be in sight. He cried and cried, and finally said to the teacher, "I don't want to give you my teddy—he will drown."

CONCLUSION

Disasters of all kinds occur far too frequently, be they hurricanes, typhoons, earthquakes, fires, flooding, and so forth. The potential for young children to be impacted is great because, even when prepared, it is not possible to anticipate when a disaster may occur. When a disaster does occur, not only is the child impacted but also the parent or caregiver, whose role is to keep the child safe and provide protection and nurturance, may be affected and often traumatized. Furthermore, with displacement, there is disruption and loss of property, sometimes loss of lives, and certainly interruption of routines that are so helpful for the stability and positive growth of young children. Young children in particular can be profoundly impacted by disasters because they lack the cognitive and emotional maturity and skills to cope that are present even in older children. In addition, young children are more reliant upon parents and other caregivers to support their development and meet their needs. Parents and caregivers coping with disasters may not have available the physical or emotional resources to meet the young children's needs. Furthermore, if there is separation of the child from significant caregivers, such as occurs routinely in first responder families, there may be a dramatic impact on the established relationship between the child and his or her parents and extended family of trusted adults. Disaster response can be much improved, with more attention to the developmental needs of children of different ages and particular attention to younger children, who are so much more vulnerable and dependent on adults. With better preparation and acknowledgment of difficulties, we can provide much more support for young children during disasters and their aftermath.

REFERENCES

Bal, A. (2008). Post-traumatic stress disorder in Turkish child and adolescent survivors three years after the Marmara earthquake. *Child and Adolescent Mental Health, 13,* 134–139.

Becker-Blease, K. A., Turner, H. A., & Finkelhor, D. (2010). Disasters, victimization and children's mental health. *Child Development, 81,* 1040–1052.

Blos, P. (1967). *The adolescent passage.* New York: International Universities Press.

Bonanno, G. A. (2004). Loss, trauma, and human resilience: Have we under-estimated the human capacity to thrive after extremely aversive events? *American Psychologist, 59,* 20–28.

Bonanno, G. A., & Mancini, A. D. (2008). The human capacity to thrive in the face of potential trauma. *Pediatrics, 121,* 369–375.

Bowlby, J. (1973). *Attachment and loss: Vol. 2. Separation: Anxiety and anger.* New York: Basic Books.

Bronfenbrenner, U. (1986). Ecology of the family as a context for human development: Research perspectives. *Developmental Psychology, 22,* 723–742.

Brymer, M., Layne, C., Pynoos, R., Ruzek, J. I., Steinberg, A., Vernberg, E., et al. (2006). *Psychological first aid: Field operations guide.* Washington, DC: U.S. Department of Health and Human Services.

Burlingham, D., & Freud, A. (1942). *Young children in wartime.* London: Allen & Unwin.

Chemtob, C. M., Nomura, Y., Rajendran, K., Yehuda, R., Schwartz, D., & Abramovitz, R. (2010). Impact of maternal posttraumatic stress disorder and depression following exposure to the September 11 attacks on preschool children's behavior. *Child Development, 81,* 1129–1141.

Crick, N. R., & Zahn-Waxler, C. (2003). The development of psychopathology in females and males: Current progress and future challenges. *Developmental Psychopathology, 15,* 719–742.

Felitti, V. (2009). Adverse childhood experiences and adult health [Editorial]. *Academic Pediatrics, 9,* 131–132.

Fernando, G. A., Miller, K. E., & Berger, D. E. (2010). Growing pains: The impact of disaster related and daily stressors on the psychological and psychosocial functioning of youth in Sri Lanka. *Child Development, 81,* 1192–1210.

Foster, D., Davies, S., & Steele, H. (2003). The evacuation of British children during World War II: A preliminary investigation into the long-term psychological effects. *Aging and Mental Health, 7,* 398–408.

Garrison, C. Z., Weinrich, M. W., Hardin, S. B., Weinrich, S., & Wang, L. (1993).

Post-traumatic stress disorder in adolescents after a hurricane. *American Journal of Epidemiology, 138,* 522–530.

Giannopoulou, I., Strouthos, M., Smith, P., Dikaiakou, A., Galanopoulou, V., & Yule, W. (2006). Post-traumatic stress reactions of children and adolescents exposed to the Athens 1999 earthquake. *European Psychiatry: The Journal of the Association of European Psychiatrists, 21,* 160–166.

Goenjian, A., Molina, L., Steinberg, A., Fairbanks, L., Alvarez, M., Goenjian, H., et al. (2001). Posttraumatic stress and depressive reactions among Nicaraguan adolescents after Hurricane Mitch. *American Journal of Psychiatry, 158,* 788–794.

Goenjian, A., Walling, D., Steinberg, A., Karayan, I., Najarian, L., & Pynoos, R. (2005). A prospective study of posttraumatic stress and depressive reactions among treated and untreated adolescents 5 years after a catastrophic disaster. *American Journal of Psychiatry, 162,* 2302–2308.

Hamada, R., Kameoka, V., Yanagida, E., & Chemtob, C. (2003). Assessment of elementary school children for disaster-related posttraumatic stress disorder symptoms: The Kauai recovery index. *Journal of Nervous and Mental Disease, 191,* 268–272.

John, P., Russell, S., & Russell, P. (2007). The prevalence of posttraumatic stress disorder among children and adolescents affected by tsunami disaster in Tamil Nadu. *Disaster Management and Response: An Official Publication of the Emergency Nurses Association, 5,* 3–7.

Kar, N., & Bastia, B. (2006). Post-traumatic stress disorder, depression and generalised anxiety disorder in adolescents after a natural disaster: A study of comorbidity. *Clinical Practice and Epidemiology in Mental Health, 26,* 17.

Kar, N., Mohapatra, P., Nayak, K., Pattanaik, P., Swain, S., & Kar, H. (2007). Posttraumatic stress disorder in children and adolescents one year after a supercyclone in Orissa, India: Exploring cross-cultural validity and vulnerability factors. *BMC Psychiatry, 14,* 8.

Kessler, R. C., Galea, S., Jones, R. T., & Parker, H. A. (2006). Mental illness and suicidality after Hurricane Katrina. *Bulletin of the World Health Organization, 84,* 930–939.

Kithakye, M., Morris, A. S., Terranova, A. M., & Myers, S. S. (2010). The Kenyan political conflict and children's adjustment. *Child Development, 81,* 1114–1128.

Klasen, F., Oettingen, G., Daniels, J., Post, M., Hoyer, C., & Adam, H. (2010). Posttraumatic resilience in former Ugandan child soldiers. *Child Development, 81,* 1096–1113.

Knabb, R., Rhome, J., & Brown, D. (2005). *Tropical Cyclone Report: Hurricane Katrina 23–30 August 2005.* Miami, FL: National Hurricane Center.

Kolaitis, G., Kotsopoulos, J., Tsiantis, J., Haritaki, S., Rigizou, F., Zacharaki, L., et al. (2003). Posttraumatic stress reactions among children following the Athens earthquake of September 1999. *European Child and Adolescent Psychiatry, 12,* 273–280.

Kronenberg, M. E., Hansel, T. C., Brennan, A. M., Lawrason, B., Osofsky, H. J., &

Osofsky, J. D. (2010). Children of Katrina: Lessons learned about post-disaster symptoms and recovery patterns. *Child Development, 81,* 1241–1259.

La Greca, A., Silverman, W., Vernberg, E., & Prinstein, M. (1996). Symptoms of posttraumatic stress in children after Hurricane Andrew: A prospective study. *Journal of Consulting and Clinical Psychology, 64,* 712–723.

Laor, N., Wolmer, L., Mayes, L. C., Gershon, A., Weizman, R., & Cohen, D. J. (1997). Israeli preschools under Scuds: A 30-month follow-up. *Journal of American Academy of Child and Adolescence Psychiatry, 36,* 349–356.

Layne, C. M., Beck, C. J., Rimmasch, H., Southwick, J. S., Moreno, M. A., & Hobfoll, S. E. (2009). Promoting "resilient" posttraumatic adjustment in childhood and beyond: "Unpacking" life events, adjustment trajectories, resources, and interventions. In D. Brom, R. Pat-Horenczyk, & J. Ford (Eds.), *Treating traumatized children: Risk, resilience, and recovery* (pp. 13–47). New York: Routledge.

Lieberman, A. F., & Van Horn, P. (2004). Assessment and treatment of young children exposed to traumatic events. In J. D. Osofsky (Ed.), *Young children and trauma: Interventions and treatment* (pp. 111–138). New York: Guilford Press.

Lieberman, A. F., & Van Horn, P. (2008). *Psychotherapy with infants and young children: Repairing the effects of stress and trauma on early attachment.* New York: Guilford Press.

Lonigan, C. J., Shannon, M. P., Taylor, C. M, Finch, A. J., Jr., & Sallee, F. (1994). Children exposed to disaster: II. Risk factors for the development of post-traumatic symptomatology. *Journal of the American Academy of Child and Adolescent Psychiatry, 33,* 94–105.

Marsee, M. A. (2008). Reactive aggression and posttraumatic stress in adolescents affected by Hurricane Katrina. *Journal of Clinical Child and Adolescent Psychiatry, 39,* 519–529.

Masten, A. S. (2007). Resilience in developing systems: Progress and promise as the fourth wave rises. *Development and Psychopathology, 19,* 921–930.

Masten, A. S. (in press). Risk and resilience in development. In P. D. Zelazo (Ed.), *Oxford handbook of developmental psychology.* New York: Oxford University Press.

Masten, A. S., & Obradović, J. (2008). Disaster preparation and recovery: Lessons from research on resilience in human development. *Ecology and Society, 13*(1), 9.

Masten, A. S., & Osofsky, J. D. (2010). Disasters and their impact on child development: Introduction to the Special Section. *Child Development, 81,* 1029–1039.

Neuner, F., Schauer, E., Catani, C., Ruf, M., & Elbert, T. (2006). Post-tsunami stress: A study of posttraumatic stress disorder in children living in three severely affected regions in Sri Lanka. *Journal of Traumatic Stress, 19,* 339–347.

O'Connor, E., & McCartney, K. (2007). Attachment and cognitive skills: An investigation of mediating mechanisms. *Journal of Applied Developmental Psychology, 28,* 458–476.

Osofsky, J. D. (Ed.). (2004). *Young children and trauma: Interventions and treatment.* New York: Guilford Press.

Osofsky, J. D., Osofsky, H. J., & Harris, W. W. (2007). Katrina's children: Social policy considerations for children in disasters. *Social Policy Report, 21*(1), 3–18.

Osofsky, H., Osofsky, J., Kronenberg, M., Brennan, A., & Hansel, T. (2009). Posttraumatic stress symptoms in children after Hurricane Katrina: Predicting the need for mental health services. *American Journal of Orthopsychiatry, 79,* 212–220.

Pfefferbaum, B. (1997). Posttraumatic stress disorder in children: A review of the past 10 years. *Journal of the American Academy of Child and Adolescent Psychiatry, 36,* 1503–1511.

Picou, J. S., & Gill, D. A. (1996). The *Exxon Valdez* oil spill and chronic psychological stress. *American Fisheries Society Symposium, 18,* 879–893.

Pine, D. S., Costello, J., & Masten, A. S. (2005). Trauma, proximity, and developmental psychopathology: The effects of war and terrorism on children. *Neuropsychopharmacology, 30,* 1781–1792.

Piyasil, V., Ketuman, P., Plubrukarn, R., Jotipanut, V., Tanprasert, S., Aowjinda, S., et al. (2007). Post traumatic stress disorder in children after tsunami disaster in Thailand: 2 years follow-up. *Journal of the Medical Association of Thailand, 90,* 2370–2376.

Pynoos, R. (1993). Traumatic stress and developmental psychopathology in children and adolescents. *American Psychiatric Press Review of Psychiatry, 12,* 205–238.

Pynoos, R., Goenjian, A., Tashjian, M., Karakashian, M., Manjikian, R., Manoukian, G., et al. (1993). Post-traumatic stress reactions in children after the 1988 Armenian earthquake. *British Journal of Psychiatry, 163,* 239–247.

Pynoos, R. S., Steinberg, A. M., & Goenjian, A. (1996). Traumatic stress in childhood and adolescence: Recent developments and current controversies. In B. A. van der Kolk, A. C. McFarlane, & L. Weisaeth (Eds.), *Traumatic stress: The effects of overwhelming experience on mind, body, and society* (pp. 331–358). New York: Guilford Press.

Pynoos, R., Steinberg, A., & Piacentini, J. (1999). A developmental psychopathology model of childhood traumatic stress and intersection with anxiety disorders. *Biological Psychiatry, 46,* 1542–1554.

Roussos, A., Goenjian, A., Steinberg, A., Sotiropoulou, C., Kakaki, M., Kabakos, C., et al. (2005). Posttraumatic stress and depressive reactions among children and adolescents after the 1999 earthquake in Ano Liosia, Greece. *American Journal of Psychiatry, 162,* 530–537.

Russoniello, C., Skalko, T., O'Brien, K., McGhee, S., Bingham-Alexander, D., & Beatley, J. (2002). Childhood posttraumatic stress disorder and efforts to cope after Hurricane Floyd. *Behavioral Medicine, 28,* 61–71.

Rydell, A. M., Bohlin, G., & Thorell, L. B. (2005). Representations of attachment to parents and shyness as predictors of children's relationships with teachers and peer competence in preschool. *Attachment and Human Development, 7,* 187–204.

Scheeringa, M. S., & Zeanah, C. H. (2008). Reconsideration of harm's way: Onsets and comorbidity patterns of disorders in preschool children and their caregivers following Hurricane Katrina. *Journal of Clinical Child and Adolescent Psychology, 37,* 508–518.

Shannon, M. P., Lonigan, C. J., Finch, A. J., Jr., & Taylor, C. M. (1994). Children exposed to disaster: I. Epidemiology of post-traumatic symptoms and symptom profiles. *Journal of the American Academy of Child and Adolescent Psychiatry, 33,* 80–93.

Shaw, J. (2000). Children, adolescents and trauma. *Psychiatric Quarterly, 71,* 227–243.

Spell, A. W., Kelley, M. L., Wang, J., Self-Brown, S., Davidson, K. L., Pellegrin, A., et al. (2008). The moderating effects of maternal psychopathology on children's adjustment post-Hurricane Katrina. *Journal of Clinical Child and Adolescent Psychology, 37,* 553–563.

Steinberg, A. M., Brymer, M. J., Decker, K. B., & Pynoos, R. S. (2004). The University of California at Los Angeles Post-traumatic Stress Disorder Reaction Index. *Current Psychiatry Reports, 6,* 96–100.

Terranova, A. M., Boxer, P., & Morris, A. S. (2009). Factors influencing the course of posttraumatic stress following a natural disaster: Children's reactions to Hurricane Katrina. *Journal of Applied Developmental Psychology, 30,* 344–355.

Thienkrua, W., Cardozo, B. L., Chakkraband, M. L., Guadamuz, T. E., Pengjuntr, W., & Tantipiwatanaskul, P. (for the Thailand Post-Tsunami Mental Health Study Group). (2006). Symptoms of posttraumatic stress disorder and depression among children in tsunami-affected areas in southern Thailand. *Journal of the American Medical Association, 296,* 549–559.

Tolin, D. F., & Foa, E. B. (2006). Sex differences in trauma and posttraumatic stress disorder: A quantitative review of 25 years of research. *Psychological Bulletin, 132,* 959–992.

Vogel, J. M., & Vernberg, E. M. (1993). Psychological responses of children to natural and human-made disasters: I. Children's psychological responses to disasters. *Journal of Clinical Child Psychology, 22,* 464–484.

Weems, C., Watts, S., Marsee, M., Taylor, L., Costa, N., Cannon, M., et al. (2007). The psychosocial impact of Hurricane Katrina: Contextual differences in psychological symptoms, social support, and discrimination. *Behaviour Research and Therapy, 45,* 2295–2306.

Weems, C., Taylor, L., Cannon, M., Marino, R., Romano, D., Scott, B., et al. (2009). Post traumatic stress, context, and the lingering effects of the Hurricane Katrina disaster among ethnic minority youth. *Journal of Abnormal Child Psychology, 38,* 49–56.

CHAPTER 16

■ ■ ■ ■

The Role of Pediatric Practitioners in Identifying and Responding to Traumatized Children

Betsy McAlister Groves
Marilyn Augustyn

For many parents, the pediatrician is the first—and often most trusted—professional to seek if their child has experienced an adverse event and if they are worried about the child's behavior. Thus, pediatric clinicians are on the front lines of learning about child or family traumatic experiences, and they serve as sentinels in the effort to provide early identification and intervention for childhood trauma. Because young children depend almost exclusively on their parents for emotional support and protection, many experts believe that an essential strategy for helping the young child affected by trauma is to help the parent by providing education, advocacy, and support. This chapter focuses on early childhood trauma and its common presentation in outpatient pediatric primary care settings. We make the case for early identification of childhood trauma as a powerful form of prevention. We consider the potential of pediatric health practitioners[1] to identify and respond to early childhood trauma, and the importance of mental health–pediatric collaboration in enabling these settings to better serve families with young children affected by traumatic stress. Finally, we

313

outline interventions and suggest implications for policy and program development.

Proponents of early identification and intervention point out that pediatric clinicians are perhaps the only professionals to see virtually all children at some point in the first 6 years of life. Sixty to seventy percent of school-age children visit pediatricians annually (Fairbrother, Stuber, Galea, Pfefferbaum, & Fleischman, 2004), and rates for children under age six are likely higher because of their required visit schedule. The pediatric health setting provides a critical opportunity for family screening of a number of social and health risks, including exposure to trauma. In addition, many primary care pediatricians serve as "de facto" mental health providers, especially those who practice in areas with a significant shortage of mental health resources. One study focusing on physician-identified psychosocial problems from 1979 to 1996 found a threefold increase in the numbers of children identified, with associated increases in the use of psychotropic medications, counseling, and referrals (Kelleher, McInerny, Gardner, Childs, & Wasserman, 2000). This increase became the focus of a policy statement from the American Academy of Pediatrics (AAP) in 2001, affirming its commitment to "prevention, early detection and management of behavioral, developmental and social problems as a focus of pediatric practice" (p. 1227). In addition in 2009, the AAP released a Policy Statement—The Future of Pediatrics: Mental Health Competencies for Pediatric Primary Care—proposed that there is a need for increased mental health competency among pediatric clinicians.

As recently as the mid-1980s, there was controversy in the child psychiatric literature about children's responses to traumatic stress—whether the responses are transient, or whether children are vulnerable to trauma in ways similar to adults, and whether, in fact, it is appropriate to diagnose a child with posttraumatic stress disorder (PTSD) (Benedek, 1985). It is now commonly accepted that all children—even very young children—can be affected by highly stressful events. Psychiatric research over the last two decades has enabled professionals to diagnose mental health disorders in children age 2 (Angold & Egger, 2007; Osofsky, 2004) or younger (Scheeringa, 2008; Scheeringa, Zeanah, Myers, & Putnam, 2005). Other studies have enumerated infant and toddler social–emotional problems and how these relate to overall child functioning (Briggs-Cowan, Carter, Skuban, & Horwitz, 2001). A study of 3,600 children in a pediatric primary care sample found that 21% of preschool-age children suffered from emotional disorders (Lavigne et al., 1993, 1996)—a rate that is similar to the prevalence in older children. In the recently released proposals for additional diagnoses in the fifth edition of the *Diagnostic and Statistical Manual of Mental Disorders* (DSM-V), a new diagnosis, "Posttraumatic stress disorder in preschool children," is included (American Psychological Association; see *www.dsm5.org/proposedrevisions/pages/proposedrevision.aspx?rid=396*). This proposal is the outcome of years of solid research on the impact of trauma on children under the age of 6, with now clear definitions of traumatic stressors, common symptoms, and resulting impairment to functioning in this age group.

Responding to the growing knowledge about the impact of early childhood trauma and the critical importance of the early years of a child's development, advocacy organizations have raised public awareness about the risks of trauma for young children.[2] A number of clinical intervention programs now identify and treat very young children who are affected by trauma. Federal funding has supported research and demonstration programs to develop effective components of intervention.[3]

DEFINITIONS

"Trauma" or "psychological trauma" is a broad term that potentially encompasses a wide range of events or occurrences. In general, traumatic events are described as those that are outside the range of normal stressors and of such magnitude as to be perceived as life threatening to self or others. Traumatic events evoke feelings of intense helplessness, fear, or horror in the child. The variable of perception is significant. A child's subjective experience of an event is as important as the objective characteristics of that event. What a young child perceives as life threatening may be quite different from what an adolescent or adult may perceive as dangerous. Because of the subjective nature of the child's appraisal of trauma, it is easier for adults to overlook the impact of a highly stressful event on a young child, assuming that it had little or no effect.

Early research to address the question of whether very young children can suffer from exposure to traumatic stress was carried out by Scheeringa and Zeanah in the mid-1990s. Their study of children under the age of 4 with significant histories of abuse and neglect found that young children's symptoms were similar to the symptoms displayed by older children diagnosed with PTSD, with some variations for developmental age and stage (Scheeringa & Zeanah, 1995). In 1994, a diagnosis of traumatic stress disorder for children under the age of 3 was proposed in a new publication, *Diagnostic Classification of Mental Health and Developmental Disorders of Infancy and Early Childhood* (Zero to Three/National Center for Clinical Infant Programs, 1994). Since then, many other studies have added to this growing body of knowledge about early childhood trauma. Among them are studies on the impact of war on preschoolers (Laor et al., 1997); the impact of dog bites treated in hospital emergency settings (Peters, Sottiaux, Appelboom, & Kahn, 2004), and the effects of motor vehicle accidents on this age group (Meiser-Stedman, Smith, Glucksman, Yule, & Dalgleish, 2007).

In the proposed DSM-V revisions to include the diagnosis of PTSD in preschool children, trauma is described as "death or threatened death, actual or threatened serious injury, or actual or threatened violation that the child was exposed to" in one or more of the following ways: experiencing the event, witnessing the event, or learning that the event happened to a close relative or friend. While there is not yet consensus about these criteria, this development has provided important official recognition of the impact of traumatic stress on very young children.

PREVALENCE OF YOUNG CHILDREN'S EXPOSURE TO TRAUMATIC STRESSORS

In a study of children ages 2–5, more than half (52.5%) had experienced a severe stressor in their lifetime (Egger & Angold, 2004). In a clinical sample of children receiving outpatient mental health treatment, 78% of children had experienced more than one trauma type and, on average, the initial trauma exposure occurred at age 5 (Cook, Blaustein, Spinazzola, & van der Kolk, 2003). Data from more than 10,000 cases of children receiving trauma-focused services from sites in the NCTSN reveal that in this cohort, one-fifth of children are ages 0–6. The traumas for which these children most often received services included exposure to domestic violence, sexual abuse, physical abuse, neglect, and traumatic loss/bereavement (National Child Traumatic Stress Network, 2009). Other common traumas include accidents, painful medical procedures, medical trauma, natural disasters, and war or political terrorism.

Direct victimization or exposure to violence within the home is the most frequently occurring traumatic stressor in children age 6 and younger. Victims ages 0–3 constituted 31.9% of all maltreatment victims reported to authorities in 2007 (*www.hhs.gov*). With regard to child fatalities, the youngest children were the most vulnerable. Children younger than 1 year old accounted for 44% of child fatalities, and 85% of child fatalities were younger than 6 years of age (National Clearinghouse on Child Abuse and Neglect Information, 2002). Forty percent of all child abuse victims were under the age of 6 (Children's Defense Fund, 2000).

A recent study found that approximately 15.5 million American children (ages 0–17) live in dual-parent families in which some form of intimate partner violence has occurred at least once in the previous year; this estimate represents almost 30% of the total number of children in the United States living in married or cohabiting opposite-sex households (McDonald, Jouriles, Ramisetty-Mikler, Caetano, & Green, 2006). Two studies highlight the high number of young children in families affected by domestic violence. One study that examined police data of domestic violence calls in five cities found that young children (age 5 years and under) were disproportionately represented in homes where there was domestic violence (Fantuzzo, Boruch, Beriama, Atkins, & Marcus, 1997). A second study reviewed restraining order data for the presence of children at the time of a threatened or actual assault, and found that 65% of children were 8 years old or younger (Massachusetts Department of Probation, 1995).

Several studies have reported on rates of children's exposure to community violence. In general, children who live in urban areas with high crime rates are at greater risk for exposure to violence in the community. However, as the spate of high-profile school shootings has made clear, no community is free from the risk of public violent incidents. A recent study by Finkelhor showed that exposure of children and adolescents to violence seems to have decreased between 2003 and 2008 (Finkelhor, Turner, Ormrod, & Hamby, 2010); nonetheless, both years showed high exposure rates among children and adolescents. For example, a clear majority (60.6%) of the children and youth in this nationally representative sample had experienced at least one direct or witnessed victimization in the previous year (Finkelhor, Turner, Ormrod, & Hamby, 2009). In a study of 6-year-old children in Baltimore, 54% witnessed some form of violence either in or outside the home (Schuler & Nair, 2001). A study of Head Start mothers in Los Angeles revealed that 71% had witnessed assaults and drug-related violence, and 65% had been direct victims of community violence. Their experiences were highly correlated with the reports of their children's direct exposure to these events (Farver, Xu, Eppe, Fernandez, & Schwartz, 2005). In another study of Head Start children, nearly two-thirds had either witnessed or been victimized by community violence, according to parent reports (Shahinfar, Fox, & Leavitt, 2000). A hospital-based study sampling families who used outpatient pediatric health services in an urban hospital serving low-income families focused on prevalence of exposure to violence in children age 6 and under, using reports from parents (Taylor, Harik, Zuckerman, & Groves, 1994). These researchers found that 10% of the children had witnessed a knifing or shooting by the age of 6; an additional 18% had witnessed "pushing, kicking, hitting or shoving"; parents reported that nearly half the violence their children had witnessed occurred in the home, and half in the community.

Studies of accidents in this young age group reveal that children ages 0–5 are hospitalized or die from drowning, burns, falls, choking, and poisoning more frequently than do children in any other age group (Grossman, 2000). Children are particularly vulnerable to burn injuries, in some studies accounting for almost 50% of all burn patients. A majority of pediatric burns are scald injuries usually affecting very young children below the age of 5 (Dissanaike & Rahimi, 2009).

THE IMPACT OF TRAUMA
ON CHILD HEALTH AND FUNCTIONING

Numerous studies have linked childhood traumatic stress with poor emotional and physical health outcomes in children, while making a case for the importance of early identification of traumatic stress. In a study of 20,000 children in North Carolina, researchers found that exposure to traumatic events was common, with more than two-thirds of children experiencing at least one event. Thirteen percent reported posttraumatic stress symptoms, and 1.4% met criteria for diagnosis of PTSD. However, other impairments—including school problems, emotional difficulties, and physical problems—occurred in more than 20% of children who had been traumatized. Posttraumatic stress symptoms were predicted by previous exposure to other traumatic events, anxiety disorders, and family adversity (Copeland, Keeler, Angold, & Costello, 2007). The Adverse Childhood Experiences Study of a sample of 17,000 members of the Kaiser Health Plan in California, has yielded a wealth of data about the associations between psychological stressors in childhood and later poor health outcomes for adults. Researchers in this study selected a history of child physical abuse, sexual abuse, and exposure to violence against the mother as three of seven risk factors to be investigated for their association with health problems in later life (Chapman, Dube, & Anda, 2007; Corso, Edwards, Fang, & Mercy, 2008; Felitti et al., 1998). Twenty-eight percent of respondents reported histories of child abuse; 20% had histories of child sexual abuse, and 12.5% of respondents reported childhood exposure to domestic violence. As the number of risk factors accumulated, the risk for the health and social–emotional problems also increased. Among the health problems listed are heart disease, depression, substance abuse, liver disease, smoking, and unintended pregnancies. Both studies highlight the cumulative risks of exposure to multiple traumatic events. Other studies have described the short-term health and mental health impact of exposure to trauma (Bair-Merritt, Blackstone, & Feudtner, 2006; Graham-Behrmann & Seng, 2005) and the impact on learning and school achievement (Hurt, Malmud, Brodsky, & Giannetta, 2001; Koenan, Moffitt, Caspi, Taylor, & Purcell, 2003).

A growing body of research documents the impact of trauma on early brain development and maturation of the central nervous system (Nemeroff et al., 2006; Perry, 1997; Shonkoff, Boyce, & McEwen, 2009; Shonkoff & Phillips, 2000; Spates, Waller, Samaraweera, & Plaisier, 2003; Teicher, 2000). Studies show that from the time of their birth, infants are affected by traumatic events in their environments. This research adds to the substantial body of knowledge about the impact of direct abuse on young children (Cicchetti & Toth, 1995; Helfer, Kempe, & Krugman, 1999) and the impact of exposure to domestic violence on children (Edleson, 1999; Fantuzzo &

Mohr, 1999; Groves, 2002; Kitzmann, Gaylord, Holt, & Kenny, 2003). In summary, both research and clinical findings indicate that age does not protect a child from the effects of trauma. The assumption that a young child will "forget" or that it may be better if the child does not talk about the trauma has been shown to be inaccurate. There is virtually no age at which a child is immune from the effects of trauma, either direct trauma or violence that is witnessed.

RECOGNIZING SYMPTOMS ASSOCIATED WITH TRAUMA IN YOUNG CHILDREN

A pediatric provider may be alerted to possible exposure to trauma or violence by the child's symptoms, particularly those associated with PTSD. In a retrospective chart review of children age 6 and under who were referred to an outpatient mental health program for children who witness violence, three symptoms were mentioned most frequently by parents: increased aggression, sleep difficulties, and increased separation anxiety (Groves, Acker, & Hennessey, 2002). The proposed DSM-V diagnosis of "posttraumatic stress disorder in preschool children," released in February 2010, describes these possible symptoms: recurrent, intrusive, distressing memories; dreams, physiological reminders of the event, dissociative reactions, and psychological distress at reminders of the traumatic event; avoidance of stimuli associated with the traumatic event; symptoms of arousal or irritability, including sleep difficulties, nightmares, night terrors, hypervigilance, exaggerated startle response, decreased concentration, and increased aggression (www. dsm5.org).

Studies have shown that some children may be more affected by traumatic stress than others. Variables such as age, temperament, gender, proximity to the traumatic event, and frequency of trauma exposure may affect children's responses (Pynoos et al., 1987). In addition, children's responses may be influenced by the response of the caregiver, and characteristics of the family and the community.

IDENTIFYING EARLY CHILDHOOD TRAUMA IN PEDIATRIC SETTINGS

Despite research findings that document the vulnerability of young children to traumatic experiences and public concern about violent behavior among children, there is scant information in the pediatric literature about identifying children's psychological trauma, with the notable exception of child abuse and domestic violence. Since the publication in 1963 of Henry

Kempe and colleagues' landmark study of abused children, public recognition, social policy, and medical practice have changed dramatically with regard to identifying and responding to children traumatized through abuse or neglect (Kempe, Silverman, Steele, Droegemueller, & Silver, 1963). Pediatric practitioners are mandated reporters and, in this role, may use a variety of screening tools, both formal and informal, to assess for child abuse. Many hospitals have multidisciplinary child protection teams, providing specialized consultation and education to providers about child sexual and physical abuse. Likewise, with the publication in 1998 of the AAP position statement entitled "The Role of the Pediatrician in Recognizing and Intervening on Behalf of Abused Women," the abuse of women was declared to be an important pediatric issue (Thackeray et al., 1998). The statement presented information about the impact of domestic violence on women and children, and the obstacles women face in disclosing that they are victims of domestic violence. One of the recommendations was that "pediatricians should attempt to recognize evidence of family or intimate partner violence in the office setting" (AAP, 1998, p. 1092). The statement made a strong case for recognizing domestic violence but did not offer specific guidelines for screening or provide discussion about the policy and practice dilemmas that arise when providers implement screening protocols for exposure to domestic violence. Since the publication of that article, there has been increased emphasis on screening for domestic violence in pediatric settings (Groves, Augustyn, Lee, & Sawires, 2002). Screening instruments for assessing the impact of accidents and medical trauma have also been developed and evaluated (Pynoos, Rodriguez, Steinberg, Stuber, & Fredericks, 1999; Saylor, Swenson, Reynolds, & Taylor, 1999; Winston, Kassam-Adams, Garcia-Espana, Ittenbach, & Cnaan, 2003). These measures generally are used in the emergency room setting and not validated for use with very young children. There are fewer options for assessing other areas of childhood traumatic stress, including exposure to community violence, traumatic loss of a family member, and exposure to war or terrorism.

BARRIERS TO SCREENING FOR PSYCHOLOGICAL TRAUMA IN PEDIATRIC SETTINGS

When asked about the challenges of identifying or managing early childhood trauma, pediatric clinicians enumerate both structural and personal barriers, which can be grouped into five categories:

1. Perhaps the most often mentioned barrier is that of time constraints. As providers face increasing demands to see large numbers of patients and additional expectations about what to cover as part of anticipatory guid-

ance, they may avoid topics that lead to lengthy discussion or extensive demands for follow-up. In an evaluation of customary practices in providing domestic violence screening, pediatricians were asked to fill out questionnaires about their screening practices (Erikson, Hill, & Siegel, 2001). Nearly 60% of respondents mentioned lack of time as a specific barrier.

2. A second barrier is inadequate training. In a study of general violence prevention counseling, Borowsky and Ireland (1999) found that 76% of pediatric residents and 83% of practitioners rated their training as inadequate in this area. A statewide mail survey of pediatricians focused specifically on their knowledge and practice in terms of identifying and assessing childhood traumatic experiences (Banh, Saxe, Mangione, & Horton, 2008). Pediatricians reported that less than 8% of their patients had psychological problems that might be related to traumatic exposures—a number below the prevalence data for childhood traumatic stress. Only 18% indicated that they had adequate knowledge of the subject.

3. A third barrier is a sense of powerlessness. Violence and traumatic experiences are not easy problems to address, nor do many patients want to talk about them. In addition to experiencing trauma, many families may present with other problems: low income, inadequate housing, and other health or mental health problems. Physicians are unlikely to be able to address any of these issues easily. In one study, for example, 42% of physicians expressed frustration that although they could intervene with advice or referral to resources, ultimately what was actually done was in the hands of the parent (Sugg & Inui, 1992). Another study found that a pediatrician's perceived self-efficacy in addressing psychosocial problems was associated with his or her willingness to bring up the issue (Cheng, DeWitt, Savageau, & O'Connor, 1999). For professionals who are expected to diagnose efficiently and treat problems, violence and trauma may represent a failure or a frustration that leaves them feeling powerless and unsuccessful.

4. A fourth barrier is concern that patients and families will be offended if asked personal questions about safety, relationships, mental health, or violent events at home. Providers worry that patients will feel singled out for this line of questioning, particularly with regard to screening for domestic violence, and resent it. However, a study by Siegel, Hill, Henderson, Ernst, and Boat (1999) showed that, rather than being offended, many women appreciated being asked the question about domestic violence, and revealed partner violence when screened in the pediatric office setting. Another study found that a 30-minute curriculum on domestic violence delivered to pediatric nurses significantly reduced their fear of offending patients (Johnson et al., 2009). Other studies have focused on pediatricians' comfort and skills in identifying mental health problems in their patients. One study found that pediatricians were more comfortable identifying maternal depression than

screening for mental health problems in children (Laraque et al., 2004). Another study found that in prevention visits, pediatric practitioners' choice of topics to assess depended on their level of confidence, and that psychosocial issues, in general, were perceived as less important (Cheng et al., 1999).

5. A fifth barrier is the presence of children in the room during screening and the related question of who the patient is. This is particularly true when a practitioner is inquiring about domestic violence. The parent is not the direct patient. Pediatric providers may feel uncomfortable inquiring about parental behavior. This concern may occur less often when they are asking about exposure to community or political violence, but providers also have mixed opinions about whether to ask these sensitive questions with children present. Some recommend interviewing the parent alone, without the partner or children (King & Strauss, 2000); however, this logistical challenge may be a significant barrier for the provider. There is strong agreement that a woman should not be screened for domestic violence if her partner is in the room. However, no systematic study has examined whether the presence of children in the exam room affects a provider's comfort in screening or the parent's comfort in talking. Zink (2000) examined this issue using interviews and focus groups with family physicians and pediatricians, and found that experts disagreed on the appropriateness of general screening for domestic violence in front of children older than age 2–3 years. The majority thought that general questions were appropriate, but in-depth questioning should be done in private.

GUIDELINES FOR IDENTIFYING TRAUMATIC STRESSORS IN YOUNG CHILDREN

Although there is not yet broad agreement about the optimal way of talking with families about traumatic stressors in the context of a pediatric visit, most experts agree that the topic is essential. In a recent report titled "Identifying, Treating, and Referring Traumatized Children: The Role of Pediatric Providers" (Cohen, Kelleher, & Mannarino, 2008), the authors discuss the importance of screening for traumatic stressors in pediatric settings and suggest direct inquiry with one question that is repeated at every visit with the child: "Since the last time I saw your child, has anything really scary or upsetting happened to your child or anyone in your family?"

Significant literature on screening for domestic violence in pediatric settings has included research on direct oral assessment, written questionnaires, and computer-based screening. Each method has strengths and weaknesses. The choice depends on the setting, the patient population, and provider preference or comfort level (Groves et al., 2002; Kimberg, 2001; Kissinger et al., 1999; Siegel et al., 2003; Thompson et al., 2000).

Several steps should be undertaken to prepare pediatric clinicians for including questions about traumatic stressors in their sessions with families:

1. *Examine personal biases and beliefs about children's exposure to violence or trauma.* Practitioners' comfort levels with questions about traumatic experiences may be affected by their history of similar experiences— either personally or within their families. In addition, practitioners may be biased in their assumptions about race, social class, neighborhood, or community in terms of who is more or less likely to encounter traumatic experiences. Such biases discourage universal inquiry of all families and may result in a failure to inquire about traumatic stressors in some situations.

2. *Learn how to talk with families about trauma and/or violence.* Training on the subject of trauma and practice with asking the questions build practitioner skills and self-confidence. If a practitioner feels comfortable with the questions, he or she is more likely to ask.

3. *Integrate assessment into routine history taking and into health maintenance for children.* Questions can be asked routinely in the course of taking the social history. Sample introductions might include "I have begun to ask all of the parents in my practice about their family life as it affects their health and safety, and that of their children. May I ask you a few questions?" or "Violence is an issue that affects everyone today, and so I have begun to ask all my families about their exposure to violence or other traumas. May I ask you a few questions?" Some questions can be asked of all parents at well-child visits:

- "Has your child ever witnessed a scary or unsafe event in the neighborhood or at home?"
- "Has your child ever been the victim of a violent incident?"
- "How do you resolve conflict with other adults in your home?"
- "Do you feel safe in your home and community?"
- "Have you been hurt or threatened by anyone since our last visit?"

In some practices, these questions are asked by a nurse assistant or a social worker; in others, they are asked by the physician or nurse practitioner. There is no evidence that one way is better than the other.

4. *Know the resources in the community.* In screening for domestic violence, the AAP recommends that pediatricians have a protocol or action plan that has been reviewed with local authorities on domestic violence. In cases where a woman acknowledges that she is a victim of domestic vio-

lence, appropriate follow-up should include further assessment for safety, referrals, and documentation. For exposure to other traumatic stressors, the clinician assesses safety and the severity of symptoms, and may decide to make a referral for behavioral health follow-up. Knowledge of appropriate referral resources is essential. In some settings, a social worker or other counselor provides brief assessments and makes follow-up referrals; in others, the pediatric provider must provide it.

5. *f you know or suspect that a child is being exposed to violence, schedule follow-up care.* One of the most important messages that pediatric providers may send to a family is that they recognize the child's trauma and want to be available to help as needed. Follow-up visits allow the clinician to monitor symptoms and check for follow-through with referrals.

DILEMMAS FOR PROVIDERS WHO SCREEN
FOR TRAUMA IN YOUNG CHILDREN

When pediatric practitioners screen families for trauma, they may face dilemmas about reporting suspected abuse of children or injuries of adult victims. Although laws in most states require medical reporting of specified injuries and wounds in adults, these laws are unlikely to apply in the pediatric setting when the health provider is treating the child. In the pediatric visit, in which the parent is not the patient and is not seeking treatment, the provider likely would have no legal obligation to report parent injuries or abuse detected during routine screening. In cases where a clinician learns of suspected direct abuse to the child, laws in each state require a report to the appropriate state agency. The question of making a report of suspected child abuse/neglect to child protection services in cases where a child has witnessed domestic violence (and has not been injured) is somewhat more complicated. State laws are less clear as to whether exposure to domestic violence in the absence of injury, or serious risk of injury, requires mandated reporting. The provider should be familiar with their state laws as they pertain to reporting on cases of domestic violence. In states that allow more discretion to the reporter, it becomes important for the provider to assess carefully whether the child has been abused, the potential for dangerousness in the home, whether the abuser has made direct threats to the child, and the capacity of the mother to keep the child safe. For a full discussion of the issues of reporting either suspected abuse of children or injuries of adult victims, consult the consensus guidelines published by the Family Violence Prevention Fund for responding to domestic violence in child and adolescent health settings (Groves et al., 2002).

Another dilemma that is unique to pediatric settings is the question of whether to ask the child directly about exposure to traumatic stress, and in the case of younger children, whether to ask these questions of the parent with the child in the room. This is usually not an issue for children under the age of 3. They are less likely to understand verbal content of questions, although they may be sensitive to the reactions, emotions, and mood of their caregivers. In visits with children between the ages of 3 and 12, the questions should be asked of the parent or adult caregiver who accompanies the child. Clinicians worry that these questions may be upsetting or confusing to the child, and/or that the parent will be reluctant to discuss these issues with the child in the room. It is ideal if these questions can be asked of the parent in private. However, in many practices, this is not possible. With older children in the room, the provider must be sensitive to the parent's cues. If the parent is uncomfortable, arrange for a follow-up telephone call or visit when it is possible to talk with the parent alone.

INTERVENTION IN THE PEDIATRIC SETTING

A young mother brought her 13-month-old daughter to the pediatrician because the child "was not eating enough." The pediatrician had known the mother and child since the child's birth. Upon examination, the child was found to be of normal weight and had not lost weight since the last visit. As the pediatrician inquired about the immediate history of the mother's concerns about her child's appetite, the mother stated that she had been worried for the past 2 weeks. When asked about any stresses or particular events that may have affected the child, the mother began to cry and confided that she and her husband had just separated. Noting that the mother was upset, the pediatrician asked if he could call the mother at a convenient time to talk further about this. The doctor was concerned that the mother's emotional state might upset the child.

In a phone call later that day, the physician asked about the circumstances of the separation. The mother replied that there had been increasing tension between them, and that her husband drank heavily. "Do you have any worries about your safety?" the pediatrician inquired. The mother replied that the reason for the separation was that her husband had hit her in front of her daughter. The assault resulted in a cut and bruises on her face. She called the police, who responded and arrested the father. She had since sought a restraining order and filed for separation. She said that she had told no one other than her immediate family because she was ashamed that this had happened to her.

The pediatrician asked several detailed questions about what the child had witnessed, and what her responses had been. The child had been playing in the room when the parents began to argue and was exposed to the increasingly heated argument and the assault. The child began to scream during the altercation. The father left the home once the police were summoned, and the child did not see the arrest. The mother reported that she had blood on her face, which was quite upsetting to the child. She cleaned it up immediately and declined medical assistance offered by the police.

In addition to the concern about eating, the mother also reported that her daughter was waking at night screaming, and that it was difficult to get her back to sleep. The child also experienced intense distress when separated from her mother, even if her mother was in the next room. The mother reported that all of these symptoms began after the violent incident.

The pediatrician explained to the mother that these symptoms were common responses of young children to extremely frightening events. Although the mother assumed the symptoms were associated with the assault and the stresses of the separation, she was nonetheless reassured that these were not unusual responses, and that her doctor was familiar with them. He asked about her immediate concerns, particularly who was supporting her, and offered to refer her to the local domestic violence service agency. He reminded the mother that her emotional well-being was key to her daughter's sense of safety and reassurance. He found out that her sister was staying with them temporarily and that her family, which lived nearby, was providing assistance. He also reassured the mother that her daughter's appetite and eating habits would likely return to normal with the passage of time, particularly if the child felt that her environment had stabilized. The pediatrician discussed with the mother some specific ideas for supporting her daughter: trying to minimize prolonged separations from her and leaving a nightlight on in the child's bedroom to help with sleep (a suggestion the mother made). He scheduled a follow-up visit for 2 weeks. At the follow-up visit, the child was eating normally again and was more comfortable separating from her mother. She still had sleep difficulties, although they were less frequent.

In this case, the pediatrician identified a significant traumatic stressor and provided supportive and sensitive intervention to the parent. His inquiry about safety provided the opportunity for the mother to share a difficult and personal experience. Taking a careful history of the specifics of exposure to violence yielded important information about what the child had experienced. The doctor gave concrete information about the child's symptoms that reassured the mother. He reminded the mother that her emotional support was essential; he made sure that she had supports for herself and offered additional resources. He provided follow-up for the family.

This intervention provided early identification of the problem and a sensitive response that likely assisted this mother in feeling less stressed about the situation and better able to be attuned to her child's emotional needs.

Summarizing from the preceding case, the pediatrician's intervention has four components: assessing the child's and the parent's response to the trauma; assessing for child and family safety; providing developmental guidance and education; and making referrals and/or follow-up plans, if necessary.

1. *Assessing the child's and the parent's response to the trauma.* Basic information about the traumatic event should be obtained, including the severity and the chronicity of the stressor. It is not advisable or necessary to obtain more details, especially if the child is in the room, or if the parent is obviously upset. The clinician should ask about symptoms the child is experiencing—the intensity and duration of these symptoms, and the extent to which the child's daily functioning is impaired. The clinician should also assess the parent's reactions to the trauma. The child's response is closely linked to the parental reaction. In some instances, specialized intervention with the child may be indicated; however, the first focus of the pediatric provider should be the parent, since this is often the gateway to child intervention.

2. *Assessing for child and family safety.* The clinician should assess the immediate safety of the child and family. If the child is unsafe, this may require a report to Child Protective Services. In cases of domestic violence in which a parent is not safe, a referral to a domestic violence program might be helpful.

3. *Providing developmental guidance and education.* Pediatric providers play a vital role in providing education and anticipatory guidance to all parents about the vulnerability of infants and young children to traumatic experiences and about common responses to traumatic stress. Pediatricians can educate parents about the sensitivity of infants and young children to adults' emotional states, and also provide active support to parents. They can provide specific information about the importance of parents being able to maintain a secure and predictable routine as a way to help reduce children's anxieties and worries. The primary goal of this guidance is to stabilize the environment for the family and to support the parent's ability to provide consistent emotional support to the child. Education includes giving parents specific information about how trauma may affect young children, including a review of the common symptoms and assistance in managing specific behaviors. This can be reassuring to parents who may be alarmed by the change in behaviors that they observe in the child. Assuring parents that

symptoms associated with trauma are normal reactions to abnormal events is important.

4. *Making follow-up plans and/or referrals.* Referrals for the child and/or the parent for concrete services may be necessary. If parents need specific referrals for legal advocacy, immigration assistance, or domestic violence services, the provider should make the appropriate referrals.

REFERRALS FOR SPECIALIZED
BEHAVIORAL HEALTH SERVICES

The pediatric provider may consider referring a young child for additional mental health services in the following instances:

1. If the symptoms have lasted for longer than 1 month and are interfering substantially in the child's life/functioning.
2. If the parent is traumatized or otherwise compromised in his or her ability to respond to the child.
3. If the trauma involves the loss of a parent or significant caretaker.

There are a growing number of evidence-based therapeutic interventions for young children affected by trauma. On its website, the NCTSN lists several interventions designed and evaluated for children age 6 or younger. Mental health clinicians who are trained to use these interventions understand the developmental issues of young children, and many are experienced in working with traumatized children.

IMPLICATIONS FOR POLICY,
TRAINING, AND PROGRAM DEVELOPMENT

In this chapter we have made a case for using pediatric health settings to screen young children for trauma and have proposed guidelines to assist health providers in doing so. Both the prevalence of trauma exposure in children and the potential adverse outcomes for children lend urgency to the task of identifying children who are at risk. A comprehensive approach to identifying early childhood trauma yields important information about the extent of the problem and may fill other important gaps in the data on this topic.

At the same time, it must be recognized that systematic inquiry would also create a greater demand for services. Resources for children's mental health, especially for very young children, are woefully lacking in most states. Increased screening would further strain a fragile and inadequate system. In addition, it is likely that a greater burden would be placed on child protection systems because more children would be discovered to be at risk for abuse or neglect. As we learn more about the nature and extent of trauma in very young children, we must use that knowledge to advocate vigorously for increased services.

Finally, the ultimate success of screening depends on adequate training and education of medical providers. Pediatric providers must acquire basic knowledge about risks to early child development, as well as learn the symptoms and characteristics of trauma in children. In addition, they must acquire specific skills in talking with families about these issues. This goal is articulated by the new policy statement from the AAP (2009), advocating for increased competency in mental health. Greater efforts to provide training and support to increase competency around childhood traumatic stress would enable providers to acquire skills in interviewing and in accessing community resources to support families. Such education requires skilled teaching and a solid commitment from the medical education system.

The rewards for building capacity for early identification of children affected by trauma are potentially significant: Early identification can lead to early intervention and, we hope, to a reduction in the adverse consequences for children living with chronic violence. Screening for exposure to trauma in pediatric and family health settings is a component of quality health care that we can no longer afford to neglect.

NOTES

1. For this chapter, the term "pediatric health practitioners" includes doctors, physician's assistants, nurse practitioners, nurses, and others who work directly with families in a pediatric setting.
2. The National Scientific Council on the Developing Child and Zero to Three (*zerotothree.org*) are two examples of organizations whose websites and online publications include extensive information on early childhood trauma.
3. The U.S. Substance Abuse and Mental Health Services Administration funds the National Child Traumatic Stress Network (NCTSN), a collaboration of over 100 sites that develop and disseminate evidence-based interventions and provide direct clinical services to children who are affected by trauma. The Early Trauma Treatment Network within the NCTSN is a collaboration of four centers that provide mental health treatment to young children affected by violence. The four sites include the Child Trauma Research Project at the University of California/ San Francisco General Hospital, the Child Violence Exposure Program at Louisiana State University Health Science Center, the Child Witness to Violence Project

at Boston Medical Center; and the Jefferson Parish Human Services Authority Infant Team/Tulane University. Another well-established federal program is the Safe Start Initiative, sponsored by the Department of Justice/Office of Juvenile Justice and Delinquency Programs. This initiative focuses on children exposed to violence, promoting systems collaboration on behalf of these children and creating new services.

REFERENCES

American Academy of Pediatrics (Committee on Child Abuse and Neglect). (1998). The role of the pediatrician in recognizing and intervening on behalf of abused women. *Pediatrics, 101*(6), 1091–1092.

American Academy of Pediatrics (Committee on Psychosocial Aspects of Child and Family Health). (2001). The new morbidity revisited: A renewed commitment to the psychosocial aspects of pediatric care. *Pediatrics, 108,* 1227–1230.

American Academy of Pediatrics (Committee on Psychosocial Aspects of Child and Family Health). (2009). The future of pediatrics: Mental health competencies for pediatric primary care. *Pediatrics, 124*(1), 410–422.

Angold, A., & Egger, H. (2007). Preschool psychopathology: Lessons for the lifespan. *Journal of Child Psychology and Psychiatry, 48*(10), 961–966.

Bair-Merritt, M., Blackstone, M., & Feudtner, C. (2006). Physical health outcomes of childhood exposure to intimate partner violence: A systematic review. *Pediatrics, 117*(2), e278–e290.

Banh, M., Saxe, G., Mangione, T., & Horton, N. (2008). Physician-reported practice of managing childhood posttraumatic stress in pediatric primary care. *General Hospital Psychiatry, 30,* 536–545.

Benedek, E. (1985). Children and psychic trauma. In S. Eth & R. S. Pynoos (Eds.), *Posttraumatic stress disorders in children* (pp. 3–16). Washington, DC: American Psychiatric Press.

Borowsky, I. W., & Ireland, M. (1999). National survey of pediatricians' violence prevention counseling. *Archives of Pediatric and Adolescent Medicine, 153,* 1170–1176.

Briggs-Cowan, M., Carter, A., Skuban, E., & Horwitz, S. (2001). Prevalence of social–emotional and behavioral problems in a community sample of 1- and 2-year-old children. *Journal of the American Academy of Child Adolescent Psychiatry, 40*(7), 811–819.

Chapman, D. P., Dube, S. R., & Anda, R. F. (2007). Adverse childhood events as risk factors for negative mental health outcomes. *Psychiatric Annals, 37*(5), 359–364.

Cheng, T., DeWitt, T., Savageau, J., & O'Connor, K. (1999). Determinants of counseling in primary care pediatric practice. *Archives of Pediatrics and Adolescent Medicine, 153*(6), 629–635.

Children's Defense Fund. (2000). Child abuse and neglect. Washington, DC: Author. Retrieved May 19, 2003, from *www.childrensdefense.org/ss_chabuse_fs.php.*

Cicchetti, D., & Toth, S. L. (1995). A developmental psychology perspective on child abuse and neglect. *Journal of the American Academy of Child and Adolescent Psychiatry, 34*(5), 541–565.

Cohen, J. A., Kelleher, K. J., Mannarino, A. P. (2008). Identifying, treating, and referring traumatized children: The role of pediatric providers, *Archives of Pediatric and Adolescent Medicine, 162*(5), 447–452.

Cook, A., Blaustein, M., Spinazzola, J., & van der Kolk, B. (2003). Complex trauma in children and adolescents. Retrieved March 27, 2010, from *nctsn.org/nctsn_ assets/pdfs/edu_materials/complextrauma_all.pdf.*

Copeland, W., Keeler, G., Angold, A., & Costello, E. (2007). Traumatic events and posttraumatic stress in childhood. *Archives of General Psychiatry, 64*(5), 577–584.

Corso, P. S., Edwards, V. J., Fang, X., & Mercy, J. A. (2008). Health-related quality of life among adults who experienced maltreatment during childhood. *American Journal of Public Health, 98,* 1094–1100.

Dissanaike, S., & Rahimi, M. (2009). Epidemiology of burn injuries: Highlighting cultural and socio-demographic aspects. *Internal Review of Psychiatry, 21*(6), 505–511.

Edleson, J. (1999). Children's witnessing of adult domestic violence. *Journal of Interpersonal Violence, 14*(8), 839–870.

Egger, E. L., & Angold, A. (2004, October). *Stressful life events and pre-school age psychiatric assessment: Version 1.1.* Paper presented at the annual meeting of the American Academy of Child and Adolescent Psychiatry, Washington, DC.

Erikson, M. J., Hill, T. D., & Siegel, R. M. (2001). Barriers to domestic violence screening in the pediatric setting. *Pediatrics, 108*(1), 98–102.

Fairbrother, G., Stuber, J., Galea, S., Pfefferbaum, B., & Fleischman, A. R. (2004). Unmet need for counseling services by children in New York City after the September 11th attacks on the World Trade Center: Implications for pediatricians. *Journal of Pediatrics, 113*(5), 1367–1374.

Fantuzzo, J., Boruch, R., Beriama, A., Atkins, M., & Marcus, S. (1997). Domestic violence and children: Prevalence and risk in five major U.S. cities. *Journal of the American Academy of Child and Adolescent Psychiatry, 36*(1), 116–122.

Fantuzzo, J. W., & Mohr, W. K. (1999). Prevalence and effects of child exposure to domestic violence. *The Future of Children, 9*(3), 21–32.

Farver, J. A., Xu, L. X., Eppe, S., Fernandez, A., & Schwartz, D. (2005). Community violence, family conflict and pre-schoolers' social–emotional functioning. *Developmental Psychology, 41,* 160–170.

Felitti, V. J., Anda, R. F., Nordenberg, D., Williamson, D. F., Spitz, A. M., Edwards, et al. (1998). Relationship of childhood abuse and household dysfunction to many of the leading causes of death in adults. *American Journal of Preventive Medicine, 14*(4), 245–258.

Finkelhor, D., Turner, H., Ormrod, R., & Hamby, S. (2009). Violence, abuse and crime exposure in a national sample of children and youth. *Journal of Pediatrics, 124*(5), 1411–1423.

Finkelhor, D., Turner, H., Ormrod, R., & Hamby, S. L. (2010). Trends in childhood violence and abuse exposure: Evidence from two national surveys. *Archives of Pediatrics and Adolescent Medicine, 164*(3), 238–242.

Graham-Bermann, S., & Seng, J. (2005). Violence exposure and traumatic stress symptoms as additional predictors of health problems in high risk children. *Pediatrics, 146*(3), 349–354.

Grossman, D. C. (2000). The history of injury control and the epidemiology of child and adolescent injuries. *The Future of Children, 10*(1), 4–22.

Groves, B. M. (1995). Witness to violence. In S. Parker & B. Zuckerman (Eds.), *Behavioral and developmental pediatrics: A handbook for primary care* (pp. 334–336). Boston: Little, Brown.

Groves, B. M. (2002). *Children who see too much: Lessons from the Child Witness to Violence Project.* Boston: Beacon Press.

Groves, B. M., Acker, M., & Hennessey, C. (2002, August). *Profiles of the youngest referrals to the Child Witness to Violence Project.* Paper presented at the International Family Violence Conference, Durham, NH.

Groves, B. M., Augustyn, M., Lee, D., & Sawires, P. (2002). *Identifying and responding to domestic violence: Consensus recommendations for child and adolescent health.* San Francisco: Family Violence Prevention Fund.

Helfer, M. E., Kempe, R. S., & Krugman, R. E. (Eds.). (1999). *The battered child.* Chicago: University of Chicago Press.

Hurt, H., Malmud, E., Brodsky, N., & Giannetta, J. (2001). Exposure to violence: Psychological and academic correlates in child witnesses. *Archives of Pediatric and Adolescent Medicine, 155,* 1351–1356.

Johnson, N. L., Klingbeil, C., Melzer-Lange, M., Humphreys, C., Scanlon, M. C., & Simpson, P. (2009). Evaluation of an intimate partner violence curriculum in a pediatric hospital. *Pediatrics, 123,* 562–568.

Kelleher, K., McInerny, T., Gardner, W., Childs, G., & Wasserman, R. (2000). Increasing identification of psychosocial problems: 1979–1996. *Pediatrics, 105*(6), 1313–1321.

Kempe, C. H., Silverman, F. N., Steele, B. F., Droegemueller, W., & Silver, H. K. (1963). The battered child syndrome. *Journal of the American Medical Association, 181,* 17–24.

Kimberg, L. (2001). Addressing intimate partner violence in primary care practice. *Medscape Women's Health eJournal, 6*(1). Retrieved May 19, 2003, from *www. medscape.com/viewarticle/408937.*

King, H. S., & Strauss, M. (2000). *Routine screening for domestic violence in pediatric practice.* Newton, MA: Newton Wellesley Hospital.

Kissinger, P., Rice, J., Farley, T., Trim, S., Jewitt, K., Margavio, V., et al. (1999). Application of computer-assisted interviews to sexual behavior research. *American Journal of Epidemiology, 149,* 950–954.

Kitzmann, K. M., Gaylord, N. K., Holt, A. R., & Kenny, E. D. (2003). Child witnessing to domestic violence: A meta-analytic review. *Journal of Consulting and Clinical Psychology, 71*(2), 339–352.

Koenan, K. C., Moffitt, T. E., Caspi, A., Taylor, A., & Purcell, S. (2003). Domestic violence is associated with environmental suppression of IQ in young children. *Developmental Psychopathology, 15,* 297–311.

Laor, N., Wolmer, L., Mayes, L., Gershon, A., Weizman, R., & Cohen, D. (1997). Israeli preschool children under scuds: A 30-month follow-up. *American Academy of Child Adolescent Psychiatry, 36*(3), 349–356.

Laraque, D., Boscarino, J., Battista, A., Fleischman, A., Casalino, M., Hu, Y., et al.

(2004). Reactions and needs of tristate-area pediatricians after the events of September 11: Implications for children's mental health services. *Journal of Pediatrics, 113*(5), 1357–1374.

Lavigne, J., Binns, H., Cristoffel, K., Rosenbaur, D., Arend, R., Smith, K., et al. (1993). Behavioral and emotional problems among preschool children in pediatric primary care: Prevalence and pediatricians' recognition. *Journal of Pediatrics, 91*(3), 649–655.

Lavigne, J., Gibbons, R., Christoffel, K., Arend, R., Rosenbaum, D., Binns, H., et al. (1996). Prevalence rates and correlates of psychiatric disorders. *Journal of American Academy of Child Adolescent Psychiatry, 35*(2), 204–214.

Massachusetts Department of Probation. (1995). *The tragedies of domestic violence: A qualitative analysis of civil restraining orders in Massachusetts.* Boston: Office of the Commissioner of Probation.

McDonald, R., Jouriles, E. N., Ramisetty-Mikler, S., Caetano, R., & Green, C. E. (2006). Estimating the number of American children living with partner-violent families. *Journal of Family Psychology, 20*(1), 137–142

Meiser-Stedman, R., Smith, P., Glucksman, E., Yule, W., & Dalgleish, T. (2007). Parent and child agreement for acute stress disorder, post-traumatic stress disorder and other psychopathology in a prospective study of children and adolescents exposed to single-event trauma. *Journal of Abnormal Child Psychology, 35,* 191–201.

National Child Traumatic Stress Network. (2009). [Core data set]. Unpublished data, Durham, NC.

National Clearinghouse on Child Abuse and Neglect Information. (2002). National Child Abuse and Neglect Data System (NCANDS) summary of key findings from calendar year 2000. Retrieved May 19, 2003, from *www. calib.com/nccanch/pubs/factsheets/canstats.cfm.*

Nemeroff, C. B., Bremner, J. D., Foa, E. B., Mayberg, H. S., North, C. S., & Stein, M. B. (2006). PTSD: A state of the science review. *Journal of Psychiatric Research, 40*(1), 1–21.

Osofsky, J. D. (Ed.). (2004). *Young children and trauma: Intervention and treatment.* New York: Guilford Press.

Perry, B. D. (1997). Incubated in terror: Neurodevelopmental factors in the "cycle of violence." In J. D. Osofsky (Ed.), *Children in a violent society* (pp. 124–149). New York: Guilford Press.

Peters, V., Sottiaux, M., Appelboom, J., & Kahn, A. (2004). Posttraumatic stress disorder after dog bites in children. *Journal of Pediatrics, 144,* 121–122.

Pynoos, R. S., Frederick, C., Nader, K., Arroyo, W., Steinberg, A., Eth, S., et al. (1987). Life threat and posttraumatic stress in school-age children. *Archives of General Psychiatry, 44,* 1057–1063.

Pynoos, R. S., Rodriguez, N., Steinberg, A. M., Stuber, M., & Fredericks, C. (1999). *PTSD Reaction Index—Revised.* Unpublished psychological test, Trauma Psychiatry Service, University of California, Los Angeles.

Saylor, C. F., Swenson, C. C., Reynolds, S. S., & Taylor, M. (1999). The Pediatric Emotional Distress Scale: A brief screening measure for young children exposed to traumatic events. *Journal of Child Psychology, 28*(1), 70–81.

Shahinfar, A., Fox, N. A., & Leavitt, L. A. (2000). Preschool children's exposure to violence: Relation of behavior problems to parent and child reports. *American Journal of Orthopsychiatry, 70*(1), 115–125.

Scheeringa, M. (2008). Developmental considerations for diagnosing PTSD and acute stress disorder in preschool and school-age children. *American Journal of Psychiatry, 29*(4), 1237–1239.

Scheeringa, M., Zeanah, C., Myers, L., & Putnam, F. (2005). Predictive validity in a prospective follow-up of PTSD in pre-school children. *Journal of the American Academy of Child and Adolescent Psychiatry, 44*, 899–906.

Scheeringa, M. S., & Zeanah, C. (1995). Symptom expression and trauma variables in children under 48 months of age. *Infant Mental Health Journal, 16*, 259–270.

Schuler, M. E., & Nair, P. (2001). Witnessing violence among inner-city children of substance-abusing and non-substance-abusing women. *Archives of Pediatrics and Adolescent Medicine, 155*, 342–346.

Shonkoff, J. P., Boyce, W. T., & McEwen, B. S. (2009). Neuroscience, molecular biology, and the childhood roots of health disparities: Building a new framework for health promotion and disease prevention. *Journal of the American Medical Association, 301*(21), 2252–2259.

Shonkoff, J. P., & Phillips, D. A. (Eds.). (2000). *From neurons to neighborhoods: The science of early childhood development.* Washington, DC: National Academy Press.

Siegel, R. M., Hill, T. D., Henderson, V. A., Ernst, H. M., & Boat, B. W. (1999). Screening for domestic violence in the community pediatric setting. *Pediatrics, 104*(4), 874–877.

Siegel, R. M., Joseph, E. C., Routh, S. A., Mendel, S. G., Jones, E., Ramesh, R. B., et al. (2003). Screening for domestic violence in the pediatric office: A multipractice experience. *Clinical Pediatrics, 42*(7), 599–602.

Spates, C. R., Waller, S., Samaraweera, N., & Plaisier, B. (2003). Behavioral aspects of trauma in children and youth. *Pediatric Clinics of North America, 50*(4), 901–918.

Sugg, N. K., & Inui, T. (1992). Primary care physicians' response to domestic violence: Opening Pandora's box. *Journal of the American Medical Association, 267*, 3157–3160.

Taylor, L., Harik, V., Zuckerman, B., & Groves, B. (1994). Exposure to violence among inner-city children. *Developmental and Behavioral Pediatrics, 15*, 120–123.

Teicher, M. (2000). Wounds that won't heal: The neurobiology of child abuse. *Cerebrum: The Dana Forum on Brain Science, 2*(4), 50–67.

Thackeray, J. F., Hibbard, R., & Dowd, M. D., the Committee on Child Abuse and Neglect, and the Committee on Injury, Violence, and Poison Prevention. (2010). Intimate partner violence: The role of the pediatrician, *Pediatrics, 125*, 1094–1100.

Thompson, R. S., Rivera, F. P., Thompson, D. C., Barlow, W. E., Sugg, N. K., Maiuro, R. D., et al. (2000). Identification and management of domestic violence: A randomized trial. *American Journal of Preventive Medicine, 19*(4), 253–263.

Winston, F. K., Kassam-Adams, N., Garcia-Espana, F., Ittenbach, R., & Cnaan, A. (2003). Screening for risk of persistent posttraumatic stress in injured children and their parents. *Journal of the American Medical Association, 290*(5), 643–649.

Zero to Three/National Center for Clinical Infant Programs. (1994). *Diagnostic classification of mental health and developmental disorders of infancy and early childhood.* Arlington, VA: Zero to Three Press.

Zink, T. (2000). Should children be in the room when the mother is screened for partner violence? *Journal of Family Practice, 49*(2), 130–136.

CHAPTER 17

■ ■ ■ ■

Vicarious Traumatization and the Need for Self-Care in Working with Traumatized Young Children

Joy D. Osofsky

In this book, the issue of vicarious traumatization or compassion fatigue for individuals who work with traumatized young children and their families, including mental health evaluators and therapists, judges, lawyers, child welfare professionals, first responders, and all other adults, has not been discussed directly. However, working with traumatized young children can take its toll because it often is very difficult to witness hardship and human suffering, and at the same time, as professionals, be required to maintain boundaries and professional roles, to make decisions about children's lives, and to take actions to help vulnerable young children and their families. Individuals find different ways of coping with these difficult feelings—some may just avoid thinking about it. In this chapter, the issues of vicarious trauma and compassion fatigue are defined and discussed, examples from different disciplines are presented, and suggestions that are offered relate to individual and professional strategies for prevention and intervention, including the importance of self-care.

HOW TO UNDERSTAND VICARIOUS
TRAUMATIZATION AND COMPASSION FATIGUE

Vicarious traumatization (VT) or compassion fatigue (CF), also called secondary trauma, refers to the cumulative effect of working with survivors of traumatic life events, or perpetrators, as part of everyday work. Figley (1996) and Pearlman and Saakvitne (1995) emphasize that people who engage empathically with victims or survivors are particularly vulnerable. They also discuss risk factors for VT or CF (Figley, 1995), which include measuring one's self-worth by how much one helps others, having unrealistic expectations of oneself and others, being self-critical and a perfectionist, fear of being judged by others if one shows "weakness" (e.g., seeking help or expressing one's feelings), being unable to give or receive emotional support, overextending oneself, and letting work bleed over into one's personal time. Secondary traumatic stress (STS) reactions were studied in health care providers, journalists, attorneys, first responders, supportive services, military personnel, volunteers, and media personnel by Figley (2002), and in judges by Jaffee, Crooks, Dunford-Jackson, and Town (2003). In some settings, due to the nature and organization of the work, prevention, intervention, and coping strategies are included as part of the work environment to support and help those who may be impacted. Support may at times just be an opportunity to debrief after dealing with a traumatic situation or event. However, in many work settings, especially those with heavy caseloads and a culture of not talking about issues, VT or CF is neither admitted nor dealt with for several reasons. One problem is that many professionals are not used to talking about emotions and issues that can impact their performance. For some, talking about the daily work impacting a professional in a personal and emotional way may be perceived as a sign of weakness. Within the legal profession or among first responders, the issue of VT or CF is rarely discussed; in most settings, prevention or intervention strategies related to "psychological reactions" are not considered a part of the culture. Individuals find their own ways to cope and adjust, and if their coping strategies are maladaptive, leading to irritability, impulsiveness, insensitivity, or arbitrariness in their work, they may leave the job. At times, individuals may also be asked to leave, if their performance suffers because the situation is too stressful.

VICARIOUS TRAUMATIZATION FOR INDIVIDUALS
WORKING WITH TRAUMATIZED YOUNG CHILDREN

Issues in Juvenile Court from Multidisciplinary Perspectives

In April 2010, I attended a meeting of multidisciplinary professionals working with juvenile court systems, including judges, lawyers, and mental health professionals; and child welfare, early intervention, and child care professionals. In preparation for a presentation on VT and CF, I asked the group to fill out the Professional Quality of Life Scale assessing compassion satisfaction and CF (Stamm, 2009). The results were both interesting and informative. This group of dedicated professionals working with juvenile courts reported many positive feelings about their jobs and the work that they do. The majority reported being caring people, liking and getting satisfaction from their work, very much wanting to help other people, and being pleased that they chose to do this work. They also stated that they often feel very successful as helpers, believing they can make a difference in people's lives. However, many also reported negative feelings, including being "bogged down" by the system, overwhelmed at times by the work, and sometimes feeling worn out because of their work as a helper. A small percentage reported that it is difficult at times to separate one's personal life from one's life as a helper and feeling impacted by the traumatic stress of others. Some reported even experiencing the trauma of someone they helped. Almost half of the respondents reported sometimes feeling "on edge." The majority reported that their beliefs helped sustain them in work that, for many, appeared to be a strong protective factor. Unfortunately, for those who work with traumatized young children and families, the personal impact is not often taken into account, and the importance of providing a supportive environment to sustain both individuals and systems doing this work is crucial.

Across multidisciplinary groups, several identified areas and topics are helpful for all professional and support groups dealing with traumatized young children. All groups agreed that they could benefit from learning about developmental issues and ways to understand the effects of trauma on children of different ages, and "red flags" to identify children who may have been traumatized. Several groups have expressed interest in learning about the effects of trauma on children over time. It would be helpful to have training videos and cross-disciplinary training for judges, lawyers, mental health professionals, and child welfare workers. All agreed that learning more about evidence-based evaluations, practice, and services that support young traumatized children and their families would be helpful. These groups also suggested that it is important to learn about protective factors, risk, and resilience (Masten, 2001, in press). Finally, related to the focus of this chapter, they expressed interest in learning more about VT and CF, as well as both personal and institutional prevention and intervention strategies.

Issues for Juvenile Judges

An issue that leads to considerable stress and potential traumatization for those working with juvenile court is finding ways to support and help substance-abusing parents and caretakers. Due to the nature of their problems, these parents struggle with their recovery and may relapse as part of their recovery, leaving their children once again and failing to keep them safe. For judges, mental health professionals, caseworkers, and others, this process can be both frustrating and at times traumatizing. In discussions with judges, many shared their concerns about VT resulting from hearing about horrors every day, seeing grisly photographs, and witnessing the suffering of young children. Although the judges described their commitment to being fair and helpful, the result for some may be anger, depression, and anxiety that, without being addressed, may have the potential to impact on the judge's ability to create a supportive, problem-solving court environment. It is crucial to address the issue of VT with all who work in juvenile court and provide needed support through the institutional environment.

In 2003, Jaffee and his colleagues reported on a study of 105 judges who, while attending National Council of Juvenile and Family Court Judges (NCJFCJ) workshops, responded to a self-report measure that included symptoms of VT, coping strategies, and prevention suggestions. While it is recognized that this sample may not be representative of judges in different jurisdictions, the findings were still informative. It is noteworthy that the majority of the judges representing criminal, domestic/civil, and juvenile courts reported one or more symptoms of VT. Consistent with data on police officers' reports of traumatic symptoms, female judges reported more symptoms than male judges, and those with 7 or more years of experience reported more symptoms. The authors concluded that although judges reported different types of coping and prevention strategies, there is a need for greater awareness of these issues and more support for judges. Education about trauma and how it might impact those exposed every day is rarely included in education for any discipline doing work with traumatized children and families. While some work environments build in more support for professionals who repeatedly work with trauma, such supports are rare in the court environment. In informal focus groups held with judges, in addition to the many positive comments about satisfaction with the work, the judges also shared the following concerns: difficulties of managing large caseloads; stress level at work; the nonjudgmental role that a judge has to take; a lonely world and profession; inability to share cases and decisions, or to "take cases home" and get support; reluctance to seek help if needed; difficulty in sharing personal issues; and feelings of anger and frustration, helplessness, hopelessness, and, at times, depression about the cases.

A collaboration was developed between the National Child Traumatic Stress Network (NCTSN) and the NCJFCJ through the NCTSN Judicial Consortium that led to focus groups being held with approximately 26 judges. The participating judges worked in different court settings, including juvenile dependency and delinquency, domestic violence, and divorce/

custody cases. Based on a concurrent survey by the NCTSN, the results indicated that over half (52%) of the judges had not received training about child trauma, about how such children could be assessed, and about established evidence-based treatments. Judges expressed many concerns related to child trauma, including at times feeling overwhelmed by the prevalence of trauma in the courtroom, the amount of need and the limited availability of resources, concerns about how to ensure that placement related to the best interest of the child, ways to facilitate coordination with other services systems, and how to maintain support and confidentiality while supporting children who receive help.

One judge stated that no one who works with children who suffer abuse and neglect, or who works rehabilitatively with their parents, is immune from feeling their pain. Juvenile and family court judges strive to improve the lives of the children and parents who appear before them. However, despite passion and dedication, these families come to court with trauma that can impact the judge emotionally. The testimony relates abuse and horror. The judge can be worn down by observing broken and abused, vulnerable children. At this point the judge may be experiencing VT. This judge suggested that all courts consider offering qualitative seminars on VT, preferably co-led by a judge and a mental health professional. To deal with VT, it is necessary for judges and others working in the juvenile court to be aware and address it directly.

Issues for Mental Health Professionals

Working with Substance-Abusing Parents

For mental health professionals working with substance-abusing parents, other issues may emerge. A psychologist who works in a residential program for substance-abusing mothers and their young children shared a very difficult time in treatment with a young mother in recovery, who, during a therapy session with her young baby present, started talking intensely about her own trauma. With that, she disengaged from paying any attention to the baby, who lay quietly on the floor staring at the ceiling. The therapist experienced herself as "abandoning and neglecting" the baby in her effort to be emotionally available to the mother, and being as neglectful as the mother she was trying to help. After the session, she felt worried, sad, and guilty, but most of all she kept "second-guessing" herself, wondering what she "missed" because she could not prevent the mother from relapsing and taking the baby with her. She continued struggling with her own feelings about not being able to protect the baby. With substance-abusing parents, probably one of the most common questions of therapists is "What did I miss?"

Working in Juvenile Court

As mental health professionals, some difficult and wrenching experiences occur when we work with young traumatized children and families within the juvenile court system. Dr. Amy Dickson, a coauthor of Chapter 7 in this book, coordinates the Orleans Parish Infant Team (Orleans Parish Zero to Three Court Team), working collaboratively with the court, lawyers, child welfare, early intervention child care specialists, and others to provide evaluation and treatment services for young children and families. Yet not a week goes by without a situation arising that results in a mixture of emotions—not only wanting to help but also anger that a young child has been treated so harshly. There is also sadness for the parent, frustration that it may be difficult to work with the many systems involved, and a sense of helplessness and hopelessness about not being able to help sufficiently to "make things better" for the child. Two poignant examples of VT and CF for mental health service providers on the Louisiana State University Health Sciences Center team may illustrate problems that can come up even in settings with much support. A very skilled mental health professional had a baby during the course of her work with the Infant Team, which provides evaluations and services for traumatized young children and families adjudicated dependent due to abuse and neglect. This young woman was referred a case of a baby in foster care who was the same age as her baby, to plan permanent placement with relatives. For this new mother, although a fine professional, it was very difficult to do the necessary work with the foster family and relatives to facilitate moving this child from the foster family when she was 10 months old. Delay of placement of the child with the relatives had been related to the failure to do investigative work with the relatives right after the baby's birth. The mental health professional had difficulty with boundaries, overidentified with the foster parents, and could not imagine separating them when the baby had been living with them her whole life. All mental health professionals, child welfare professionals, and many judges know how difficult it may be for a child to form a secure attachment for almost a year, then have to interrupt that attachment relationship for the sake of a permanent placement. At the same time, the goal of the work is to achieve permanency and stability for the children, and to stay within the guidelines of the Adoption and Safe Families Act (ASFA; 1997). Another very difficult case that caused much distress to the whole Orleans Parish Infant Team (Orleans Parish Zero to Three Court Team) was learning that a 1-year-old child had been tortured to death, and that her sister, for whom we were providing services and support, weighed only 12 pounds, had permanent brain damage, and scars on her body. To carry out the important work effectively for this child and foster family, much processing and support from team members was needed, but even with that extra effort, the result was much distress, sleep lost, and other concerns for team members.

Specific Issues for Child Welfare

Those who work in the child welfare system are exposed routinely to child abuse and neglect, family violence, and multiple traumatic experiences. These children often are seen by many people, including police officers, health care professionals, social workers, and judges, all of whom provide information to the child welfare professional. In addition to all of these systems, foster parents and volunteers spend much time working with and supporting traumatized children. In the course of their day-to-day work, they are exposed to frightening accounts and situations, shocking and disturbing stories, and disheartening results. Common sources of VT for individuals in the child welfare system include the death of a child or adult on the worker's caseload; having to investigate a particularly vicious abuse or neglect report; frequent and chronic exposure to emotional and detailed accounts by children of traumatic experiences; photographic images of horrific injuries and scenes of recent injury and/or death; support of grieving family members following a child abuse death; concerns about bureaucratic issues, including continued funding and adequate resources to support the work; and concerns about being identified in a difficult case when it was not possible to intervene effectively due to lack of authority or means. These professionals could benefit from more support than is often available to support them in these situations.

Researchers have studied the effects of VT on a number of professions involved in the child welfare system, including child protection workers, police officers, nurses, and mental health therapists. For example, a Canadian study of hospital based child protection workers found that one third reported emotional exhaustion, high levels of cynicism, and low levels of professional efficacy. The risk of job turnover was great with two thirds considering changing jobs and three quarters of those who worked full time with child abuse victims considering leaving the profession. For those child protection workers who chose to retire early or leave for other work, one third reported stress as the major reason (Bennett, Plint, & Clifford, 2005). Bride (2007) found that of social workers within the child welfare system, 70% reported at least one symptom of secondary traumatization in the prior week. Over 50% met criteria for at least one posttraumatic stress disorder (PTSD) symptom cluster, and 15% met full PTSD criteria. Staff turnover was significantly higher for public child welfare workers than for other state or city government workers. A similar study showed that half of 365 child protection services workers had "high" or "very high" levels of secondary traumatization (Conrad & Keller-Guenther, 2006).

At the same time, similar to the recent survey reported by Conrad and Keller-Guenther (2006), all of the studies found that child protection services workers reported high levels of "job satisfaction" and low levels of "job burnout." This unexpected funding shows that secondary traumatization (CF, VT, etc.) is different from job burnout, which can occur in professions that may not involve exposure to victims of abuse and violence. Stamm (2002) discussed the concept of "compassion satisfaction," which may mitigate job burnout and is defined as pleasure and fulfillment from helping others, affection for colleagues, and a sense of making an important contribution to the welfare of others and society. Consistent with the authors' recent survey, compassion satisfaction does not necessarily reduce secondary traumatization because those working in child protection may endorse both measures. We can hypothesize that those workers showing more compassion satisfaction may be functioning in work environments providing more support.

While each of these groups experiences unique stressors and traumatic experiences, all share in common responses and outcomes to these situations. There are a number of common signs and symptoms of VT, and adverse effects of work-related exposure to both traumatized individuals and disturbing situations can impact both personal and professional lives. Some of these signs and symptoms are anger and irritability; anxiety and new fears, especially about the safety of one's family; emotional numbing and detachment; sadness and depression; difficulty concentrating, with intrusive thoughts about victims or perpetrators; difficulty sleeping, including nightmares; social withdrawal from family and friends; changes in beliefs about the world and more pessimism; changes in spiritual beliefs; less self-care; increased physical complaints and illness; and use of alcohol and/or drugs to "forget about work" or "relax."

VT and stress occur in individuals in both the child welfare system and systems within which they work. Each person and each system brings a specific set of stressors to the work. At the same time, many individuals are working within the context of overburdened and sometime underfunded systems, which may increase risk for secondary traumatization. Some of the organizational and work-related problems cited frequently as related to job burnout include high caseload, and excessive workload and paperwork; little support from supervisors; having to deal with situations with conflicting roles, expectations, and values; lack of peer support; inadequate resources to meet demands; concerns about personal safety; and little job recognition. Unfortunately, the secondary traumatization that results may lead to increased absenteeism, impaired judgment, unwillingness to accept extra work or assume responsibility, low motivation, lower productivity and poor quality of work, decreased compliance with work requirements, greater friction among staff members, and high staff turnover. Overall, there is little question that working in the child welfare system can be very stressful, lead to secondary traumatization and/or job burnout.

Compassion Fatigue for Those Who Work with Military Families

Most clinicians who work with military families seem to manage the challenges well. Those who have more difficulties tend to be new to the military population and may become overwhelmed with the many new experiences. As in other work with traumatized young children, increased experience helps a clinician to put the stressful demands of the work in perspective. At a group meeting of clinicians working with military families, a colleague shared concerns about the possibility of mental health professionals becoming hardened to the experiences of the patients to defend themselves against the trauma they witness. This risk is consistent across all groups who work with trauma. This sensitive clinician shared the challenging experience of a new-to-the-military clinician dealing with the family of a severely combat-injured young father of three little boys, who visited him in the hospital. Like the example of the clinician working with the Orleans Parish Infant Team, this clinician was a new father himself, so seeing this very damaged young soldier with his young children, and working with the consequent confusion, family disarray, and marital tension, created emotional disturbance for him. He had difficulty with boundaries and was too personally upset by the situation to be able to support the service man and his family. He requested that this case be transferred to another clinician because he felt he could not distance himself enough to be able to help them. This example serves as an important reminder that this work cannot be done in isolation.

GENERAL RECOMMENDATIONS FOR SUPPORT, PREVENTION, AND TREATMENT FOR INDIVIDUALS WORKING WITH TRAUMATIZED YOUNG CHILDREN

Recommendations for prevention and treatment by experts in STS can be divided into two types: personal and organizational. Personal recommendations focus on what the individual can do to recognize, reduce, or prevent STS effects. Organizational recommendations focus on what institutions and agencies can do to minimize secondary traumatization (and burnout) in their workers. At present, we know very little, however, about whether these recommendations are being implemented and, if so, the degree to which they are effective.

Individual Strategies

Recommendations aimed at helping first ask the individual systematically to assess his or her exposure to secondary traumatic stressors. A number of self-administered checklists have been published and circulated that allow people to make their own assessment of the degree to which they experience secondary traumatization (see Stamm, 2008). Measures typically ask people to rate the degree to which they experience many of the symptoms described earlier. Scores are grouped into general categories, such as mild, moderate, and severe levels of secondary traumatic stress. Higher scores on these measures are moderately correlated with standard measures of anxiety, depression, and posttraumatic stress. The intent of self-assessment measures is not to pathologize secondary traumatic stress but to help people understand that these are expectable effects of exposure to the trauma and suffering of others. These scales also provide an opportunity for people to understand their level of compassion satisfaction, which can mitigate the stress.

Individuals with moderate to high scores or other evidence of secondary traumatization are urged to learn and to utilize various self-care and stress reduction strategies. Some of these strategies involve personal lifestyle changes, such as eating regularly, getting sufficient exercise and sleep, taking more time for themselves, developing outside interests, and achieving a balance between work and home life. Strategies for psychological, emotional, and spiritual self-care are also often included as recommendations. A comprehensive list of these recommendations is available at the NCTSN website (*www.nctns.org*).

In a study of therapists who specialize in work with trauma and should know about traumatic stress effects, Bober and Regehr (2005) found that while the therapists strongly endorsed these self-care concepts and recommendations, they did not systematically practice them. Furthermore, the amount of time therapists spent working with trauma victims was most predictive of their secondary traumatization score. However, there was no relationship between the amount of time therapists devoted to coping strategies and their traumatic stress score.

Organizational Strategies

For organizations, the research indicates that organizational issues, policies, and working environment make substantial contributions to increasing employees' risk for traumatic stress. This awareness has led to recommendations designed to redress these factors, and the knowledge that organizations have much to gain by reducing or preventing secondary traumatization and negative effects. As with individuals, the first step of the organization is to recognize that secondary traumatization is possible and may be occurring. Unless administrators and managers in an agency or organization are in day-to-day contact with traumatized staff, they are often slow to recognize the problem. A number of available survey measures allow managers to gather systematic data on levels of work-related secondary traumatization and its effects on employees (White, 2006). In order to reduce the risk of VT, it is important that organizations recognize the need to implement changes, which include reducing the workloads and caseloads; providing adequate supervision to frontline workers; providing good mental health insurance coverage; acknowledging that there may be work stress and work-related secondary traumatization for staff; providing educational workshops and informal "brown bag" lunches to increase awareness; developing peer support; and encouraging self-care, adequate backup for staff in stressful positions, and discussion of possible VT among staff and administration members. The Child Welfare Trauma Training Toolkit (2008) developed by the National Child Traumatic Stress Network provides a valuable resource to address many of these issues.

CONCLUSION

Work with traumatized young children and families pulls a great deal from therapists, child welfare workers, judges, and others in the child's environment. Despite being very dedicated, they can suffer from VT, burnout, CF, and strong feelings that they at times do not understand. Sometimes the extent of exposure to others' traumatic experiences can lead to personal traumatization and resultant symptoms. A helper may find him- or herself feeling sorry for the children and wanting to rescue them; feeling as helpless and hopeless as the parents or caregivers and angry with abusive, neglectful caregivers; and feeling overwhelmed. A helper may also become frustrated when the work to help the parents become more sensitive and emotionally available to their children is slow.

It is very important for all who work with survivors of traumatic experiences to recognize that many children do well. In fact, the traumatic experiences may be short-lived, and symptoms may remit rapidly. Therapists especially must be prepared to listen, to "hold" traumatized children's concerns, and to help them and their parents or caregivers to return to normal developmental functioning. Therapists cannot right wrongs and erase scars; however, the children can be helped and supported in their development. Each clinician, therapist, judge, and child welfare worker must find his or her own way to deal with the overwhelming affects and emotions that accompany this work. And each needs to find a way to gain support through self-care, a supportive team, or some other method, to do the work effectively. I have heard of professionals who work with trauma welcoming a drive home through the country to unwind after a hard day at work. I have heard of others who take a walk or relax with friends. All professionals working with young traumatized children need to find individual ways to gain support and reduce the risk of ongoing VT to ensure that their work is effective and helpful.

REFERENCES

Adoption and Safe Families Act (ASFA) of 1997, P.L. 105-89, 111 Stat. 2115-2136.

Bennett, S., Plint, A., & Clifford, T. J. (2005). Burnout, psychological morbidity, job satisfaction, and stress: A survey of Canadian hospital-based child protection professionals. *Archives of Diseases of Children, 90,* 1112–1116.

Bober, T., & Regehr, C. (2005). Strategies for reducing secondary or vicarious trauma: Do they work? *Brief Treatment and Crisis Intervention, 6,* 1–9.

Bride, B. E. (2007). Prevalence of secondary traumatic stress among social workers. *Social Work, 52,* 63–70.

Child Welfare Trauma Training Toolkit (2008). National Child Traumatic Stress Network. Retrieved May 1, 2010, from *www.nctsn.org.*

Conrad, D., & Kellar-Guenther, Y. (2006). Compassion fatigue, burnout, and compassion satisfaction among Colorado child protection workers. *Child Abuse and Neglect, 30,* 1071–1080.

Figley, C. R. (1996). *Compassion fatigue: Coping with secondary traumatic stress disorder in those who treat the traumatized.* New York: Brunner/Mazel.

Figley, C. R. (2002). Compassion fatigue: Psychotherapists' chronic lack of self care. *Journal of Clinical Psychology, 58,* 1433–1441.

Figley, C. R. (1995). Compassion fatigue as secondary traumatic stress disorder: An overview. In *Compassion fatigue: Coping with secondary traumatic stress disorder in those who treat the traumatized* (pp. 1–20). New York: Brunner/Mazel.

Jaffe, P. G., Crooks, C. V., Dunford-Jackson, B. L., & Town, M. (2003, Fall). Vicarious trauma in judges: The personal challenge of dispensing justice. *Juvenile and Family Court Journal,* pp. 1–9.

Masten, A. S. (2001). Ordinary magic: Resilience processes in development. *American Psychologist, 56,* 227–238.

Masten, A. S. (in press). Risk and resilience in development. In P. D. Zelazo (Ed.), *Oxford handbook of developmental psychology.* New York: Oxford University Press.

Pearlman, L. A., & Saakvitne, K. W. (1995). Treating therapists with vicarious traumatization and secondary traumatic stress disorders. In C. R. Figley (Ed.), *Compassion fatigue: Coping with secondary traumatic stress disorder in those who treat the traumatized* (pp. 150–177). New York: Brunner/Mazel.

Stamm, B. H. (2002). Measuring compassion satisfaction as well as fatigue. In C.

R. Figley (Ed.), *Treating compassion fatigue* (pp. 7–119). New York: Brunner/ Routledge.

Stamm, B. H. (2008). The ProQOL. Retrieved April 10, 2010, from *www.proqol. org*.

Stamm, B. H. (2009). The concise ProQOL manual. Available at *www.proqol.org*.

White, D. (2006). The hidden costs of caring: What managers need to know. *Health Care Manager, 25,* 341–347.

Index

Page numbers followed by *f* indicate figure; *n*, note; and *t*, table.